Cancer
SOURCEBOOK
for Women

Second Edition

Health Reference Series

Second Edition

Cancer
SOURCEBOOK
for Women

*Basic Consumer Health Information about
Gynecologic Cancers and Related Concerns, Including
Cervical Cancer, Endometrial Cancer, Gestational
Trophoblastic Tumor, Ovarian Cancer, Uterine Cancer,
Vaginal Cancer, Vulvar Cancer, Breast Cancer, and
Common Non-Cancerous Uterine Conditions, with
Facts about Cancer Risk Factors, Screening and
Prevention, Treatment Options, and Reports on
Current Research Initiatives*

*Along with a Glossary of Cancer Terms and
a Directory of Resources for Additional Help
and Information*

Edited by
Karen Bellenir

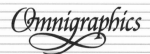

Omnigraphics

615 Griswold Street • Detroit, MI 48226

Bibliographic Note

Because this page cannot legibly accommodate all the copyright notices, the Bibliographic Note portion of the Preface constitutes an extension of the copyright notice.

Edited by Karen Bellenir

Health Reference Series

Karen Bellenir, *Managing Editor*
David A. Cooke, MD, *Medical Consultant*
Elizabeth Barbour, *Permissions Associate*
Dawn Matthews, *Verification Assistant*
Carol Munson, *Permissions Assistant*
Laura Pleva, *Index Editor*
EdIndex, Services for Publishers, *Indexers*

* * *

Omnigraphics, Inc.

Matthew P. Barbour, *Senior Vice President*
Kay Gill, *Vice President—Directories*
Kevin Hayes, *Operations Manager*
David P. Bianco, *Marketing Consultant*

* * *

Peter E. Ruffner, *President and Publicher*

Frederick G. Ruffner, Jr., *Chairman*

Copyright © 2002 Omnigraphics, Inc.

ISBN 0-7808-0226-8

Printed in the United States

Table of Contents

Part VI: Cancer Screening and Prevention

Part VII: Treatment Options

Part VIII: Recent Research and Clinical Trials

Part IX: Coping Strategies

Part X: Additional Help and Information

Preface

About This Book

Although cancer continues to claim the lives of thousands of women every year, progress against the disease has been made. According to the National Cancer Institute, cancer incidence rates fell by an average of nearly 1.3 percent per year between 1992 and 1997. Additionally, as of January 1997 there were more than five million women living in the United States who were cancer survivors. However, encouraging statistics such as these are often accompanied by grim reminders that much work remains to be done.

Cancer Sourcebook for Women, Second Edition includes general information for all women who are cancer patients, but it focuses specifically on the gynecologic cancers (those that involve a woman's reproductive organs). It provides facts about risk factors, screening methods for early detection, symptoms, diagnostic tests, and treatment options for cervical, endometrial, ovarian, and other women's cancers. It also describes some common concerns about related gynecologic issues such as pregnancy during cancer, fertility after cancer treatment, and non-cancerous uterine conditions that may be confused with cancer symptoms. Reports on current research initiatives, a glossary of terms, and a directory of resources for cancer patients are also included.

Breast cancer, which impacts significantly more women than men, is covered briefly in this volume. Readers seeking more comprehensive information on breast cancer may wish to consult Omnigraphics' *Breast Cancer Sourcebook*.

Other types of cancers also have a significant impact on women's health. For example, lung cancer which is the number one cancer killer in men, is likewise the number one cancer killer in women with more than 78,000 female deaths every year. Colorectal cancers claim nearly 30,000 women annually, and skin cancer, which has a lower death rate, is the most prevalent type of cancer in the United States. Readers seeking in-depth, disease-specific information about these and other non-gynecologic cancers may wish to consult *Cancer Sourcebook*. Other cancer-related titles in the *Health Reference Series* include *Pediatric Cancer Sourcebook* and *Prostate Cancer Sourcebook*.

How to Use This Book

This book is divided into parts and chapters. Parts focus on broad areas of interest. Chapters are devoted to single topics within a part.

Part I: Breast Cancer provides an overview of breast cancer and related concerns. More than 180,000 new cases of breast cancer are diagnosed every year and the incidence rates for breast cancer have been increasing since 1990. Death rates, however, have declined by about two percent per year. Researchers attribute this trend to early detection and better treatment. Readers with questions about the risk factors for breast cancer, screening and detection methods, prevention tips, and treatment issues will find answers in this section.

Part II: Cervical Cancer describes the risk factors, prevention, and treatment of cancer of the cervix, a type of cancer that accounts for six percent of all malignancies in women. It also includes information on the Pap test, an important screening tool for identifying cellular changes that can lead to cervical cancer. Death rates from cervical cancer have decreased by 70 percent over the last four decades, primarily as a result of early diagnosis using the Pap test.

Part III: Endometrial Cancer offers details about this type of cancer, which accounts for 38,000 annual diagnoses among American women. Although incidence rates of endometrial cancer have fallen by more than 26 percent since the early 1980s, death rates have been rising— a statistical observation often attributed to the aging population. Risk factors associated with endometrial cancer include diabetes, cigarette smoking, lack of physical activity, and estrogen therapy. These issues and others are explained in this part.

Part IV: Ovarian Cancer gives facts about what is often called a "silent killer" because it has the highest mortality of all cancers of the female reproductive system. When detected early, ovarian cancer is treatable with five-year survival rates near 95 percent. Early ovarian cancer is often without symptoms, however, and 70 percent of the more than 23,000 cases of ovarian cancer diagnosed annually in the United States are diagnosed at advanced stages. Five-year survival rates for cancer that has spread beyond the localized stage drop significantly. Readers seeking information about risk factors for ovarian cancer, screening methods, and treatment approaches will find these details and more in this part.

Part V: Other Gynecologic Cancers and Related Concerns provides information about gestational trophoblastic tumor, uterine sarcoma, vaginal cancer, and vulvar cancer. It includes facts about metastatic cancer and describes pregnancy-related concerns in women being treated for Hodgkin's disease and non-Hodgkin's lymphoma. Details about common non-cancerous gynecologic conditions with symptoms that women may confuse with cancer warning signs are also provided.

Part VI: Cancer Screening and Prevention describes commonly used cancer screening tests, identifies known and controversial risk factors, and offers information about cancer prevention.

Part VII: Treatment Options provides information about commonly used cancer treatments, including chemotherapy and radiation therapy. It offers descriptions of some newer tools being used in the cancer-fighting arsenal and offers suggestions for women considering complimentary and alternative therapies.

Part VIII: Recent Research and Clinical Trials offers a review of some of the most promising areas of current investigation in women's cancer prevention, screening, and treatment.

Part IX: Coping Strategies provides suggestions for cancer patients, their families, and loved ones, including home care issues, helps for children, nutrition facts, and tips for managing fatigue, depression, and cancer pain. It also provides information about how cancer treatment can affect sexuality and fertility.

Part X: Additional Help and Information offers a glossary of important terms related to cancer in women, an explanation of the Family and Medical Leave Act, and a directory of helpful resources.

Bibliographic Note

This volume contains documents and excerpts from publications issued by the following government agencies: Agency for Healthcare Research and Quality (AHRQ); Centers for Disease Control and Prevention (CDC); National Cancer Institute (NCI); National Heart, Lung, and Blood Institute (NHLBI); National Institute of Child Health and Human Development (NICHD); National Women's Health Information Center; U.S. Department of Labor (DoL); and the U.S. Food and Drug Administration (FDA).

In addition, this volume contains copyrighted articles from the American Academy of Family Physicians; American Cancer Society; American Social Health Association; College of American Pathologists; *Journal of Gynecologic Oncology Nursing*; Lippincott, Williams, and Wilkins; Medical College of Wisconsin; OncoLink (sponsored by the University of Pennsylvania); University of Iowa Hospitals and Clinics; University of Wisconsin; and the Women's Cancer Network.

Full citation information is provided on the first page of each chapter. Every effort has been made to secure all necessary rights to reprint the copyrighted material. If any omissions have been made, please contact Omnigraphics to make corrections for future editions.

Acknowledgements

In addition to the organizations listed above, special thanks are due to document engineer Bruce Bellenir, verification assistant Dawn Matthews, permissions associate Elizabeth Barbour, and production coordinator Kevin Hayes.

Note from the Editor

This book is part of Omnigraphics' *Health Reference Series*. The series provides basic information about a broad range of medical concerns. It is not intended to serve as a tool for diagnosing illness, in prescribing treatments, or as a substitute for the physician/patient relationship. All persons concerned about medical symptoms or the possibility of disease are encouraged to seek professional care from an appropriate health care provider.

Our Advisory Board

The *Health Reference Series* is reviewed by an Advisory Board comprised of librarians from public, academic, and medical libraries. We would like to thank the following board members for providing guidance to the development of this series:

Dr. Lynda Baker, Associate Professor of Library and Information Science, Wayne State University, Detroit, MI

Nancy Bulgarelli, William Beaumont Hospital Library, Royal Oak, MI

Karen Imarasio, Bloomfield Township Public Library, Bloomfield Township, MI

Karen Morgan, Mardigian Library, University of Michigan-Dearborn, Dearborn, MI

Rosemary Orlando, St. Clair Shores Public Library, St. Clair Shores, MI

Medical Consultant

Medical consultation services are provided to the *Health Reference Series* editors by David A. Cooke, MD. Dr. Cooke is a graduate of Brandeis University, and he received his M.D. degree from the University of Michigan. He completed residency training at the University of Wisconsin Hospital and Clinics. He is board-certified in Internal Medicine. Dr. Cooke currently works as part of the University of Michigan Health System and practices in Brighton, MI. In his free time, he enjoys writing, science fiction, and spending time with his family.

Health Reference Series *Update Policy*

The inaugural book in the *Health Reference Series* was the first edition of *Cancer Sourcebook* published in 1992. Since then, the Series has been enthusiastically received by librarians and in the medical community. In order to maintain the standard of providing high-quality health information for the layperson the editorial staff at Omnigraphics felt it was necessary to implement a policy of updating volumes when warranted.

Medical researchers have been making tremendous strides, and it is the purpose of the *Health Reference Series* to stay current with the most recent advances. Each decision to update a volume will be made on an individual basis. Some of the considerations will include how much new information is available and the feedback we receive from people who use the books. If there is a topic you would like to see added to the update list, or an area of medical concern you feel has not been adequately addressed, please write to:

Editor
Health Reference Series
Omnigraphics, Inc.
615 Griswold
Detroit, MI 48226

The commitment to providing on-going coverage of important medical developments has also led to some format changes in the *Health Reference Series*. Each new volume on a topic is individually titled and called a "First Edition." Subsequent updates will carry sequential edition numbers. To help avoid confusion and to provide maximum flexibility in our ability to respond to informational needs, the practice of consecutively numbering each volume has been discontinued.

Part One

Breast Cancer

Chapter 1

Understanding Breast Cancer

Introduction

Other than skin cancer, breast cancer is the most common type of cancer among women in the United States. More than 180,000 women are diagnosed with breast cancer each year. The National Cancer Institute (NCI) has written this text to help patients with breast cancer and their families and friends better understand this disease. We hope others will read it as well to learn more about breast cancer.

This chapter discusses screening and early detection, symptoms, diagnosis, treatment, and rehabilitation. It also has information to help patients cope with breast cancer.

Research has led to progress against breast cancer—better treatments, a lower chance of death from the disease, and improved quality of life. Through research, knowledge about breast cancer keeps increasing. Scientists are learning more about what causes breast cancer and are exploring new ways to prevent, detect, diagnose, and treat this disease.

Male Breast Cancer

Breast cancer affects more than 1,000 men in this country each year. Although this chapter was written mainly for women, much of the information on symptoms, diagnosis, treatment, and living with

National Cancer Institute (NCI), NIH Pub. No. 00-1556, updated December 2000.

the disease applies to men as well. However, the "Detecting Breast Cancer" section does not apply to men. Experts do not recommend routine screening for men.

The Breasts

Each breast has 15 to 20 sections called lobes. Within each lobe are many smaller lobules. Lobules end in dozens of tiny bulbs that can produce milk. The lobes, lobules, and bulbs are all linked by thin tubes called ducts. These ducts lead to the nipple in the center of a dark area of skin called the areola. Fat surrounds the lobules and ducts. There are no muscles in the breast, but muscles lie under each breast and cover the ribs.

Each breast also contains blood vessels and lymph vessels. The lymph vessels carry colorless fluid called lymph, and lead to small bean-shaped organs called lymph nodes. Clusters of lymph nodes are found near the breast in the axilla (under the arm), above the collarbone, and in the chest. Lymph nodes are also found in many other parts of the body.

Understanding the Cancer Process

Cancer is a group of many related diseases that begin in cells, the body's basic unit of life. To understand cancer, it is helpful to know what happens when normal cells become cancerous.

The body is made up of many types of cells. Normally, cells grow and divide to produce more cells only when the body needs them. This orderly process helps keep the body healthy. Sometimes, however, cells keep dividing when new cells are not needed. These extra cells form a mass of tissue, called a growth or tumor. Tumors can be benign or malignant.

- **Benign tumors** are not cancer. They can usually be removed, and in most cases, they do not come back. Cells from benign tumors do not spread to other parts of the body. Most important, benign breast tumors are not a threat to life.

- **Malignant tumors** are cancer. Cells in these tumors are abnormal. They divide without control or order, and they can invade and damage nearby tissues and organs. Also, cancer cells can break away from a malignant tumor and enter the bloodstream or the lymphatic system. That is how cancer spreads from the original (primary) cancer site to form new tumors in other organs. The spread of cancer is called metastasis.

4

When cancer arises in breast tissue and spreads (metastasizes) outside the breast, cancer cells are often found in the lymph nodes under the arm (axillary lymph nodes). If the cancer has reached these nodes, it means that cancer cells may have spread to other parts of the body—other lymph nodes and other organs, such as the bones, liver, or lungs. When cancer spreads from its original location to another part of the body, the new tumor has the same kind of abnormal cells and the same name as the primary tumor. For example, if breast cancer spreads to the brain, the cancer cells in the brain are actually breast cancer cells. The disease is called metastatic breast cancer. (It is not brain cancer.) Doctors sometimes call this "distant" disease.

This chapter deals with breast cancer. For information about benign breast lumps and other benign breast changes, read NCI's booklet, *Understanding Breast Changes: A Health Guide for All Women.*

Breast Cancer: Who's at Risk?

The exact causes of breast cancer are not known. However, studies show that the risk of breast cancer increases as a woman gets older. This disease is very uncommon in women under the age of 35. Most breast cancers occur in women over the age of 50, and the risk is especially high for women over age 60. Also, breast cancer occurs more often in white women than African American or Asian women.

Research has shown that the following conditions increase a woman's chances of getting breast cancer:

- **Personal history of breast cancer.** Women who have had breast cancer face an increased risk of getting breast cancer in their other breast.

- **Family history.** A woman's risk for developing breast cancer increases if her mother, sister, or daughter had breast cancer, especially at a young age.

- **Certain breast changes.** Having a diagnosis of atypical hyperplasia or lobular carcinoma *in situ* (LCIS) may increase a woman's risk for developing cancer.

- **Genetic alterations.** Changes in certain genes (BRCA1, BRCA2, and others) increase the risk of breast cancer. In families in which many women have had the disease, gene testing can sometimes show the presence of specific genetic changes that increase the risk of breast cancer. Doctors may suggest ways to try to delay or prevent breast cancer, or to improve the detection of this disease in women who have these changes in their genes. For more information about gene testing, read the "Causes and Prevention" section under "The Promise of Cancer Research."

Other factors associated with an increased risk for breast cancer include:

- **Estrogen.** Evidence suggests that the longer a woman is exposed to estrogen (estrogen made by the body, taken as a drug, or delivered by a patch), the more likely she is to develop breast cancer. For example, the risk is somewhat increased among women who began menstruation at an early age (before age 12), experienced menopause late (after age 55), never had children, or took hormone replacement therapy for long periods of time. Each of these factors increases the amount of time a woman's body is exposed to estrogen.

  DES (diethylstilbestrol) is a synthetic form of estrogen that was used between the early 1940s and 1971. Women who took DES during pregnancy to prevent certain complications are at a slightly higher risk for breast cancer. This does not appear to be the case for their daughters who were exposed to DES before birth. However, more studies are needed as these daughters enter the age range when breast cancer is more common.

- **Late childbearing.** Women who have their first child late (after about age 30) have a greater chance of developing breast cancer than women who have a child at a younger age.

- **Breast density.** Breasts that have a high proportion of lobular and ductal tissue appear dense on mammograms. Breast cancers nearly always develop in lobular or ductal tissue (not fatty tissue). That's why cancer is more likely to occur in breasts that have a lot of lobular and ductal tissue (that is, dense tissue) than in breasts with a lot of fatty tissue. In addition, when breasts are dense, it is more difficult for doctors to see abnormal areas on a mammogram.

- **Radiation therapy.** Women whose breasts were exposed to radiation during radiation therapy before age 30, especially those who were treated with radiation for Hodgkin's disease, are at an increased risk for developing breast cancer. Studies show that the younger a woman was when she received her treatment, the higher her risk for developing breast cancer later in life.

- **Alcohol.** Some studies suggest a slightly higher risk of breast cancer among women who drink alcohol.

Most women who develop breast cancer have none of the risk factors listed above, other than the risk that comes with growing older. Scientists are conducting research into the causes of breast cancer to learn more about risk factors and ways of preventing this disease.

Detecting Breast Cancer

Women should talk with their doctor about factors that can increase their chance of getting breast cancer. Women of any age who are at higher risk for developing this disease should ask their doctor when to start and how often to be checked for breast cancer. Breast cancer screening has been shown to decrease the risk of dying from breast cancer.

Women can take an active part in the early detection of breast cancer by having regularly scheduled screening mammograms and clinical breast exams (breast exams performed by health professionals). Some women also perform breast self-exams.

A screening mammogram is the best tool available for finding breast cancer early, before symptoms appear. A mammogram is a special kind of x-ray. Screening mammograms are used to look for breast changes in women who have no signs of breast cancer.

Mammograms can often detect a breast lump before it can be felt. Also, a mammogram can show small deposits of calcium in the breast. Although most calcium deposits are benign, a cluster of very tiny specks of calcium (called microcalcifications) may be an early sign of cancer.

If an area of the breast looks suspicious on the screening mammogram, additional (diagnostic) mammograms may be needed. Depending on the results, the doctor may advise the woman to have a biopsy.

Although mammograms are the best way to find breast abnormalities early, they do have some limitations. A mammogram may miss some cancers that are present (false negative) or may find things that turn out not to be cancer (false positive). And detecting a tumor early does not guarantee that a woman's life will be saved. Some fast-growing breast cancers may already have spread to other parts of the body before being detected.

Nevertheless, studies show that mammograms reduce the risk of dying from breast cancer. Most doctors recommend that women in their forties and older have mammograms regularly, every 1 to 2 years.

Some women perform monthly breast self-exams to check for any changes in their breasts. When doing a breast self-exam, it's important to remember that each woman's breasts are different, and that changes can occur because of aging, the menstrual cycle, pregnancy, menopause, or taking birth control pills or other hormones. It is normal for the breasts to feel a little lumpy and uneven. Also, it is common for a woman's breasts to be swollen and tender right before or during her menstrual period. Women in their forties and older should be aware that a monthly breast self-exam is not a substitute for regularly scheduled screening mammograms and clinical breast exams by a health professional.

Recognizing Symptoms

Early breast cancer usually does not cause pain. In fact, when breast cancer first develops, there may be no symptoms at all. But as the cancer grows, it can cause changes that women should watch for:

- A lump or thickening in or near the breast or in the underarm area;
- A change in the size or shape of the breast;
- Nipple discharge or tenderness, or the nipple pulled back (inverted) into the breast;
- Ridges or pitting of the breast (the skin looks like the skin of an orange); or
- A change in the way the skin of the breast, areola, or nipple looks or feels (for example, warm, swollen, red, or scaly).

A woman should see her doctor about any symptoms like these. Most often, they are not cancer, but it's important to check with the doctor so that any problems can be diagnosed and treated as early as possible.

Diagnosing Breast Cancer

To help find the cause of any sign or symptom, a doctor does a careful physical exam and asks about personal and family medical history. In addition, the doctor may do one or more breast exams:

- **Clinical breast exam.** The doctor can tell a lot about a lump by carefully feeling it and the tissue around it. Benign lumps often feel different from cancerous ones. The doctor can examine the size and texture of the lump and determine whether the lump moves easily.

- **Mammography.** X-rays of the breast can give the doctor important information about a breast lump.

- **Ultrasonography.** Using high-frequency sound waves, ultrasonography can often show whether a lump is a fluid-filled cyst (not cancer) or a solid mass (which may or may not be cancer). This exam may be used along with mammography.

Based on these exams, the doctor may decide that no further tests are needed and no treatment is necessary. In such cases, the doctor may need to check the woman regularly to watch for any changes.

Biopsy

Often, fluid or tissue must be removed from the breast so the doctor can make a diagnosis. A woman's doctor may refer her for further evaluation to a surgeon or other health care professional who has experience with breast diseases. These doctors may perform:

- **Fine-needle aspiration.** A thin needle is used to remove fluid and/or cells from a breast lump. If the fluid is clear, it may not need to be checked by a lab.

- **Needle biopsy.** Using special techniques, tissue can be removed with a needle from an area that looks suspicious on a mammogram but cannot be felt. Tissue removed in a needle biopsy goes to a lab to be checked by a pathologist for cancer cells.

- **Surgical biopsy.** In an incisional biopsy, the surgeon cuts out a sample of a lump or suspicious area. In an excisional biopsy, the surgeon removes all of a lump or suspicious area and an area of healthy tissue around the edges. A pathologist then examines the tissue under a microscope to check for cancer cells.

When a woman needs a biopsy, these are some questions she may want to ask her doctor:

- What type of biopsy will I have? Why?
- How long will it take? Will I be awake? Will it hurt?
- How soon will I know the results?
- If I do have cancer, who will talk with me about treatment? When?

When Cancer Is Found

The most common type of breast cancer is ductal carcinoma. It begins in the lining of the ducts. Another type, called lobular carcinoma, arises in the lobules. When cancer is found, the pathologist can tell what kind of cancer it is (whether it began in a duct or a lobule) and whether it is invasive (has invaded nearby tissues in the breast).

Special lab tests of the tissue help the doctor learn more about the cancer. For example, hormone receptor tests (estrogen and progesterone receptor tests) can help determine whether hormones help the cancer to grow. If test results show that hormones do affect the cancer's growth (a positive test result), the cancer is likely to respond to hormonal therapy. This therapy deprives the cancer cells of estrogen. More information about hormonal therapy can be found in the "Planning Treatment" section.

Other tests are sometimes done to help the doctor predict whether the cancer is likely to progress. For example, the doctor may order x-rays and lab tests. Sometimes a sample of breast tissue is checked for a gene (the human epidermal growth factor receptor-2 or HER-2 gene) that is associated with a higher risk that the breast cancer will come back. The doctor may also order special exams of the bones, liver, or lungs because breast cancer may spread to these areas.

If the diagnosis is breast cancer, a woman may want to ask these questions:

- What kind of breast cancer do I have?

- What did the hormone receptor test show? What other lab tests were done on the tumor tissue, and what did they show?

- How will you determine whether the disease has spread?

- How will this information help in deciding what type of treatment or further tests will be best for me?

Planning Treatment

Many women with breast cancer want to take an active part in decisions about their medical care. They want to learn all they can about their disease and their treatment choices. However, the shock and stress that people often feel after a diagnosis of cancer can make it hard for them to think of everything they want to ask the doctor. Often it is helpful to prepare a list of questions in advance. To help remember what the doctor says, patients may take notes or ask whether they may use a tape recorder. Some people also want to have a family member or friend with them when they talk to the doctor— to take part in the discussion, to take notes, or just to listen.

The patient's doctor may refer her to doctors who specialize in treating cancer, or she may ask for a referral. Treatment generally begins within a few weeks after the diagnosis. There will be time for the woman to talk with the doctor about her treatment choices, to get a second opinion, and to prepare herself and her loved ones.

Second Opinion

Before starting treatment, the patient might want a second opinion about the diagnosis and the treatment plan. Some insurance companies require a second opinion; others may cover a second opinion if the woman requests it. It may take a little while to arrange to see another doctor. In most cases, a brief delay (up to 3 or 4 weeks) between biopsy and treatment does not make breast cancer treatment less effective. There are a number of ways to find a doctor for a second opinion:

- The patient's doctor may refer her to one or more specialists. Specialists who treat women with breast cancer include surgeons, medical oncologists, plastic surgeons, and radiation oncologists. At cancer centers or special centers for breast diseases, these doctors often work together as a team.

- The Cancer Information Service, at 1-800-4-CANCER, can tell callers about treatment facilities, including cancer centers and other NCI-supported programs, in their area.

- Patients can get the names of specialists from their local medical society, a nearby hospital, or a medical school.

- The Official ABMS Directory of Board Certified Medical Specialists lists doctors' names along with their specialty and their educational background. This resource, produced by the American Board of Medical Specialties (ABMS), is available in most public libraries. The ABMS also provides an online service to help people locate doctors (http://www.certifieddoctor.org/).

Methods of Treating Breast Cancer

Breast cancer may be treated with local or systemic therapy. Some patients have both kinds of treatment.

Local therapy is used to remove or destroy breast cancer in a specific area. Surgery and radiation therapy are local treatments. They are used to treat the disease in the breast. When breast cancer has spread to other parts of the body, local therapy may be used to control cancer in those specific areas, such as in the lung or bone.

Systemic treatments are used to destroy or control cancer throughout the body. Chemotherapy, hormonal therapy, and biological therapy are systemic treatments. Some patients have systemic therapy to shrink the tumor before local therapy. Others have systemic therapy to prevent the cancer from coming back, or to treat cancer that has spread.

Surgery is the most common treatment for breast cancer, and there are several types of surgery. The doctor can explain each type, discuss and compare their benefits and risks, and describe how each will affect the patient's appearance.

- An operation to remove the cancer but not the breast is called breast-sparing surgery or breast-conserving surgery. Lumpectomy and segmental mastectomy (also called partial mastectomy) are types of breast-sparing surgery. After breast-sparing surgery, most women receive radiation therapy to destroy cancer cells that remain in the area.

- An operation to remove the breast (or as much of the breast as possible) is a mastectomy. Breast reconstruction is often an option at the same time as the mastectomy, or later on.

- In most cases, the surgeon also removes lymph nodes under the arm to help determine whether cancer cells have entered the lymphatic system. This is called an axillary lymph node dissection.

Breast reconstruction (surgery to rebuild the shape of a breast) is often an option after mastectomy. Women considering reconstruction should discuss this with a plastic surgeon before having a mastectomy.

Here are some questions a woman may want to ask her doctor before having surgery:

- What kinds of surgery can I consider? Is breast-sparing surgery an option for me? Which operation do you recommend for me? What are the risks of surgery?

- Should I store some of my own blood in case I need a transfusion?

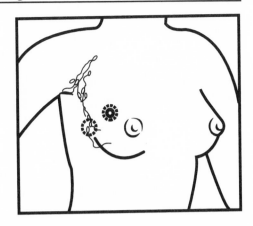

Figure 1.1. In **lumpectomy**, the surgeon removes the breast cancer and some normal tissue around it. *(Sometimes an excisional biopsy serves as a lumpectomy.)* Often, some of the lymph nodes under the arm are removed.

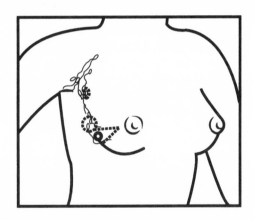

Figure 1.2. In **segmental mastectomy**, the surgeon removes the cancer and a larger area of normal breast tissue around it. Occasionally, some of the lining over the chest muscles below the tumor is removed as well. Some lymph nodes under the arm may also be removed.

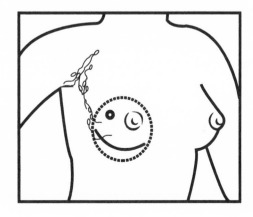

Figure 1.3. In **total (simple) mastectomy**, the surgeon removes the whole breast. Some lymph nodes under the arm may also be removed.

Figure 1.4. In **modified radical mastectomy**, *the surgeon removes the whole breast, most of the lymph nodes under the arm, and, often, the lining over the chest muscles. The smaller of the two chest muscles also may be taken out to help in removing the lymph nodes.*

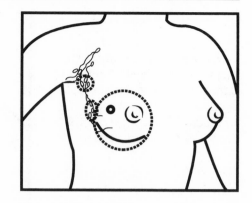

Figure 1.5. In **radical mastectomy** *(also called Halsted radical mastectomy), the surgeon removes the breast, both chest muscles, all of the lymph nodes under the arm, and some additional fat and skin. For many years, this operation was considered the standard one for women with breast cancer, but it is almost never used today. In rare cases, radical mastectomy may be suggested if the cancer has spread to the chest muscles.*

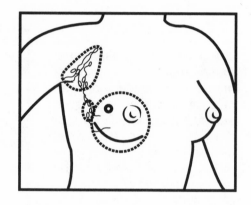

- Do I need my lymph nodes removed? How many? Why? What special precautions will I need to take if lymph nodes are removed?

- How will I feel after the operation?

- Will I need to learn how to do special things to take care of myself or my incision when I get home?

- Where will the scars be? What will they look like?

- If I decide to have plastic surgery to rebuild my breast, how and when can that be done? Can you suggest a plastic surgeon for me to contact?

- Will I have to do special exercises?

- When can I get back to my normal activities?
- Is there someone I can talk with who has had the same treatment I'll be having?

Radiation therapy (also called radiotherapy) is the use of high-energy rays to kill cancer cells. The radiation may be directed at the breast by a machine (external radiation). The radiation can also come from radioactive material placed in thin plastic tubes that are placed directly in the breast (implant radiation). Some women have both kinds of radiation therapy.

For external radiation therapy, the patient goes to the hospital or clinic, generally 5 days a week for several weeks. For implant radiation, a patient stays in the hospital. The implants remain in place for several days. They are removed before the woman goes home.

Sometimes, depending on the size of the tumor and other factors, radiation therapy is used after surgery, especially after breast-sparing surgery. The radiation destroys any breast cancer cells that may remain in the area.

Before surgery, radiation therapy, alone or with chemotherapy or hormonal therapy, is sometimes used to destroy cancer cells and shrink tumors. This approach is most often used in cases in which the breast tumor is large or not easily removed by surgery.

Before having radiation therapy, a patient may want to ask her doctor these questions:

- Why do I need this treatment?
- What are the risks and side effects of this treatment?
- Are there any long-term effects?
- When will the treatments begin? When will they end?
- How will I feel during therapy?
- What can I do to take care of myself during therapy?
- Can I continue my normal activities?
- How will my breast look afterward?
- What are the chances that the tumor will come back in my breast?

Chemotherapy is the use of drugs to kill cancer cells. Chemotherapy for breast cancer is usually a combination of drugs. The drugs may be given in a pill or by injection. Either way, the drugs enter the bloodstream and travel throughout the body.

Most patients have chemotherapy in an outpatient part of the hospital, at the doctor's office, or at home. Depending on which drugs are given and her general health, however, a woman may need to stay in the hospital during her treatment.

Hormonal therapy keeps cancer cells from getting the hormones they need to grow. This treatment may include the use of drugs that change the way hormones work, or surgery to remove the ovaries, which make female hormones. Like chemotherapy, hormonal therapy can affect cancer cells throughout the body.

Biological therapy is a treatment designed to enhance the body's natural defenses against cancer. For example, Herceptin® (trastuzumab) is a monoclonal antibody that targets breast cancer cells that have too much of a protein known as human epidermal growth factor receptor-2 (HER-2). By blocking HER-2, Herceptin slows or stops the growth of these cells. Herceptin may be given by itself or along with chemotherapy.

Patients may want to ask these questions about systemic therapy (chemotherapy, hormonal therapy, or biological therapy):

- Why do I need this treatment?
- If I need hormonal treatment, which would be better for me, drugs or an operation?
- What drugs will I be taking? What will they do?
- Will I have side effects? What can I do about them?
- How long will I be on this treatment?

Treatment Choices

Women with breast cancer now have many treatment options. Many women want to learn all they can about the disease and their treatment choices so that they can take an active part in decisions about their medical care. They are likely to have many questions and concerns about their treatment options.

The doctor is the best person to answer questions about treatment for a particular patient: what her treatment choices are and how successful her treatment is expected to be. Most patients also want to know how they will look after treatment and whether they will have to change their normal activities. A woman should not feel that she needs to ask all her questions or understand all the answers at once. She will have many chances to ask the doctor to explain things that are not clear and to ask for more information.

A woman may want to talk with her doctor about taking part in a clinical trial, a research study of new treatment methods. Clinical trials are an important option for women with all stages of breast cancer. The Promise of Cancer Research section has more information.

A woman's treatment options depend on a number of factors. These factors include her age and menopausal status; her general health; the size and location of the tumor and the stage of the cancer; the results of lab tests; and the size of her breast. Certain features of the tumor cells (such as whether they depend on hormones to grow) are also considered. In most cases, the most important factor is the stage of the disease. The stage is based on the size of the tumor and whether the cancer has spread. The following are brief descriptions of the stages of breast cancer and the treatments most often used for each stage. (Other treatments may sometimes be appropriate.)

- **Stage 0** is sometimes called noninvasive carcinoma or carcinoma *in situ*.

  Lobular carcinoma *in situ* (LCIS) refers to abnormal cells in the lining of a lobule. These abnormal cells seldom become invasive cancer. However, their presence is a sign that a woman has an increased risk of developing breast cancer. This risk of cancer is increased for both breasts. Some women with LCIS may take a drug called tamoxifen, which can reduce the risk of developing breast cancer. Others may take part in studies of other promising new preventive treatments. Some women may choose not to have treatment, but to return to the doctor regularly for checkups. And, occasionally, women with LCIS may decide to have surgery to remove both breasts to try to prevent cancer from developing. (In most cases, removal of underarm lymph nodes is not necessary.)

  Ductal carcinoma *in situ* (DCIS) refers to abnormal cells in the lining of a duct. DCIS is also called intraductal carcinoma. The abnormal cells have not spread beyond the duct to invade the surrounding breast tissue. However, women with DCIS are at an increased risk of getting invasive breast cancer. Some women with DCIS have breast-sparing surgery followed by radiation therapy. Or they may choose to have a mastectomy, with or without breast reconstruction (plastic surgery) to rebuild the breast. Underarm lymph nodes are not usually removed. Also, women with DCIS may want to talk with their doctor about tamoxifen to reduce the risk of developing invasive breast cancer.

- **Stage I** and **stage II** are early stages of breast cancer in which the cancer has spread beyond the lobe or duct and invaded nearby tissue. Stage I means that the tumor is no more than about an inch across and cancer cells have not spread beyond the breast. Stage II means one of the following: the tumor in the breast is less than 1 inch across and the cancer has spread to the lymph nodes under the arm; or the tumor is between 1 and 2 inches (with or without spread to the lymph nodes under the arm); or the tumor is larger than 2 inches but has not spread to the lymph nodes under the arm.

  Women with early stage breast cancer may have breast-sparing surgery followed by radiation therapy to the breast, or they may have a mastectomy, with or without breast reconstruction to rebuild the breast. These approaches are equally effective in treating early stage breast cancer. (Sometimes radiation therapy is also given after mastectomy.)

  The choice of breast-sparing surgery or mastectomy depends mostly on the size and location of the tumor, the size of the woman's breast, certain features of the cancer, and how the woman feels about preserving her breast. With either approach, lymph nodes under the arm usually are removed.

  Many women with stage I and most with stage II breast cancer have chemotherapy and/or hormonal therapy after primary treatment with surgery or surgery and radiation therapy. This added treatment is called adjuvant therapy. If the systemic therapy is given to shrink the tumor before surgery, this is called neoadjuvant therapy. Systemic treatment is given to try to destroy any remaining cancer cells and prevent the cancer from recurring, or coming back, in the breast or elsewhere.

- **Stage III** is also called locally advanced cancer. In this stage, the tumor in the breast is large (more than 2 inches across) and the cancer has spread to the underarm lymph nodes; or the cancer is extensive in the underarm lymph nodes; or the cancer has spread to lymph nodes near the breastbone or to other tissues near the breast.

Inflammatory breast cancer is a type of locally advanced breast cancer. In this type of cancer the breast looks red and swollen (or inflamed) because cancer cells block the lymph vessels in the skin of the breast.

Patients with stage III breast cancer usually have both local treatment to remove or destroy the cancer in the breast and systemic treatment to stop the disease from spreading. The local treatment may be surgery and/or radiation therapy to the breast and underarm. The systemic treatment may be chemotherapy, hormonal therapy, or both. Systemic therapy may be given before local therapy to shrink the tumor or afterward to prevent the disease from recurring in the breast or elsewhere.

- **Stage IV** is metastatic cancer. The cancer has spread beyond the breast and underarm lymph nodes to other parts of the body.

  Women who have stage IV breast cancer receive chemotherapy and/or hormonal therapy to destroy cancer cells and control the disease. They may have surgery or radiation therapy to control the cancer in the breast. Radiation may also be useful to control tumors in other parts of the body.

- **Recurrent cancer** means the disease has come back in spite of the initial treatment. Even when a tumor in the breast seems to have been completely removed or destroyed, the disease sometimes returns because undetected cancer cells remained somewhere in the body after treatment.

  Most recurrences appear within the first 2 or 3 years after treatment, but breast cancer can recur many years later. Cancer that returns only in the area of the surgery is called a local recurrence. If the disease returns in another part of the body, the distant recurrence is called metastatic breast cancer. The patient may have one type of treatment or a combination of treatments for recurrent cancer.

Side Effects of Treatment

It is hard to protect healthy cells from the harmful effects of breast cancer treatment. Because treatment does damage healthy cells and tissues, it causes side effects. The side effects of cancer treatment depend mainly on the type and extent of the treatment. Also, the effects may not be the same for each person, and they may be different from one treatment to the next. An important part of the treatment plan is the management of side effects.

A patient's reaction to treatment is closely monitored by physical exams, blood tests, and other tests. Doctors and nurses will explain the possible side effects of treatment, and they can suggest ways to deal with problems that may occur during and after treatment. The NCI provides helpful, informative booklets about cancer treatments and coping with side effects. Patients may want to read *Understanding Breast Cancer Treatment: A Guide for Patients*, as well as *Radiation Therapy and You*, *Chemotherapy and You*, and *Eating Hints for Cancer Patients*.

Surgery

Surgery causes short-term pain and tenderness in the area of the operation, so women may need to talk with their doctor about pain management. Any kind of surgery also carries a risk of infection, poor wound healing, bleeding, or a reaction to the anesthesia used during surgery. Women who experience any of these problems should tell their doctor or nurse right away.

Removal of a breast can cause a woman's weight to be out of balance—especially if she has large breasts. This imbalance can cause discomfort in her neck and back. Also, the skin in the area where the breast was removed may be tight, and the muscles of the arm and shoulder may feel stiff. After a mastectomy, some women have some permanent loss of strength in these muscles, but for most women, reduced strength and limited movement are temporary. The doctor, nurse, or physical therapist can recommend exercises to help a woman regain movement and strength in her arm and shoulder.

Because nerves may be injured or cut during surgery, a woman may have numbness and tingling in the chest, underarm, shoulder, and upper arm. These feelings usually go away within a few weeks or months, but some women have permanent numbness.

Removing the lymph nodes under the arm slows the flow of lymph. In some women, this fluid builds up in the arm and hand and causes swelling (lymphedema). Women need to protect the arm and hand on the treated side from injury or pressure, even long after surgery. They should ask the doctor how to handle any cuts, scratches, insect bites, or other injuries to the arm or hand. Also, they should contact the doctor if an infection develops in that arm or hand.

Radiation Therapy

During radiation therapy, patients may become extremely tired, especially after several treatments. This feeling may continue for a while after treatment is over. Resting is important, but doctors usually advise their patients to try to stay reasonably active, matching their activities to their energy level. It is also common for the skin in the treated area to become red, dry, tender, and itchy. The breast may feel heavy and hard, but these conditions will clear up with time. Toward the end of treatment, the skin may become moist and "weepy." Exposing this area to air as much as possible will help the skin heal. Because bras and some types of clothing may rub the skin and cause irritation, patients may want to wear loose-fitting cotton clothes. Gentle skin care is important at this time, and patients should check with their doctor before using any deodorants, lotions, or creams on the treated area. These effects of radiation therapy on the skin are temporary, and the area gradually heals once treatment is over. However, there may be a permanent change in the color of the skin.

Chemotherapy

As with radiation, chemotherapy affects normal as well as cancer cells. The side effects of chemotherapy depend mainly on the specific drugs and the dose. In general, anticancer drugs affect rapidly dividing cells. These include blood cells, which fight infection, help the blood to clot, and carry oxygen to all parts of the body. When blood cells are affected, patients are more likely to get infections, may bruise or bleed easily, and may feel unusually weak and very tired. Rapidly dividing cells in hair roots and cells that line the digestive tract may also be affected. As a result, side effects may include loss of hair, poor appetite, nausea and vomiting, diarrhea, or mouth and lip sores. Many of these side effects can now be controlled, thanks to new or improved drugs. Side effects generally are short-term and gradually go away. Hair grows back, but it may be different in color and texture.

Some anticancer drugs can damage the ovaries. If the ovaries fail to produce hormones, the woman may have symptoms of menopause, such as hot flashes and vaginal dryness. Her periods may become irregular or may stop, and she may not be able to become pregnant. Other long-term side effects are quite rare, but there have been cases in which the heart is weakened, and second cancers such as leukemia (cancer of the blood cells) have occurred.

Women who are still menstruating may still be able to get pregnant during treatment. Because the effects of chemotherapy on an unborn child are not known, it is important for a woman to talk with her doctor about birth control before treatment begins. After treatment, some women regain their ability to become pregnant, but in women over the age of 35, infertility is likely to be permanent.

Hormonal Therapy

The side effects of hormonal therapy depend largely on the specific drug or type of treatment. Tamoxifen is the most common hormonal treatment. This drug blocks the cancer cells' use of estrogen but does not stop estrogen production. Tamoxifen may cause hot flashes, vaginal discharge or irritation, nausea, and irregular periods. Women who are still menstruating and having irregular periods may become pregnant more easily when taking tamoxifen. They should discuss birth control methods with their doctor.

Serious side effects of tamoxifen are rare. It can cause blood clots in the veins, especially in the legs and in the lungs, and in a small number of women, it can slightly increase the risk of stroke. Also, tamoxifen can cause cancer of the lining of the uterus. Any unusual vaginal bleeding should be reported to the doctor. The doctor may do a pelvic exam, as well as a biopsy of the lining of the uterus, or other tests. (This does not apply to women who have had a hysterectomy, surgery to remove the uterus.)

Young women whose ovaries are removed to deprive the cancer cells of estrogen experience menopause immediately. Their symptoms are likely to be more severe than symptoms associated with natural menopause.

Biological Therapy

The side effects of biological therapy differ with the types of substances used, and from patient to patient. Rashes or swelling where the biological therapy is injected are common. Flu-like symptoms also may occur.

Herceptin may cause these and other side effects, but these effects generally become less severe after the first treatment. Less commonly, Herceptin can also cause damage to the heart that can lead to heart failure. It can also affect the lungs, causing breathing problems that require immediate medical attention. For these reasons, women are checked carefully for heart and lung problems before taking Herceptin. Patients who do take it are watched carefully during treatment.

Breast Reconstruction

After a mastectomy, some women decide to wear a breast form (prosthesis). Others prefer to have breast reconstruction, either at the same time as the mastectomy or later on. Each option has its pros and cons, and what is right for one woman may not be right for another. What is important is that nearly every woman treated for breast cancer has choices. It is best to consult with a plastic surgeon before the mastectomy, even if reconstruction will be considered later on.

Various procedures are used to reconstruct the breast. Some use implants (either saline or silicone); others use tissue moved from another part of the woman's body. The safety of silicone breast implants has been under review by the Food and Drug Administration (FDA) for several years. Women interested in having silicone implants should talk with their doctor about the FDA's findings and the availability of silicone implants. Which type of reconstruction is best depends on a woman's age, body type, and the type of surgery she had. A woman should ask the plastic surgeon to explain the risks and benefits of each type of reconstruction. The National Cancer Institute booklet *Understanding Breast Cancer Treatment: A Guide for Patients* contains more information about breast reconstruction. The Cancer Information Service at 1-800-4-CANCER can suggest other sources of information about breast reconstruction and can talk with callers about breast cancer support groups.

Rehabilitation

Rehabilitation is a very important part of breast cancer treatment. The health care team makes every effort to help women return to their normal activities as soon as possible. Recovery will be different for each woman, depending on the extent of the disease, the type of treatment, and other factors.

Exercising the arm and shoulder after surgery can help a woman regain motion and strength in these areas. It can also reduce pain and stiffness in her neck and back. Carefully planned exercises should be started as soon as the doctor says the woman is ready, often within a day or so after surgery. Exercising begins slowly and gently and can even be done in bed. Gradually, exercising can be more active, and regular exercise becomes part of a woman's normal routine. (Women who have a mastectomy and immediate breast reconstruction need special exercises, which the doctor or nurse will explain.)

Often, lymphedema after surgery can be prevented or reduced with certain exercises and by resting with the arm propped up on a pillow. If lymphedema occurs, the doctor may suggest exercises and other ways to deal with this problem. For example, some women with lymphedema wear an elastic sleeve or use an elastic cuff to improve lymph circulation. The doctor also may suggest other approaches, such as medication, manual lymph drainage (massage), or use of a machine that gently compresses the arm. The woman may be referred to a physical therapist or another specialist.

Followup Care

Regular followup exams are important after breast cancer treatment. Regular checkups ensure that changes in health are noticed. Followup exams usually include examination of the breasts, chest, neck, and underarm areas, as well as periodic mammograms. If a woman has a breast implant, special mammogram techniques can be used. Sometimes the doctor may order other imaging procedures or lab tests.

A woman who has had cancer in one breast should report any changes in the treated area or in the other breast to her doctor right away. Because a woman who has had breast cancer is at risk of getting cancer in the other breast, mammograms are an important part of followup care.

Also, a woman who has had breast cancer should tell her doctor about other physical problems, such as pain, loss of appetite or weight, changes in menstrual cycles, unusual vaginal bleeding, or blurred vision. She should also report headaches, dizziness, shortness of breath, coughing or hoarseness, backaches, or digestive problems that seem unusual or that don't go away. These symptoms may be a sign that the cancer has returned, but they can also be signs of various other problems. It's important to share these concerns with a doctor.

Support for Women with Breast Cancer

The diagnosis of breast cancer can change a woman's life and the lives of those close to her. These changes can be hard to handle. It is common for the woman and her family and friends to have many different and sometimes confusing emotions. Having helpful information and support services can make it easier to cope with these problems.

People living with cancer may worry about caring for their families, keeping their jobs, or continuing daily activities. Concerns about tests, treatments, hospital stays, and medical bills are also common. Doctors, nurses, and other members of the health care team can answer questions about treatment, working, or other activities. Meeting with a social worker, counselor, or member of the clergy can be helpful to people who want to talk about their feelings or discuss their concerns. Often, a social worker can suggest resources for help with rehabilitation, emotional support, financial aid, transportation, or home care.

Friends and relatives can be very supportive. Also, it helps many patients to discuss their concerns with others who have cancer. Women with breast cancer often get together in support groups, where they can share what they have learned about coping with their disease and the effects of their treatment. It is important to keep in mind, however, that each person is different. Treatments and ways of dealing with cancer that work for one person may not be right for another — even if they both have the same kind of cancer. It is always a good idea to discuss the advice of friends and family members with the doctor.

Several organizations offer special programs for patients with breast cancer. Trained volunteers, who have had breast cancer themselves, may talk with or visit patients, provide information, and lend emotional support before and after treatment. They often share their experiences with breast cancer treatment, rehabilitation, and breast reconstruction.

Sometimes women who have had breast cancer are afraid that changes to their body will affect not only how they look but how other people feel about them. They may be concerned that breast cancer and its treatment will affect their sexual relationships. Many couples find that talking about these concerns helps them find ways to express their love during and after treatment. Some seek counseling or a couples' support group.

The Promise of Cancer Research

Doctors all over the country are conducting many types of clinical trials (research studies in which people take part voluntarily). These include studies of ways to prevent, detect, diagnose, and treat breast cancer; studies of the psychological effects of the disease; and studies of ways to improve comfort and quality of life. Research already has led to significant advances in these areas, and researchers continue to search for more effective approaches.

People who take part in clinical trials have the first chance to benefit from new approaches. They also make important contributions to medical science. Although clinical trials may pose some risks, researchers take very careful steps to protect people who take part.

Women who are interested in being part of a clinical trial should talk with their doctor. They may want to read the National Cancer Institute booklets *Taking Part in Clinical Trials: What Cancer Patients Need To Know* or *Taking Part in Clinical Trials: Cancer Prevention Studies*, which describe how research studies are carried out and explain their possible benefits and risks. NCI's cancerTrials™ Web site at http://cancertrials.nci.nih.gov/ provides general information about clinical trials. It also offers detailed information about specific ongoing studies of breast cancer by linking to PDQ®, a cancer information database developed by the NCI.

Causes and Prevention

Doctors can seldom explain why one woman gets breast cancer and another doesn't. It is clear, however, that breast cancer is not caused by bumping, bruising, or touching the breast. And this disease is not contagious; no one can "catch" breast cancer from another person.

Scientists are trying to learn more about factors that increase the risk of developing this disease. For example, they are looking at whether the risk of breast cancer might be affected by environmental factors. So far, scientists do not have enough information to know whether any factors in the environment increase the risk of this disease. (The main known risk factors are listed in the "Breast Cancer: Who's at Risk?" section.)

Some aspects of a woman's lifestyle may affect her chances of developing breast cancer. For example, recent studies suggest that regular exercise may decrease the risk in younger women. Also, some evidence suggests a link between diet and breast cancer. Ongoing studies are looking at ways to prevent breast cancer through changes in diet or with dietary supplements. However, it is not yet known whether specific dietary changes will actually prevent breast cancer. These are active areas of research.

Scientists are trying to learn whether having a miscarriage or an abortion increases the risk of breast cancer. Thus far, studies have produced conflicting results, and this question is still unresolved.

Research has led to the identification of changes (mutations) in certain genes that increase the risk of developing breast cancer. Women with a strong family history of breast cancer may choose to have a blood test to see if they have inherited a change in the BRCA1 or BRCA2 gene. Women who are concerned about an inherited risk for breast cancer should talk to their doctor. The doctor may suggest seeing a health professional trained in genetics. Genetic counseling can help a woman decide whether testing would be appropriate for her. Also, counseling before and after testing helps women understand and deal with the possible results of a genetic test. Counseling can also help with concerns about employment or about health, life, and disability insurance. The Cancer Information Service can supply additional material on genetic testing.

Scientists are looking for drugs that may prevent the development of breast cancer. In one large study, the drug tamoxifen reduced the number of new cases of breast cancer among women at an increased risk for the disease. Doctors are now studying how another drug called raloxifene compares to tamoxifen. This study is called STAR (Study of Tamoxifen and Raloxifene). For more information about prevention clinical trials, call the Cancer Information Service.

Detection and Diagnosis

At present, mammograms are the most effective tool we have to detect breast cancer. Researchers are looking for ways to make mammography more accurate, such as using computers to read mammograms (digital mammography). They are also exploring other techniques, such as magnetic resonance imaging (MRI), breast ultrasonography, and positron emission tomography (PET), to produce detailed pictures of the tissues in the breast.

In addition, researchers are studying tumor markers. These are substances that may be present in abnormal amounts in people with cancer. Tumor markers may be found in blood or urine, or in fluid from the breast (nipple aspirate). Some of these markers may be used to check women who have already been diagnosed with breast cancer. At this time, however, no tumor marker test is reliable enough to be used routinely to detect breast cancer.

Treatment

Through research, doctors try to find new, more effective ways to treat cancer. Many studies of new approaches for patients with breast cancer are under way. When laboratory research shows that a new treatment method has promise, cancer patients receive the new approach in treatment clinical trials. These studies are designed to answer important questions and to find out whether the new approach is safe and effective. Often, clinical trials compare a new treatment with a standard approach.

Researchers are testing new anticancer drugs, doses, and treatment schedules. They are working with various drugs and drug combinations, as well as with several types of hormonal therapy. They also are looking at the effectiveness of using chemotherapy before surgery (called neoadjuvant chemotherapy) and at new ways of combining treatments, such as adding hormonal therapy or radiation therapy to chemotherapy.

New biological approaches also are under study. For example, several cancer vaccines have been designed to stimulate the immune system to mount a response against breast cancer cells. Combinations of biological treatments with other agents are also undergoing clinical study.

Researchers are exploring ways to reduce the side effects of treatment (such as lymphedema from surgery), improve the quality of patients' lives, and reduce pain. One procedure under study is called sentinel lymph node biopsy. Researchers are trying to learn whether this procedure may reduce the number of lymph nodes that must be removed during breast cancer surgery. Before surgery, the doctor injects a radioactive substance near the tumor. The substance flows through the lymphatic system to the first lymph node or nodes where cancer cells are likely to have spread (the "sentinel" node or nodes). The doctor uses a scanner to locate the radioactive substance in the sentinel nodes. Sometimes the doctor also injects a blue dye near the tumor. The dye travels through the lymphatic system to collect in the sentinel nodes. The surgeon makes a small incision and removes only the nodes with radioactive substance or blue dye. A pathologist checks the sentinel lymph nodes for cancer cells. If no cancer cells are detected, it may not be necessary to remove additional nodes. If sentinel lymph node biopsy proves to be as effective as the standard axillary lymph node dissection, the new procedure could prevent lymphedema.

Chemotherapy can reduce the ability of bone marrow to make blood cells. That is why researchers are studying ways to help the blood cells recover so that high doses of chemotherapy can be given. These studies use biological therapies (known as colony-stimulating factors), autologous bone marrow transplants, or peripheral stem cell transplants.

Chapter 2

Screening for Breast Cancer

What Is Screening?

Screening for cancer is examination (or testing) of people for early stages in the development of cancer even though they have no symptoms. Scientists have studied patterns of cancer in the population to learn which people are more likely to get certain types of cancer. They have also studied what things around us and what things we do in our lives may cause cancer. This information sometimes helps doctors recommend who should be screened for certain types of cancer, what types of screening tests people should have, and how often these tests should be done. Not all screening tests are helpful, and they often have risks. For this reason, scientists at the National Cancer Institute are studying many screening tests to find out how useful they are and to determine the relative benefits and harms.

If your doctor suggests certain cancer screening tests as part of your health care plan, this does not mean he or she thinks you have cancer. Screening tests are done when you have no symptoms. Since decisions about screening can be difficult, you may want to discuss them with your doctor and ask questions about the potential benefits and risks of screening tests and whether they have been proven to decrease the risk of dying from cancer.

If your doctor suspects that you may have cancer, he or she will order certain tests to see whether you do. These are called diagnostic

CancerNet, National Cancer Institute, November 2000.

tests. Some tests are used for diagnostic purposes, but are not suitable for screening people who have no symptoms.

Purposes of This Summary

The purposes of this summary on breast cancer screening are to:

- give information on breast cancer and what makes it more likely to occur (risk factors)

- describe breast cancer screening methods and what is known about their effectiveness

You can talk to your doctor or health care professional about cancer screening and whether it would be likely to help you.

Breast Cancer Screening

The breast consists of lobes, lobules, and bulbs that are connected by ducts. The breast also contains blood and lymph vessels. These lymph vessels lead to structures that are called lymph nodes. Clusters of lymph nodes are found under the arm, above the collarbone, in the chest, and in other parts of the body. Together, the lymph vessels and lymph nodes make up the lymphatic system, which circulates a fluid called lymph throughout the body. Lymph contains cells that help fight infection and disease.

When breast cancer spreads outside the breast, cancer cells are most often found under the arm in the lymph nodes. In many cases, if the cancer has reached the lymph nodes, cancer cells may have also spread to other parts of the body via the lymphatic system or through the bloodstream.

Risk of Breast Cancer

More women in the United States get breast cancer than any other type of cancer (except for skin cancer). The number of cases per 1,000 women has increased slightly every year over the last 50 years. It is the second leading cause of death from cancer in women (lung cancer causes the most deaths from cancer in women). Breast cancer occurs in men also, but the number of new cases is small.

Anything that increases a person's chance of developing a disease is called a risk factor. Some of these risk factors for breast cancer are as follows:

Age—Breast cancer is more likely to develop as you grow older. Beginning menstruation at an early age and late age at first birth may also increase the risk of development of breast cancer.

History of Breast Cancer—If you have already had breast cancer, you are more likely to develop breast cancer again.

Family History—If your mother or sister had breast cancer, you are more likely to develop breast cancer, especially if they had it at an early age.

Radiation Therapy—Radiation therapy to the chest that was given more than 10 years ago, especially in women younger than 30 years old, may increase a woman's risk of developing breast cancer.

Other Breast Diseases—If you have had a breast biopsy specimen that showed certain types of benign breast conditions, you may be more likely to develop breast cancer. For most women, however, the ordinary "lumpiness" they feel in their breasts does not increase their risk of breast cancer.

Studies have found that race, social status, income, education, and access to screening and treatment services may affect a woman's risk of developing breast cancer.

Screening Tests for Breast Cancer

Breast Self-Examination—When you examine your own breasts it is called breast self-examination (BSE). Studies so far have not shown that BSE alone reduces the number of deaths from breast cancer. Therefore, it should not be used in place of clinical breast examination and mammography.

Clinical Breast Examination—During your routine physical examination, your doctor or health care professional may do a clinical breast examination (CBE). During a CBE, your doctor will carefully feel your breasts and under your arms to check for lumps or other unusual changes.

Mammogram—A mammogram is a special x-ray of the breast that can often find tumors that are too small for you or your doctor to feel.

Your doctor may suggest that you have a mammogram, especially if you have any of the risk factors listed above.

The ability of mammography to detect cancer depends on such factors as the size of the tumor, the age of the woman, breast density, and the skill of the radiologist. Studies have found that screening mammography is beneficial in women aged 50 to 69. Screening in women younger than 50 years or older than 69 years may or may not be helpful.

Ultrasonography—During ultrasonography, sound waves (called ultrasound) are bounced off tissues and the echoes are converted into a picture (sonogram). Ultrasound is used to evaluate lumps that have been identified by BSE, CBE, or mammography. Studies have not shown that ultrasonography is of any proven benefit in detecting breast cancer.

Magnetic Resonance Imaging (MRI)—A procedure in which a magnet linked to a computer is used to create detailed pictures of areas inside the body. MRIs are used to evaluate breast masses that have been found by BSE or CBE and to recognize the difference between cancer and scar tissue. The role of MRI in breast cancer screening has not yet been established.

Other screening methods are being studied. Your doctor can talk to you about what screening tests would be best for you.

To Learn More

For more information, call the National Cancer Institute's Cancer Information Service at 1-800-4-CANCER (1-800-422-6237); TTY at 1-800-332-8615. The call is free and a trained information specialist is available to answer your questions.

Chapter 3

Prevention of Breast Cancer

What Is Prevention?

Doctors can not always explain why one person gets cancer and another does not. However, scientists have studied general patterns of cancer in the population to learn what things around us and what things we do in our lives may increase our chance of developing cancer.

Anything that increases a person's chance of developing a disease is called a risk factor; anything that decreases a person's chance of developing a disease is called a protective factor. Some of the risk factors for cancer can be avoided, but many can not. For example, although you can choose to quit smoking, you can not choose which genes you have inherited from your parents. Both smoking and inheriting specific genes could be considered risk factors for certain kinds of cancer, but only smoking can be avoided. Prevention means avoiding the risk factors and increasing the protective factors that can be controlled so that the chance of developing cancer decreases.

Although many risk factors can be avoided, it is important to keep in mind that avoiding risk factors does not guarantee that you will not get cancer. Also, most people with a particular risk factor for cancer do not actually get the disease. Some people are more sensitive than others to factors that can cause cancer. Talk to your doctor about methods of preventing cancer that might be effective for you.

National Cancer Institute, PDQ®, August 2000.

The purposes of this summary on breast cancer prevention are to:

- give information on breast cancer and how often it occurs
- describe breast cancer prevention methods
- give current facts about which people or groups of people would most likely be helped by following breast cancer prevention methods

You can talk to your doctor or health care professional about cancer prevention methods and whether they would be likely to help you.

Breast Cancer Prevention

The breast consists of lobes, lobules, and bulbs that are connected by ducts. The breast also contains blood and lymph vessels. These lymph vessels lead to structures that are called lymph nodes. Clusters of lymph nodes are found under the arm, above the collarbone, in the chest, and in other parts of the body. Together, the lymph vessels and lymph nodes make up the lymphatic system, which circulates a fluid called lymph throughout the body. Lymph contains cells that help fight infection and disease.

When breast cancer spreads outside the breast, cancer cells are most often found under the arm in the lymph nodes. In many cases, if the cancer has reached the lymph nodes, cancer cells may have also spread to other parts of the body via the lymphatic system or through the bloodstream.

Breast cancer is second only to lung cancer as the leading cause of cancer death among women in the United States. Breast cancer occurs in men also, but the number of new cases is small. Early detection and effective treatment is expected to reduce the number of women who die from breast cancer, and development of new methods of prevention continue to be studied.

Breast cancer can sometimes be associated with known risk factors for the disease. Many risk factors are modifiable though not all can be avoided.

Tamoxifen for Prevention of Breast Cancer

Tamoxifen is a drug that blocks the effect of estrogen on breast cancer cells. A large study has shown that tamoxifen lowers the risk of getting breast cancer in women who are at elevated risk of getting breast cancer. However, tamoxifen may also increase the risk of getting some other serious diseases, including endometrial cancer, stroke, and blood clots in veins and in the lungs. Women who are concerned that they may be at an increased risk of developing breast cancer should talk with their doctor about whether to take tamoxifen to prevent breast cancer. It is important to consider both the benefits and risks of taking tamoxifen.

Hormonal Factors

Hormones produced by the ovaries appear to increase a woman's risk for developing breast cancer. The removal of one or both ovaries reduces the risk. The use of drugs that suppress the production of estrogen may inhibit tumor cell growth. The use of hormone replacement therapy may be associated with an increased risk of developing breast cancer, mostly in recent users. The use of oral contraceptives may also be associated with a slight increase in breast cancer risk.

Beginning to menstruate at an older age and having a full-term pregnancy reduces breast cancer risk. Also, a woman who has her first child before the age of 20 experiences a greater decrease in breast cancer risk than a woman who has never had children or who has her first child after the age of 35. Beginning menopause at a later age increases a woman's risk of developing breast cancer.

Radiation

Studies have shown that reducing the number of chest x-rays, especially at a young age, decreases the risk of breast cancer. Radiation treatment for childhood Hodgkin's disease may put women at a greater risk for breast cancer later in life. A small number of breast cancer cases can be linked to radiation exposure.

Diet and Lifestyle

Diet is being studied as a risk factor for breast cancer. Studies show that in populations that consume a high-fat diet, women are more likely to die of breast cancer than women in populations that consume a low-fat diet. It is not known if a diet low in fat will prevent breast cancer. Studies also show that certain vitamins may decrease a woman's risk of breast cancer, especially premenopausal women at high risk. Exercise, especially in young women, may decrease hormone levels and contribute to a decreased breast cancer risk. Breast feeding may also decrease a woman's risk of breast cancer. Studies suggest that the consumption of alcohol is associated with a slight increase in the risk of developing breast cancer. Postmenopausal weight gain, especially after natural menopause and/or after age 60, may increase breast cancer risk.

Prophylactic Mastectomy

Following cancer risk assessment and counseling, the removal of both breasts may reduce the risk of breast cancer in women with a family history of breast cancer.

Genetics

Women who inherit specific genes are at a greater risk for developing breast cancer. Research is underway to develop methods of identifying high-risk genes.

Drugs Being Studied

Fenretinide and raloxifene are two other drugs that are being studied for their usefulness as potential breast cancer prevention agents.

Chapter 4

Breast Cancer: Better Treatments Save More Lives

Two different women. The same deadly disease. One thought she couldn't get it. The other was told she didn't have it. Both opinions were wrong.

In 1994, one week before turning 35, Cathy Young received the devastating news. "I thought people had to be in their 50s to get cancer," the Oak Grove, Mo., resident says. "And then it happened to me."

Linda Hunter, 42, recalls that in January 1995, her mammogram results came back normal. But skin changes on one of her breasts compelled her to seek a second, third and fourth opinion—all of which supported the initial mammogram findings. Her tenacity finally paid off when a fifth doctor she visited detected a rare form of the disease.

Every three minutes a woman in the United States learns she has breast cancer. It is the most common cancer among women, next to skin cancers, and is second only to lung cancer in cancer deaths in women. Only 5 to 10 percent of breast cancers occur in women with a clearly defined genetic predisposition for the disease. The overall risk for developing breast cancer increases as a woman gets older.

Although treatment is initially successful for many women, the American Cancer Society (ACS) says that breast cancer will return in about 50 percent of these cases.

"Breast Cancer: Better Treatments Save More Lives," by Carol Lewis, *FDA Consumer*, July-August 1999; this version is from Publication No. (FDA) 00-1306 and contains revisions made in October 1999 and June 2000.

"It's hard to say that things are back to normal when one survives breast cancer," says Young, "because a survivor always has a fear that one day the cancer may return."

New drugs, new treatment regimens, and better diagnostic techniques have improved the outlook for many, and are responsible, according to ACS, for breast cancer death rates going down.

"Women have greater options in breast cancer treatment compared to a decade ago," says Harman Eyre, M.D., chief medical officer for ACS. "New drugs and procedures open up a whole new era of effective treatment."

Breast Cancer Treatments

Breast cancer can be treated with surgery, radiation and drugs (chemotherapy and hormonal therapy). Doctors may use one of these or a combination, depending on factors such as the type and location of the cancer, whether the disease has spread, and the patient's overall health.

Most women with breast cancer will have some type of surgery, depending on the stage of the breast cancer. (See "Stages of Breast Cancer.") The least invasive, lumpectomy (breast-conserving surgery), removes only the cancerous tissue and a surrounding margin of normal tissue. Removal of the entire breast is a mastectomy. A modified radical mastectomy includes the entire breast and some of the underarm lymph nodes. The very disfiguring radical mastectomy, in which the breast, lymph nodes, and chest wall muscles under the breast are removed, is rarely performed today because doctors believe that a modified radical mastectomy is just as effective.

While removing underarm lymph nodes after surgery is important in order to determine if the cancer has spread, this procedure may add chronic arm swelling and restricted shoulder motion to the discomforts of the overall treatment. But a new method, sentinel node biopsy, still under investigation, allows physicians to pinpoint the first lymph node into which a tumor drains (the sentinel node), and remove only the nodes most likely to contain cancer cells.

To locate the sentinel node, the physician injects a radioactive tracer in the area around the tumor before the mastectomy. The tracer travels the same path to the lymph nodes that cancer cells would take, making it possible for the surgeon to determine the one or two nodes most likely to test positive. The surgeon will then remove the nodes most likely to be cancerous.

Radiation therapy is treatment with high-energy rays or particles given to destroy cancer. In almost all cases, lumpectomy is followed by six to seven weeks of radiation, an integral part of breast-conserving treatment. Although radiation therapy damages both normal cells and cancerous cells, most of the normal cells are able to repair themselves and function properly.

Radiation therapy can cause side effects such as swelling and heaviness in the breast, sunburn-like skin changes in the treated area, and lymphedema (swelling of the arm due to fluid buildup) if the underarm lymph nodes were treated after a node dissection.

Drug Options Expand

Drugs are used to reach cancer cells that may have spread beyond the breast—in many cases even if no cancer is detected in the lymph nodes after surgery.

While doctors once believed that the spread of breast cancer could be controlled with extensive surgery, they now believe that cancer cells may break away from the primary tumor and spread through the bloodstream, even in the earliest stages of the disease. These cells cannot be felt by examination or seen on x-rays or other imaging methods, and they cause no symptoms. But they can establish new tumors in other organs or the bones. The goal of drug treatment, even if there's no detectable cancer after surgery, is to kill these hidden cells. This treatment, known as adjuvant therapy, is not needed by every patient. Doctors will make recommendations regarding specific types of therapy based on the stage of the breast cancer.

FDA has approved several new drugs and new uses for older drugs in recent years that improve the chances of successfully treating breast cancer. These drugs include:

Herceptin: About 30 percent of women with breast cancer have an excess of a protein called HER2, which makes tumors grow quickly. A genetically engineered drug, Herceptin (trastuzumab), binds to HER2 and kills the excess cancer cells, theoretically leaving healthy cells alone.

Herceptin, made by Genentech Inc., San Francisco, California., and approved by FDA in September 1998, is an intravenous treatment that is used alone in patients who have had little success with other drugs, or as a first-line treatment in combination with the drug Taxol (paclitaxel).

Recent follow-up research shows that Herceptin, in combination with chemotherapy, also may modestly extend the lives of terminal breast cancer patients. Updated survival figures reported from a two-year study by one of the drug's key developers from the University of California at Los Angeles showed an improvement in survival (about 4 months on average) in those getting Herceptin. Scientists say that while the improvement is small—about four months on average—it is especially noteworthy in a disease that until now has eluded many efforts to slow its progression to death.

Selection of patients who are most likely to benefit from Herceptin is important because of the possible serious risks from the drug, including weakening of the heart muscle that can lead to congestive heart failure. It is not known whether Herceptin has beneficial effects in women with normal levels of the HER2 protein.

FDA also approved in September 1998 a test called DAKO Hercep-Test to measure HER2 protein in tumors.

Nolvadex: A drug that has been used as a breast cancer treatment for more than 20 years, Nolvadex (tamoxifen citrate) was approved by FDA in October 1998 for breast cancer risk reduction in high-risk women.

Doctors know that estrogen promotes the growth of breast cancer cells. Tamoxifen interferes with the activity of estrogen by slowing or stopping the growth of cancer cells already present in the body. As adjuvant therapy, tamoxifen has been shown to help prevent both the original breast cancer from returning, and also the development of new cancers in the other breast.

A National Cancer Institute study showed that the drug reduced the short-term chance of getting breast cancer by 44 percent in women who were judged to be at increased risk for the disease. FDA emphasizes, however, that tamoxifen, manufactured by AstraZeneca Pharmaceuticals, Wilmington, Del., will not eliminate breast cancer risk completely, and should be used only following a medical evaluation of individual risk factors.

Due to potentially serious side effects, including endometrial (lining of the uterus) cancer and blood clots in major veins and the lungs, the American Society of Clinical Oncology recommends that patients talk with their regular health-care providers to determine whether individual medical circumstances and histories are appropriate for considering use of tamoxifen.

Xeloda: Xeloda (capecitabine), made by Hoffmann-La Roche, Nutley, New Jersey, was approved by FDA in April 1998 for the treatment of breast cancer that has spread to other parts of the body (metastasized) and is resistant to both paclitaxel and an anthracycline-containing regimen. Xeloda does not kill the cancer cells directly. Instead, once the drug enters the cancer cells, it is metabolized to 5-fluorouracil (5-FU), a drug routinely used for breast cancer. The advantage of Xeloda, in addition to the convenience of its pill form, is that cancer cells actively convert it to 5-FU, but normal cells convert very little to 5-FU.

Taxotere: In May 1996, FDA gave accelerated approval to Taxotere (docetaxel) to treat patients whose locally advanced or metastasized breast cancer has progressed despite treatment with other drugs. The approval was conditional on the manufacturer, Rhone-Poulenc Rorer Pharmaceuticals, Inc., Collegeville, Pa., conducting additional studies. In June 1998, after additional studies confirmed its safety and effectiveness, the drug was granted full FDA approval.

In addition to these newer drugs, combinations of the anticancer drugs Cytoxan (cyclophosphamide) and Adriamycin (doxorubicin), with or without Adrucil (fluorouracil), may be used to treat breast cancer.

Chemotherapy (drug treatment) is given in cycles, with each period of treatment followed by a recovery period. The total course of chemotherapy can last three to six months, depending on the drugs and how far the cancer has spread.

Kelly Munsell of Tucson, Arizona., took the combination Adriamycin and Cytoxan in six cycles, spaced three weeks apart, after doctors diagnosed her breast cancer in 1996 at age 27.

"Chemo for me was torture," Munsell recalls, describing profuse vomiting and severe weight gain as two of the serious side effects. But despite the discomfort, Munsell, whose mother and grandmother both died of breast cancer, is glad she underwent the grueling treatment two years ago. "My recent battery of tests came back negative for cancer," she says.

In addition to the drugs actually battling the disease, there also is help for patients in severe pain from cancer. FDA approved Actiq (oral transmucosal fentanyl citrate) in November 1998 as a treatment specifically for cancer patients with severe pain that breaks through their regular narcotic therapy. A narcotic more potent than morphine, Actiq is in the form of a flavored sugar lozenge that dissolves slowly in the mouth. Actiq is approved for patients already taking at least 60 milligrams of morphine per day for their underlying persistent cancer pain.

Looking Ahead

It is important for every woman to consider herself at risk for breast cancer, ACS says, simply because she's female. At the same time, however, studies continue to uncover lifestyle factors and habits that can alter that risk, and many new chemotherapy drugs and drug combinations continue to be developed and tested in clinical trials. Drugs and procedures currently under investigation include bisphosphonates (a group of drugs routinely used to treat osteoporosis), monoclonal antibodies (similar to Herceptin), and angiogenesis inhibitors (drugs that block the development of blood vessels that nourish cancer cells).

"While death rates from breast cancer are falling, and while there are a number of exciting new strategies being developed," says Michael A. Friedman, M.D., former FDA deputy commissioner and cancer research specialist, "we recognize that a great deal more needs to be done."

Mammography: A Lifesaving Step

The American Cancer Society says that the best strategy for successfully beating breast cancer is to follow guidelines for early detection. Currently, the most effective technique for early detection is screening mammography, an x-ray procedure that can detect small tumors and breast abnormalities up to two years before they can be felt and when they are most treatable.

Studies show that regular screening mammograms can help decrease the chance of dying from breast cancer. Finding a breast tumor early may mean that a woman can choose breast-saving surgery. Furthermore, she may not have to undergo chemotherapy.

To find a certified mammography facility near you, go to www.fda. gov/cdrh/mammography/certified.html on FDA's Website, or call the National Cancer Institute at 1-800-4-CANCER (1-800-422-6237).

Cancer Liaison Program

FDA's Cancer Liaison Program answers questions from patients, their friends and family members, and patient advocates about therapies for life-threatening diseases. The staff works closely with cancer patients, other federal agencies (including the National Cancer Institute), and cancer patient advocacy programs, listening to their concerns and educating them about the FDA drug approval process, cancer clinical trials, and access to investigational therapies.

For more information on the Cancer Liaison Program, call 301-827-4460 or visit www.fda.gov/oashi/cancer/cancer.html on FDA's Website.

Stages of Breast Cancer

Stages of breast cancer, according to the American Cancer Society, indicate the size of a tumor and how far the cancer has spread within the breast, to nearby tissues, and to other organs. Specific treatment is most often determined by the following stages of the disease:

Carcinoma *in situ*: Cancer is confined to the lobules (milk-producing glands) or ducts (passages connecting milk-producing glands to the nipple) and has not invaded nearby breast tissue.

Stage I: Tumor is smaller than or equal to 2 centimeters in diameter and underarm (axillary) lymph nodes test negative for cancer.

Stage II: Tumor is between 2 and 5 centimeters in diameter with or without positive lymph nodes, or tumor is greater than 5 centimeters without positive lymph nodes.

Stage III: This stage is divided into substages known as IIIA and IIIB:

- **IIIA:** Tumor is larger than 5 centimeters with positive movable lymph nodes, or tumor is any size with lymph nodes that adhere to one another or surrounding tissue.

- **IIIB:** Tumor of any size has spread to the skin, chest wall, or internal mammary lymph nodes (located beneath the breast and inside the chest).

Stage IV: Tumor, regardless of size, has metastasized (spread) to distant sites such as bones, lungs, or lymph nodes not near the breast.

Recurrent breast cancer: The disease has returned in spite of initial treatment.

— by Carol Lewis

Carol Lewis is a staff writer for FDA Consumer.

For More Information

Contact any of these organizations for more on breast cancer and support groups.

American Cancer Society
1599 Clifton Road, N.E.
Atlanta, GA 30329-4251
1-800-ACS-2345 (1-800-227-2345)
www.cancer.org

Komen (Susan G.) Breast Cancer Foundation
5005 LBJ Freeway
Suite 250
Dallas, TX 75244
1-800-IM-AWARE or 1-800-462-9273
www.komen.org

National Alliance of Breast Cancer Organizations (NABCO)
9 E. 37th St., 10th Floor
New York, NY 10016
1-888-806-2226
www.nabco.org

National Cancer Institute
31 Center Drive, MSC 2580
Bethesda, MD 20892-2580
1-800-4-CANCER (1-800-422-6237)
www.nci.nih.gov
cancertrials.nci.nih.gov

Y-ME National Breast Cancer Hotline
212 West Van Buren Street
Chicago, IL 60607-3908
1-800-221-2141 (English)
1-800-986-9505 (Spanish)
www.y-me.org

Part Two

Cervical Cancer

Chapter 5

Cancer of the Cervix

Introduction

Each year, about 15,000 women in the United States learn that they have cancer of the cervix. This chapter will give you some important information about cancer of the cervix and about some conditions that may lead to this disease. You can read about prevention, symptoms, diagnosis, and treatment. This chapter also has information to help you deal with cancer of the cervix if it affects you or someone you know.

Our knowledge about cancer of the cervix keeps increasing. The National Cancer Institute's Cancer Information Service (CIS) provides accurate, up-to-date information on cancer to patients and their families, health professionals, and the general public. Information specialists translate the latest scientific information into understandable language and respond in English, Spanish, or on TTY equipment.

Telephone 1-800-4-CANCER (1-800-422-6237)

TTY: 1-800-332-8615 (for deaf and hard of hearing callers)

The Cervix

The cervix is the lower, narrow part of the uterus (womb). The uterus, a hollow, pear-shaped organ, is located in a woman's lower abdomen, between the bladder and the rectum. The cervix forms a canal that opens into the vagina, which leads to the outside of the body.

National Cancer Institute, NIH Pub. No. 95-2047, December 2000

What Is Cancer?

Cancer is a group of more than 100 different diseases. They all affect the body's basic unit, the cell. Cancer occurs when cells become abnormal and divide without control or order.

Like all other organs of the body, the cervix is made up of many types of cells. Normally, cells divide to produce more cells only when the body needs them. This orderly process helps keep us healthy.

If cells keep dividing when new cells are not needed, a mass of tissue forms. This mass of extra tissue, called a growth or tumor, can be benign or malignant.

- **Benign tumors** are not cancer. They can usually be removed and, in most cases, they do not come back. Most important, cells from benign tumors do not spread to other parts of the body. Benign tumors are not a threat to life. Polyps, cysts, and genital warts are types of benign growths of the cervix.

- **Malignant tumors** are cancer. Cancer cells can invade and damage tissues and organs near the tumor. Cancer cells also can break away from a malignant tumor and enter the lymphatic system or the bloodstream. This is how cancer of the cervix can spread to other parts of the body, such as nearby lymph nodes, the rectum, the bladder, the bones of the spine, and the lungs. The spread of cancer is called metastasis.

Cancer of the cervix also may be called cervical cancer. Like most cancers, it is named for the part of the body in which it begins. Cancers of the cervix also are named for the type of cell in which they begin. Most cervical cancers are squamous cell carcinomas. Squamous cells are thin, flat cells that form the surface of the cervix.

When cancer spreads to another part of the body, the new tumor has the same kind of abnormal cells and the same name as the original (primary) cancer. For example, if cervical cancer spreads to the bones, the cancer cells in the bones are cervical cancer cells. The disease is called metastatic cervical cancer (it is not bone cancer).

Note: Cancer of the cervix is different from cancer that begins in other parts of the uterus and requires different treatment. The most common type of cancer of the uterus begins in the endometrium, the lining of the organ. Endometrial cancer is discussed in the booklet *What You Need To Know About Cancer of the Uterus.* This booklet may be ordered by calling the Cancer Information Service at 1-800-4-CANCER.

Precancerous Conditions and Cancer of the Cervix

Cells on the surface of the cervix sometimes appear abnormal but not cancerous. Scientists believe that some abnormal changes in cells on the cervix are the first step in a series of slow changes that can lead to cancer years later. That is, some abnormal changes are precancerous; they may become cancerous with time.

Over the years, doctors have used different terms to refer to abnormal changes in the cells on the surface of the cervix. One term now used is squamous intraepithelial lesion (SIL). (The word lesion refers to an area of abnormal tissue; intraepithelial means that the abnormal cells are present only in the surface layer of cells.) Changes in these cells can be divided into two categories:

- **Low-grade SIL** refers to early changes in the size, shape, and number of cells that form the surface of the cervix. Some low-grade lesions go away on their own. However, with time, others may grow larger or become more abnormal, forming a high-grade lesion. Precancerous low-grade lesions also may be called mild dysplasia or cervical intraepithelial neoplasia 1 (CIN 1). Such early changes in the cervix most often occur in women between the ages of 25 and 35 but can appear in other age groups as well.

- **High-grade SIL** means there are a large number of precancerous cells; they look very different from normal cells. Like low-grade SIL, these precancerous changes involve only cells on the surface of the cervix. The cells will not become cancerous and invade deeper layers of the cervix for many months, perhaps years. High-grade lesions also may be called moderate or severe dysplasia, CIN 2 or 3, or carcinoma *in situ*. They develop most often in women between the ages of 30 and 40 but can occur at other ages as well.

If abnormal cells spread deeper into the cervix or to other tissues or organs, the disease is then called cervical cancer, or invasive cervical cancer. It occurs most often in women over the age of 40.

Early Detection

If all women had pelvic exams and Pap tests regularly, most precancerous conditions would be detected and treated before cancer develops.

That way, most invasive cancers could be prevented. Any invasive cancer that does occur would likely be found at an early, curable stage.

In a pelvic exam, the doctor checks the uterus, vagina, ovaries, fallopian tubes, bladder, and rectum. The doctor feels these organs for any abnormality in their shape or size. A speculum is used to widen the vagina so that the doctor can see the upper part of the vagina and the cervix.

The Pap test is a simple, painless test to detect abnormal cells in and around the cervix. A woman should have this test when she is not menstruating; the best time is between 10 and 20 days after the first day of her menstrual period. For about 2 days before a Pap test, she should avoid douching or using spermicidal foams, creams, or jellies or vaginal medicines (except as directed by a physician), which may wash away or hide any abnormal cells.

A Pap test can be done in a doctor's office or a health clinic. A wooden scraper (spatula) and/or a small brush is used to collect a sample of cells from the cervix and upper vagina. The cells are placed on a glass slide and sent to a medical laboratory to be checked for abnormal changes.

The way of describing Pap test results is changing. The newest method is the Bethesda System. Changes are described as low-grade or high-grade SIL. Many doctors believe that the Bethesda System provides more useful information than an older system, which uses numbers ranging from class 1 to class 5. (In class 1, the cells in the sample are normal, while class 5 refers to invasive cancer.) Women should ask their doctor to explain the system used for their Pap test.

Women should have regular checkups, including a pelvic exam and a Pap test, if they are or have been sexually active or if they are age 18 or older. Those who are at increased risk of developing cancer of the cervix should be especially careful to follow their doctor's advice about checkups. (For a discussion of risk factors for cervical cancer see the Cause and Prevention section.) Women who have had a hysterectomy (surgery to remove the uterus, including the cervix) should ask their doctor's advice about having pelvic exams and Pap tests.

Symptoms

Precancerous changes of the cervix usually do not cause pain. In fact, they generally do not cause any symptoms and are not detected unless a woman has a pelvic exam and a Pap test.

Symptoms usually do not appear until abnormal cervical cells become cancerous and invade nearby tissue. When this happens, the most common symptom is abnormal bleeding. Bleeding may start and stop between regular menstrual periods, or it may occur after sexual intercourse, douching, or a pelvic exam. Menstrual bleeding may last longer and be heavier than usual. Bleeding after menopause also may be a symptom of cervical cancer. Increased vaginal discharge is another symptom of cervical cancer.

These symptoms may be caused by cancer or by other health problems. Only a doctor can tell for sure. It is important for a woman to see her doctor if she is having any of these symptoms.

Diagnosis

The pelvic exam and Pap test allow the doctor to detect abnormal changes in the cervix. If these exams show that an infection is present, the doctor treats the infection and then repeats the Pap test at a later time. If the exam or Pap test suggests something other than an infection, the doctor may repeat the Pap test and do other tests to find out what the problem is.

Colposcopy is a widely used method to check the cervix for abnormal areas. The doctor applies a vinegar-like solution to the cervix and then uses an instrument much like a microscope (called a colposcope) to look closely at the cervix. The doctor may then coat the cervix with an iodine solution (a procedure called the Schiller test). Healthy cells turn brown; abnormal cells turn white or yellow. These procedures may be done in the doctor's office.

The doctor may remove a small amount of cervical tissue for examination by a pathologist. This procedure is called a biopsy. In one type of biopsy, the doctor uses an instrument to pinch off small pieces of cervical tissue. Another method used to do a biopsy is called loop electrosurgical excision procedure (LEEP). In this procedure, the doctor uses an electric wire loop to slice off a thin, round piece of tissue. These types of biopsies may be done in the doctor's office using local anesthesia.

The doctor also may want to check inside the opening of the cervix, an area that cannot be seen during colposcopy. In a procedure called endocervical curettage (ECC), the doctor uses a curette (a small, spoon-shaped instrument) to scrape tissue from inside the cervical opening.

These procedures for removing tissue may cause some bleeding or other discharge. However, healing usually occurs quickly. Women also often experience some pain similar to menstrual cramping, which can be relieved with medicine.

These tests may not show for sure whether the abnormal cells are present only on the surface of the cervix. In that case, the doctor will then remove a larger, cone-shaped sample of tissue. This procedure, called conization or cone biopsy, allows the pathologist to see whether the abnormal cells have invaded tissue beneath the surface of the cervix. Conization also may be used as treatment for a precancerous lesion if the entire abnormal area can be removed. This procedure requires either local or general anesthesia and may be done in the doctor's office or in the hospital.

In a few cases, it may not be clear whether an abnormal Pap test or a woman's symptoms are caused by problems in the cervix or in the endometrium (the lining of the uterus). In this situation, the doctor may do dilation and curettage (D and C). The doctor stretches the cervical opening and uses a curette to scrape tissue from the lining of the uterus as well as from the cervical canal. Like conization, this procedure requires local or general anesthesia and may be done in the doctor's office or in the hospital.

Treating Precancerous Conditions

Treatment for a precancerous lesion of the cervix depends on a number of factors. These factors include whether the lesion is low or high grade, whether the woman wants to have children in the future, the woman's age and general health, and the preference of the woman and her doctor. A woman with a low-grade lesion may not need further treatment, especially if the abnormal area was completely removed during biopsy, but she should have a Pap test and pelvic exam regularly. When a precancerous lesion requires treatment, the doctor may use cryosurgery (freezing), cauterization (burning, also called diathermy), or laser surgery to destroy the abnormal area without harming nearby healthy tissue. The doctor also can remove the abnormal tissue by LEEP or conization. Treatment for precancerous lesions may cause cramping or other pain, bleeding, or a watery discharge.

In some cases, a woman may have a hysterectomy, particularly if abnormal cells are found inside the opening of the cervix. This surgery is more likely to be done when the woman does not want to have children in the future.

Treating Cancer of the Cervix

Staging

The choice of treatment for cervical cancer depends on the location and size of the tumor, the stage (extent) of the disease, the woman's age and general health, and other factors.

Staging is a careful attempt to find out whether the cancer has spread and, if so, what parts of the body are affected. Blood and urine tests usually are done. The doctor also may do a thorough pelvic exam in the operating room with the patient under anesthesia. During this exam, the doctor may do procedures called cystoscopy and proctosigmoidoscopy. In cystoscopy, the doctor looks inside the bladder with a thin, lighted instrument. Proctosigmoidoscopy is a procedure in which a lighted instrument is used to check the rectum and the lower part of the large intestine. Because cervical cancer may spread to the bladder, rectum, lymph nodes, or lungs, the doctor also may order x-rays or tests to check these areas. For example, the woman may have a series of x-rays of the kidneys and bladder, called an intravenous pyelogram. The doctor also may check the intestines and rectum using a barium enema. To look for lymph nodes that may be enlarged because they contain cancer cells, the doctor may order a CT or CAT scan, a series of x-rays put together by a computer to make detailed pictures of areas inside the body. Other procedures that may be used to check organs inside the body are ultrasonography and MRI.

Getting a Second Opinion

Before starting treatment, the patient may want a second pathologist to review the diagnosis and another specialist to review the treatment plan. Some insurance companies require a second opinion; others may cover a second opinion if the patient requests it. It may take a week or two to arrange for a second opinion. This short delay will not reduce the chance that treatment will be successful. There are a number of ways to find a doctor who can give a second opinion:

- The woman's doctor may be able to suggest pathologists and specialists to consult.

- The Cancer Information Service, at 1-800-4-CANCER, can tell callers about treatment facilities, including cancer centers and other programs supported by the National Cancer Institute.

- Women can get the names of specialists from their local medical society, a nearby hospital, or a medical school.

Preparing for Treatment

Most women with cervical cancer want to learn all they can about their disease and treatment choices so they can take an active part in decisions about their medical care. Doctors and others on the medical team can help women learn what they need to know.

When a person is diagnosed with cancer, shock and stress are natural reactions. These feelings may make it difficult for patients to think of everything they want to ask the doctor. Often it helps to make a list of questions. Also, to help remember what the doctor says, patients may take notes or ask whether they may use a tape recorder. Some people also want to have a family member or friend with them when they talk to the doctor—to take part in the discussion, to take notes, or just to listen.

Patients should not feel they need to ask all their questions or remember all the answers at one time. They will have other chances to ask the doctor to explain things and to get more information.

Here are some questions a woman with cervical cancer may want to ask the doctor before her treatment begins:

- What is the stage (extent) of my disease?

- What are my treatment choices? Which do you recommend for me? Why?

- What are the chances that the treatment will be successful?

- Would a clinical trial be appropriate for me?

- What are the risks and possible side effects of each treatment?

- How long will treatment last?

- Will it affect my normal activities?

- What is the treatment likely to cost?

- What is likely to happen without treatment?

- How often will I need to have checkups?

Methods of Treatment

Most often, treatment for cervical cancer involves surgery and radiation therapy. Sometimes, chemotherapy or biological therapy is used. Patients are often treated by a team of specialists. The team may include gynecologic oncologists and radiation oncologists. The doctors may decide to use one treatment method or a combination of methods. Some patients take part in a clinical trial (research study) using new treatment methods. Such studies are designed to improve cancer treatment. More information about clinical trials is in the Clinical Trials section.

Surgery is local therapy to remove abnormal tissue in or near the cervix. If the cancer is only on the surface of the cervix, the doctor may destroy the cancerous cells in ways similar to the methods used to treat precancerous lesions. If the disease has invaded deeper layers of the cervix but has not spread beyond the cervix, the doctor may perform an operation to remove the tumor but leave the uterus and the ovaries. In other cases, however, a woman may need to have a hysterectomy or may choose to have this surgery, especially if she is not planning to have children in the future. In this procedure, the doctor removes the entire uterus, including the cervix; sometimes the ovaries and fallopian tubes also are removed. In addition, the doctor may remove lymph nodes near the uterus to learn whether the cancer has spread to these organs.

Here are some questions a woman may want to ask the doctor before surgery:

- What kind of operation will it be?
- How will I feel after the operation?
- If I have pain, how will you help me?
- When can I return to my normal activities?
- How will this treatment affect my sex life?

Radiation therapy (also called radiotherapy) uses high-energy rays to damage cancer cells and stop them from growing. Like surgery, radiation therapy is local therapy; the radiation can affect cancer cells only in the treated area. The radiation may come from a large machine (external radiation) or from radioactive materials placed directly into the cervix (implant radiation). Some patients receive both types of radiation therapy.

A woman receiving external radiation therapy goes to the hospital or clinic each day for treatment. Usually treatments are given 5 days a week for 5 to 6 weeks. At the end of that time, the tumor site very often gets an extra "boost" of radiation.

For internal or implant radiation, a capsule containing radioactive material is placed directly in the cervix. The implant puts cancer-killing rays close to the tumor while sparing most of the healthy tissue around it. It is usually left in place for 1 to 3 days, and the treatment may be repeated several times over the course of 1 to 2 weeks. The patient stays in the hospital while the implants are in place.

The National Cancer Institute booklet *Radiation Therapy and You*, contains more information about this form of treatment.

Here are some questions a woman may want to ask the doctor before radiation therapy:

- What is the goal of this treatment?

- How will the radiation be given?

- How long will treatment last?

- How will I feel during therapy?

- What can I do to take care of myself during therapy?

- Can I continue my normal activities?

- How will this treatment affect my sex life?

Chemotherapy is the use of drugs to kill cancer cells. It is most often used when cervical cancer has spread to other parts of the body. The doctor may use just one drug or a combination of drugs.

Anticancer drugs used to treat cervical cancer may be given by injection into a vein or by mouth. Either way, chemotherapy is systemic treatment, meaning that the drugs flow through the body in the bloodstream.

Chemotherapy is given in cycles: a treatment period followed by a recovery period, then another treatment period, and so on. Most patients have chemotherapy as an outpatient (at the hospital, at the doctor's office, or at home). Depending on which drugs are given and the woman's general health, however, she may need to stay in the hospital during her treatment.

Here are some questions a woman may want to ask the doctor before chemotherapy begins:

- What is the goal of this treatment?

- What drugs will I be taking?

- Do the drugs have side effects? What can I do about them?

- How long will I need to take this treatment?

Biological therapy is treatment using substances to improve the way the body's immune system fights disease. It may be used to treat cancer that has spread from the cervix to other parts of the body. Interferon is the most common form of biological therapy for this disease; it may be used in combination with chemotherapy. Most patients who receive interferon are treated as outpatients.

56

Clinical Trials

Some women with cervical cancer are treated in clinical trials. Doctors conduct clinical trials to find out whether a new treatment is both safe and effective and to answer scientific questions. Patients who take part in these studies may be the first to receive treatments that have shown promise in laboratory research. Some patients may receive the new treatment while others receive the standard approach. In this way, doctors can compare different therapies. Patients who take part in a trial make an important contribution to medical science and may have the first chance to benefit from improved treatment methods.

Clinical trials of new treatments for cervical cancer are under way. Doctors are studying new types and schedules of radiation therapy. They also are looking for new drugs, drug combinations, and ways to combine various types of treatment.

Women with cervical cancer may want to read the National Cancer Institute booklet called *Taking Part in Clinical Trials: What Cancer Patients Need To Know*, which explains the possible benefits and risks of treatment studies. Those who are interested in taking part in a trial should talk with their doctor.

One way to learn about clinical trials is through PDQ, a computerized resource developed by the National Cancer Institute. This resource contains information about cancer treatment and about clinical trials in progress all over the country. The Cancer Information Service can provide PDQ information to doctors, patients, and the public.

Side Effects of Treatment

It is hard to limit the effects of therapy so that only cancer cells are removed or destroyed. Because treatment also damages healthy cells and tissues, it often causes unpleasant side effects.

The side effects of cancer treatment depend mainly on the type and extent of the treatment. Also, each patient reacts differently. Doctors and nurses can explain the possible side effects of treatment, and they can help relieve symptoms that may occur during and after treatment. It is important to let the doctor know if any side effects occur. The booklets *Radiation Therapy and You* and *Chemotherapy and You* also have helpful information about cancer treatment and coping with side effects.

Surgery

Methods for removing or destroying small cancers on the surface of the cervix are similar to those used to treat precancerous lesions.

Treatment may cause cramping or other pain, bleeding, or a watery discharge.

Hysterectomy is major surgery. For a few days after the operation, the woman may have pain in her lower abdomen. The doctor can order medicine to control the pain. A woman may have difficulty emptying her bladder and may need to have a catheter inserted into the bladder to drain the urine for a few days after surgery. She also may have trouble having normal bowel movements. For a period of time after the surgery, the woman's activities should be limited to allow healing to take place. Normal activities, including sexual intercourse, usually can be resumed in 4 to 8 weeks.

Women who have had their uterus removed no longer have menstrual periods. However, sexual desire and the ability to have intercourse usually are not affected by hysterectomy. On the other hand, many women have an emotionally difficult time after this surgery. A woman's view of her own sexuality may change, and she may feel an emotional loss because she is no longer able to have children. An understanding partner is important at this time. Women may want to discuss these issues with their doctor, nurse, medical social worker, or member of the clergy. They also may find it helpful to read the National Cancer Institute booklet called *Taking Time*.

Radiation Therapy

Patients are likely to become very tired during radiation therapy, especially in the later weeks of treatment. Resting is important, but doctors usually advise patients to try to stay as active as they can.

With external radiation, it is common to lose hair in the treated area and for the skin to become red, dry, tender, and itchy. There may be permanent darkening or "bronzing" of the skin in the treated area. This area should be exposed to the air when possible but protected from the sun, and patients should avoid wearing clothes that rub the treated area. Patients will be shown how to keep the area clean. They should not use any lotion or cream on their skin without the doctor's advice.

Usually, women are told not to have intercourse during radiation therapy or while an implant is in place. However, most women can have sexual relations within a few weeks after treatment ends. Sometimes, after radiation treatment, the vagina becomes narrower and less flexible, and intercourse may be painful. Patients may be taught how to use a dilator as well as a water-based lubricant to help minimize these problems.

Patients who receive external or internal radiation therapy also may have diarrhea and frequent, uncomfortable urination. The doctor can make suggestions or order medicines to control these problems.

Chemotherapy

The side effects of chemotherapy depend mainly on the drugs and the doses the patient receives. In addition, as with other types of treatment, side effects vary from person to person. Generally, anticancer drugs affect cells that divide rapidly. These include blood cells, which fight infection, help the blood to clot, or carry oxygen to all parts of the body. When blood cells are affected by anticancer drugs, patients are more likely to get infections, may bruise or bleed easily, and may have less energy. Cells in hair roots and cells that line the digestive tract also divide rapidly. When chemotherapy affects these cells, patients may lose their hair and may have other side effects, such as poor appetite, nausea, vomiting, or mouth sores. The doctor may be able to give medicine to help with side effects. Side effects gradually go away during the recovery periods between treatments or after treatment is over.

Biological Therapy

The side effects caused by biological therapies vary with the type of treatment the patient receives. These treatments may cause flu-like symptoms such as chills, fever, muscle aches, weakness, loss of appetite, nausea, vomiting, and diarrhea. Sometimes patients get a rash, and they may bleed or bruise easily. These problems can be severe, but they gradually go away after the treatment stops.

Nutrition for Cancer Patients

Some patients find it hard to eat well during cancer treatment. They may lose their appetite. In addition to loss of appetite, the common side effects of treatment, such as nausea, vomiting, or mouth sores, can make eating difficult. For some patients, foods taste different. Also, people may not feel like eating when they are uncomfortable or tired.

Eating well during cancer treatment means getting enough calories and protein to help prevent weight loss and regain strength. Patients who eat well often feel better and have more energy. In addition, they may be better able to handle the side effects of treatment.

Doctors, nurses, and dietitians can offer advice for healthy eating during cancer treatment. Patients and their families also may want to read the National Cancer Institute booklet *Eating Hints for Cancer Patients*, which contains many useful suggestions.

Followup Care

Regular followup exams—including a pelvic exam, a Pap test, and other laboratory tests—are very important for any woman who has been treated for precancerous changes or for cancer of the cervix. The doctor will do these tests and exams frequently for several years to check for any sign that the condition has returned.

Cancer treatment may cause side effects many years later. For this reason, patients should continue to have regular checkups and should report any health problems that appear.

Support for Cancer Patients

Living with a serious disease is not easy. Cancer patients and those who care about them face many problems and challenges. Coping with these problems is often easier when people have helpful information and support services. Several useful booklets, including the National Cancer Institute booklet *Taking Time*, are available from the Cancer Information Service.

Cancer patients may worry about holding their job, caring for their family, keeping up with daily activities, or starting a new relationship. Worries about tests, treatments, hospital stays, and medical bills are common. Doctors, nurses, and other members of the health care team can answer questions about treatment, working, or other activities. Also, meeting with a social worker, counselor, or member of the clergy can be helpful to patients who want to talk about their feelings or discuss their concerns.

Friends and relatives can be very supportive. Also, it helps many patients to discuss their concerns with others who have cancer. Cancer patients often get together in support groups, where they can share what they have learned about coping with cancer and the effects of treatment. It is important to keep in mind, however, that each patient is different. Treatments and ways of dealing with cancer that work for one person may not be right for another—even if they both have the same kind of cancer. It is always a good idea to discuss the advice of friends and family members with the doctor.

Often, a social worker at the hospital or clinic can suggest groups that can help with rehabilitation, emotional support, financial aid, transportation, or home care. For example, the American Cancer

Society has many services for patients and their families. They also offer many free booklets, including one on sexuality and cancer. Local offices of the American Cancer Society are listed in the white pages of the telephone directory.

What the Future Holds

The outlook for women with precancerous changes of the cervix or very early cancer of the cervix is excellent; nearly all patients with these conditions can be cured. Researchers continue to look for new and better ways to treat invasive cervical cancer.

Patients and their families are naturally concerned about what the future holds. Sometimes patients use statistics to try to figure out their chances of being cured. It is important to remember, however, that statistics are averages based on large numbers of patients. They cannot be used to predict what will happen to a particular woman because no two patients are alike; treatments and responses vary greatly. The doctor who takes care of the patient and knows her medical history is in the best position to talk with her about her chance of recovery (prognosis).

Doctors often talk about surviving cancer, or they may use the term remission rather than cure. Although many women with cervical cancer recover completely, doctors use these terms because the disease can recur. (The return of cancer is called a recurrence.)

Cause and Prevention

By studying large numbers of women all over the world, researchers have identified certain risk factors that increase the chance that cells in the cervix will become abnormal or cancerous. They believe that, in many cases, cervical cancer develops when two or more risk factors act together.

Research has shown that women who began having sexual intercourse before age 18 and women who have had many sexual partners have an increased risk of developing cervical cancer. Women also are at increased risk if their partners began having sexual intercourse at a young age, have had many sexual partners, or were previously married to women who had cervical cancer.

Scientists do not know exactly why the sexual practices of women and their partners affect the risk of developing cervical cancer. However, research suggests that some sexually transmitted viruses can cause cells in the cervix to begin the series of changes that can lead to cancer. Women who have had many sexual partners or whose partners have had many sexual partners may have an increased risk for cervical cancer at least in part because they are more likely to get a sexually transmitted virus.

Scientists are studying the effects of sexually transmitted human papillomaviruses (HPVs). Some sexually transmitted HPVs cause genital warts (condylomata acuminata). In addition, scientists believe that some of these viruses may cause the growth of abnormal cells in the cervix and may play a role in cancer development. They have found that women who have HPV or whose partners have HPV have a higher-than-average risk of developing cervical cancer. However, most women who are infected with HPV do not develop cervical cancer, and the virus is not present in all women who have this disease. For these reasons, scientists believe that other factors act together with HPVs. For example, the genital herpes virus also may play a role. Further research is needed to learn the exact role of these viruses and how they act together with other factors in the development of cervical cancer.

Smoking also increases the risk of cancer of the cervix, although it is not clear exactly how or why. The risk appears to increase with the number of cigarettes a woman smokes each day and with the number of years she has smoked.

Women whose mothers were given the drug diethylstilbestrol (DES) during pregnancy to prevent miscarriage also are at increased risk. (This drug was used for this purpose from about 1940 to 1970.) A rare type of vaginal and cervical cancer has been found in a small number of women whose mothers used DES.

Several reports suggest that women whose immune systems are weakened are more likely than others to develop cervical cancer. For example, women who have the human immunodeficiency virus (HIV), which causes AIDS, are at increased risk. Also, organ transplant patients, who receive drugs that suppress the immune system to prevent rejection of the new organ, are more likely than others to develop precancerous lesions.

Some researchers believe that there is an increased risk of cervical cancer in women who use oral contraceptives (the pill). However, scientists have not found that the pill directly causes cancer of the cervix. This relationship is hard to prove because the two main risk factors for cervical cancer—intercourse at an early age and multiple sex partners—may be more common among women who use the pill than among those who do not. Still, oral contraceptive labels warn of this possible risk and advise women who use them to have yearly Pap tests.

Some research has shown that vitamin A may play a role in stopping or preventing cancerous changes in cells like those on the surface of the cervix. Further research with forms of vitamin A may help scientists learn more about preventing cancer of the cervix.

At present, early detection and treatment of precancerous tissue remain the most effective ways of preventing cervical cancer. Information about early detection appears in the Early Detection section. Women should talk with their doctors about an appropriate schedule of checkups. The doctor's advice will be based on such factors as the women's age, medical history, and risk factors.

Chapter 6

Cervical Cancer and Older Women

Older Women Continue to Be at Risk for Developing Cervical Cancer

Women ages 65 and older account for nearly 25 percent of all cervical cancer cases and 41 percent of cervical cancer deaths in the United States.[1] Women ages 65 and older have a cervical cancer incidence rate of 16.8 per 100,000, compared to 7.4 for women younger than 65.[2] The incidence rate is the number of newly diagnosed cancers per 100,000 population during a specific period of time (usually one year).

Women ages 65 and older have a cervical cancer mortality rate of 9.3 per 100,000, compared to 2.2 for women younger than 65. The mortality rate is the number of deaths due to a certain type of cancer per 100,000 population during a specific period of time (usually one year).

More than one-half (51%) of all women ages 65 and older have not had a Pap test in the past 3 years.[3] Many older women experience barriers to regular Pap test screening, which include: lack of knowledge about testing frequency; anxiety that the test might be painful or embarrassing; underestimation of personal risk for cervical cancer; fear of test results; language and cultural barriers;[4] and cost.[5]

"Cervical Cancer and Older Women: Tip Sheet," National Cancer Institute, [1998].

Older Women Representing Minority Populations Are at Particular Risk for Developing Cervical Cancer

- The incidence rate and the mortality rate of cervical cancer for African American women ages 65 and older are more than two times greater than those for white women of the same age group (34.4 and 23.3 per 100,000 women, respectively, compared to 14.7 and 8.0 for white women).[2]

- Hispanic women ages 65 and older also have a higher incidence rate and mortality rate of cervical cancer than do white women (27.6 and 11.6 per 100,000 women, respectively).[2]

Women Can Take Steps to Help Prevent Cervical Cancer

- Every woman who is 18 or older, or is sexually active, should get regular Pap tests and pelvic exams. Older women continue to be at risk for cervical cancer and should continue to have Pap tests at least once every three years.

- The Pap test is the most effective screening procedure for detecting abnormal changes in the cervix, including precancerous conditions. If an abnormality is detected, it is important to get any needed follow up tests and/or treatment. Appropriate treatment of precancerous conditions prevents the development of cervical cancer.

- Recent advances in Pap test technology are under evaluation and may improve the test's sensitivity.

Older and Medically Underserved Women Can Get Free or Low-Cost Pap Tests

- Older women should have a Pap test at least once every three years.

- As of January 1998, Medicare covers Pap tests once every 3 years for all Medicare beneficiaries. For more information about Medicare coverage for cervical cancer screening examinations, please call the Medicare toll-free hotline at 1-800-638-6833.

- Women and health care providers can call the National Cancer Institute's Cancer Information Service (CIS) at 1-800-4-CANCER

(1-800-422-6237) or TTY: 1-800-332-8615 (for deaf and hard of hearing callers) to find out the latest, most accurate information about cervical cancer and cervical cancer screening. Information specialists translate the latest scientific information into understandable language and respond in English, Spanish, or on TTY equipment. The CIS also provides referrals for free and low-cost cervical cancer screening through the Centers for Disease Control and Prevention's (CDC) Breast and Cervical Cancer Early Detection Program (BCCEDP), which targets medically underserved, low-income women, particularly members of racial and ethnic minorities.

Cervical Cancer Remains a Major Public Health Concern

- Worldwide, cervical cancer is the second most common cancer among women; in many developing countries, it is the number one killer of women.[1]

- For women of all ages in the United States, the incidence rate of cervical cancer is 8.3 per 100,000 women and the mortality rate is 2.9 per 100,000 women.[2] The highest incidence rate occurs among Vietnamese women (43 per 100,000 women), many of whom are recent immigrants to the U.S. and have not benefited from cervical cancer screening. Incidence rates of 15 per 100,000 women or higher also occur among Alaska Native, Korean, and Hispanic women.[6] The lowest incidence rate is 5.8 per 100,000 among Japanese women.

- It is estimated that approximately 13,700 women in the United States will develop invasive cervical cancer, and 4,900 women will die from this disease in 1998.[7]

- One-half of the women with newly diagnosed invasive cervical cancer have never had a Pap test, and another 10 percent have not had a Pap test in the past 5 years.[1]

Notes

1. NIH Consensus Panel. *NIH Consensus Conference: Cervical Cancer*, Vol. 14, No. 1, 1996.

2. National Cancer Institute Cancer Statistics Branch, Surveillance, Epidemiology, and End Results (SEER) data, 1990-1994.

3. Breen, N. Report for Pap screenings within 0-36 months, Division of Cancer Control and Population Sciences, *National Health Interview Survey, 1992 data.* February 18, 1997.

4. Breast and Cervical Cancer Screening: Barriers and Use Among Specific Population, *AMC Cancer Research Center, Supplement 3,* January 1995.

5. Healthstyles, 1997.

6. *Racial/Ethnic Patterns of Cancer in the United States 1988-1992,* National Cancer Institute.

7. *Cancer Facts and Figures: 1998.* American Cancer Society.

Chapter 7

Prevention of Cervical Cancer

Prevention

Doctors can not always explain why one person gets cancer and another doesn't. However, scientists have studied general patterns of cancer in the population to learn what things around us and what things we do in our lives may increase our chance of developing cancer.

Anything that increases a person's chance of developing a disease is called a risk factor; anything that decreases a person's chance of developing a disease is called a protective factor. Some of the risk factors for cancer can be avoided, but many can not. For example, although you can choose to quit smoking, you can not choose which genes you have inherited from your parents. Both smoking and inheriting specific genes could be considered risk factors for certain kinds of cancer, but only smoking can be avoided. Prevention means avoiding the risk factors and increasing the protective factors that can be controlled so that the chance of developing cancer decreases.

Although many risk factors can be avoided, it is important to keep in mind that avoiding risk factors does not guarantee that you will not get cancer. Also, most people with a particular risk factor for cancer do not actually get the disease. Some people are more sensitive than others to factors that can cause cancer. Talk to your doctor about methods of preventing cancer that might be effective for you.

CancerNet, National Cancer Institute (www.nci.nih.gov), August 2000.

69

Purposes of This Summary

The purposes of this summary on cervical cancer prevention are to:

- give information on cervical cancer and how often it occurs
- describe cervical cancer prevention methods
- give current facts about which people or groups of people would most likely be helped by following cervical cancer prevention methods

You can talk to your doctor or health care professional about cancer prevention methods and whether they would be likely to help you.

Cervical Cancer Prevention

The uterine cervix is the lower, narrow part of the uterus (womb) that connects the uterus with the vagina. It is part of the female reproductive system.

Significance of Cervical Cancer

Thanks to widespread screening with the Pap test (smear), the number of deaths due to cervical cancer has been decreasing.

Cervical Cancer Prevention

Many cases of cervical cancer are associated with known risk factors for the disease. Many risk factors are modifiable though not all can be avoided.

Screening history. Women who have not regularly had a Pap test (smear) are at increased risk of cervical cancer. In particular, many women over age 60 have not had regular Pap tests and are at increased risk. Receiving regular gynecological exams and Pap tests are the most important steps in preventing cervical cancer. Abnormal changes in the cervix can be detected by the Pap test and treated before cancer develops.

HPV infection. There are over 80 types of human papillomavirus (HPV). Approximately 30 types are transmitted sexually and can infect the cervix. About half of these have been linked to cervical cancer.

Cervical infection with HPV is the primary risk factor for cervical cancer. However, HPV infection is very common and only a very small percentage of women infected with untreated HPV will develop cervical cancer.

Sexual history. Women who begin having sexual intercourse before they are 16 years old, and women who have had many sexual partners, are at a greater risk of HPV infection and developing cervical cancer. A number of health professional groups recommend that all women receive regular gynecological exams at the onset of sexual activity or by 18 years of age. The prevention of sexually transmitted diseases reduces the risk of cervical cancer.

Smoking. Cigarette smoking may be associated with an increased risk of cervical cancer. Many studies have shown an association while other studies have not.

HIV infection. Women who have been infected with HIV have a higher-than-average risk of developing cervical cancer.

Diet. Several studies have suggested that various micronutrients, such as carotene and vitamins C and E, may reduce the risk of cervical cancer.

Educating women about the risk factors for cervical cancer may lead to lifestyle and behavioral changes that result in decreased exposure to these factors.

Chapter 8

Factors that Affect Your Risk of Developing Cervical Cancer

Factors that Increase Your Risk

Failure to Have Routine Pelvic Examinations with Cervical Screening

The Pap test (or Pap smear) is the most important weapon we have in the fight against cervical cancer. If you do not have a regular examination with a Pap test, you are at higher risk for having a preinvasive abnormality develop into cancer.

Intercourse at an Early Age

If you started having sexual relations at a young age, you are at higher risk for developing a cervical cancer when compared to those who wait.

Infection with HPV (Human Papillomavirus)

HPV is a sexually transmitted virus that can cause genital warts. If you have had genital warts or other evidence of HPV infection, you are at higher risk for developing cervical cancer. Most women who are infected with HPV never have visible warts and do not know they have the virus. Fortunately, in the great majority of cases this viral infection produces no problems and does not result in cancer. Only a small number of cases will progress to cancer.

Excerpted from "Cervical Cancer," © 2000 Women's Cancer Network; reprinted with permission. Full text available at http://www.wcn.org.

73

Having Multiple Sexual Partners

Because cervical cancer is almost always caused by HPV which is sexually transmitted, having a greater number of sexual partners will increase your risk of becoming infected with HPV.

Sex with a High-Risk Male

Even if you have had only one sexual partner, if that man has had many other sexual partners, he is at high-risk for transmitting HPV to you. This increases your risk for developing cervical cancer. A man who has had a partner who has developed cervical cancer presents risk.

Sexually Transmitted Diseases

If you have had other sexually transmitted illnesses such as chlamydia, gonorrhea, herpes, or syphilis, you are at higher risk for also having acquired an HPV infection.

Cigarette Smoking

Using tobacco products increases your risk of developing either a preinvasive abnormality or invasive cervical cancer. If you stop smoking, your risk of developing cervical cancer probably will be lower.

Lower Socioeconomic Status

Women from lower income groups have a higher risk of developing cervical cancer. This may be due to their lack of access to good health care and Pap tests. African American women are also at higher risk, but it is not known if this is unique to these women or due to poor access to Pap testing.

Factors that Decrease Your Risk of Cervical Cancer

- **Regular pelvic examinations with a Pap test.** The Pap test can accurately identify an abnormality in the cervix long before it turns into an actual cancer. This simple, painless screening test is the most powerful tool in a woman's arsenal to prevent cervical cancer. During the pelvic exam, a small sample of cells is taken from the outer portion of the cervix. The sample is later viewed under a microscope and results are reported within a few days. If the cells prove to be abnormal, close follow-up is necessary. Women should begin getting an annual Pap test at the age of 18 or earlier if they are sexually active. If three consecutive tests are normal and the woman is in a low risk group, the doctor may decide that less frequent screening is required. A Pap test can be performed by an obstetrician gynecologist, a family practitioner, or a nurse practitioner.

- **Regular use of condoms.** Use of a latex condom during intercourse can prevent transmission of HPV and other sexually transmitted diseases.

- **Becoming a non-smoker.** Women who quit smoking can lower their risk of developing cervical cancer.

For More Information

Women's Cancer Network
c/o Gynecologic Cancer Foundation
401 N. Michigan Avenue
Chicago, IL 60611
Toll Free: 800-444-4441 (for a referral to a gynecologic cancer specialist)
Phone: 312-644-6610
Internet: www.wcn.org
E-mail: gcf@sba.com

Chapter 9

Screening for Cervical Cancer

What Is Screening?

Screening for cancer is examination (or testing) of people for early stages in the development of cancer even though they have no symptoms. Scientists have studied patterns of cancer in the population to learn which people are more likely to get certain types of cancer. They have also studied what things around us and what things we do in our lives that may cause cancer. This information sometimes helps doctors recommend who should be screened for certain types of cancer, what types of screening tests people should have, and how often these tests should be done. Not all screening tests are helpful, and they often have risks. For this reason, scientists at the National Cancer Institute are studying many screening tests to find out how useful they are and to determine the relative benefits and harms.

If your doctor suggests certain cancer screening tests as part of your health care plan, this does not mean he or she thinks you have cancer. Screening tests are done when you have no symptoms. Since decisions about screening can be difficult, you may want to discuss them with your doctor and ask questions about the potential benefits and risks of screening tests and whether they have been proven to decrease the risk of dying from cancer.

If your doctor suspects that you may have cancer, he or she will order certain tests to see whether you do. These are called diagnostic

CancerNet, National Cancer Institute (www.nci.nih.gov), November 2000.

tests. Some tests are used for diagnostic purposes, but are not suitable for screening people who have no symptoms.

Cervical Cancer Screening

The uterine cervix is the lower, narrow part of the uterus (womb) that connects the uterus with the vagina. It is part of the female reproductive system.

Screening Test for Cervical Cancer

Pap Test (Smear): This test is performed during a regular office visit to a doctor. A doctor uses a wooden scraper and/or a small brush to collect a sample of cells from the cervix and upper vagina. These cells are placed on a slide and sent to a laboratory to check for abnormalities. Studies suggest that the death rate of cervical cancer will decrease if women who are or have been sexually active or who are in their late teens or older have regular Pap tests.

Chapter 10

Treatment of Cervical Cancer

What Is Cancer of the Cervix?

Cancer of the cervix, a common kind of cancer in women, is a disease in which cancer (malignant) cells are found in the tissues of the cervix. The cervix is the opening of the uterus (womb). The uterus is the hollow, pear-shaped organ where a baby develops. The cervix connects the uterus to the vagina (birth canal).

Cancer of the cervix usually grows slowly over a period of time. Before cancer cells are found on the cervix, the tissues of the cervix go through changes in which cells that are not normal begin to appear (known as dysplasia). A Pap smear will usually find these cells. Later, cancer cells start to grow and spread more deeply into the cervix and to surrounding areas.

Since there are usually no symptoms associated with cancer of the cervix, a doctor should do a series of tests to look for it. The first of these is a Pap smear, which is done by using a piece of cotton, a brush, or a small wooden stick to gently scrape the outside of the cervix in order to pick up cells. Pressure is sometimes felt and it is usually not accompanied by pain.

If cells that are not normal are found, the doctor will need to cut a sample of tissue (this procedure is called a biopsy) from the cervix and look at it under a microscope to see if there are any cancer cells. A biopsy that needs only a small amount of tissue may be done in the

CancerNet, National Cancer Institute (www.nci.nih.gov), November 2000.

doctor's office. A person may need to go to the hospital if the doctor needs to remove a larger, cone-shaped biopsy specimen (conization).

The prognosis (chance of recovery) and choice of treatment depend on the stage of the cancer (whether it is just in the cervix or has spread to other places) and the patient's general health.

Stages of Cancer of the Cervix

Once cancer of the cervix is found (diagnosed), more tests will be done to find out if cancer cells have spread to other parts of the body. This testing is called staging. To plan treatment, a doctor needs to know the stage of the disease. The following stages are used for cancer of the cervix.

Stage 0 or carcinoma *in situ*: Carcinoma *in situ* is very early cancer. The abnormal cells are found only in the first layer of cells of the lining of the cervix and do not invade the deeper tissues of the cervix.

Stage I: Cancer involves the cervix but has not spread nearby.

Stage IA: A very small amount of cancer that is only visible under a microscope is found deeper in the tissues of the cervix.

Stage IB: A larger amount of cancer is found in the tissues of the cervix.

Stage II: Cancer has spread to nearby areas but is still inside the pelvic area.

Stage IIA: Cancer has spread beyond the cervix to the upper two thirds of the vagina.

Stage IIB: Cancer has spread to the tissue around the cervix.

Stage III: Cancer has spread throughout the pelvic area. Cancer cells may have spread to the lower part of the vagina. The cells also may have spread to block the tubes that connect the kidneys to the bladder (the ureters).

Stage IV: Cancer has spread to other parts of the body.

Stage IVA: Cancer has spread to the bladder or rectum (organs close to the cervix).

Stage IVB: Cancer has spread to faraway organs such as the lungs.

Recurrent: Recurrent disease means that the cancer has come back (recurred) after it has been treated. It may come back in the cervix or in another place.

How Cancer of the Cervix Is Treated

There are treatments for all patients with cancer of the cervix. Three kinds of treatment are used:

- surgery (removing the cancer in an operation)

- radiation therapy (using high-dose x-rays or other high-energy rays to kill cancer cells)

- chemotherapy (using drugs to kill cancer cells)

Surgery. A doctor may use one of several types of surgery for carcinoma *in situ* to destroy the cancerous tissue:

- Cryosurgery kills the cancer by freezing it.

- Laser surgery is the use of a narrow beam of intense light to kill cancerous cells.

A doctor may remove the cancer using one of these operations:

- Conization is the removal of a cone-shaped piece of tissue where the abnormality is found. Conization may be used to take out a piece of tissue for biopsy, but it can also be used to treat early cancers of the cervix.

- Alternatively, a doctor may perform a loop electrosurgical excision procedure (LEEP) to remove the abnormal tissue. LEEP uses an electrical current passed through a thin wire loop to act as a knife.

- A laser beam can also be used as a knife to remove the tissue.

- A hysterectomy is an operation in which the uterus and cervix are taken out along with the cancer. If the uterus is taken out through the vagina, the operation is called a vaginal hysterectomy. If the uterus is taken out through a cut (incision) in the abdomen, the operation is called a total abdominal hysterectomy. Sometimes the ovaries and fallopian tubes are also removed, which is called a bilateral salpingo-oophorectomy.

81

- A radical hysterectomy is an operation in which the cervix, uterus, and part of the vagina are removed. Lymph nodes in the area are also removed. This is called lymph node dissection. (Lymph nodes are small bean-shaped structures that are found throughout the body. They produce and store cells that fight infection).

- If the cancer has spread outside the cervix or the female organs, a doctor may take out the lower colon, rectum, or bladder (depending on where the cancer has spread) along with the cervix, uterus, and vagina. This is called an exenteration and is rarely needed. Plastic surgery may be needed to make an artificial vagina after this operation.

Radiation therapy is the use of x-rays or other high-energy rays to kill cancer cells and shrink tumors. Radiation may come from a machine outside the body (external radiation) or from putting materials that produce radiation (radioisotopes) through thin plastic tubes into the area where the cancer cells are found (internal radiation). Radiation may be used alone or in addition to surgery.

Chemotherapy is the use of drugs to kill cancer cells. Chemotherapy may be taken by pill, or it may be put into the body by a needle inserted into a vein. Chemotherapy is called a systemic treatment because the drugs enter the bloodstream, travel through the body, and can kill cancer cells outside the cervix.

Treatment by Stage

Treatments for cancer of the cervix depend on the stage of the disease, the size of the tumor, and the patient's age, overall condition, and desire to have children.

Treatment of cervical cancer during pregnancy may be delayed depending on the stage of the cancer and how many months a patient has been pregnant.

Standard treatment may be considered because of its effectiveness in patients in past studies, or participation in a clinical trial may be considered. Not all patients are cured with standard therapy and some standard treatments may have more side effects than are desired. For these reasons, clinical trials are designed to find better ways to treat cancer patients and are based on the most up-to-date information. Clinical trials are ongoing in most parts of the country for most stages of cancer of the cervix. To learn more about clinical trials, call the Cancer Information Service at 1-800-4-CANCER (1-800-422-6237); TTY at 1-800-332-8615.

Stage 0 Cervical Cancer: Stage 0 cervical cancer is sometimes called carcinoma *in situ*. Treatment may be one of the following:

- Conization.
- Laser surgery.
- Loop electrosurgical excision procedure (LEEP).
- Cryosurgery.
- Surgery to remove the cancerous area, cervix, and uterus (total abdominal or vaginal hysterectomy) for those women who cannot or no longer want to have children.

Stage I Cervical Cancer: Treatment may be one of the following depending on how deep the tumor cells have invaded into the normal tissue:

For stage IA cancer:

- Surgery to remove the cancer, uterus, and cervix (total abdominal hysterectomy). The ovaries may also be taken out (bilateral salpingo-oophorectomy), but are usually not removed in younger women.
- Conization.
- For tumors with deeper invasion (3-5 millimeters): Surgery to remove the cancer, the uterus and cervix, and part of the vagina (radical hysterectomy) along with the lymph nodes in the pelvic area (lymph node dissection).
- Internal radiation therapy.

For stage IB cancer:

- Internal and external radiation therapy.
- Radical hysterectomy and lymph node dissection.
- Radical hysterectomy and lymph node dissection followed by radiation therapy plus chemotherapy.
- Radiation therapy plus chemotherapy.

Stage II Cervical Cancer: Treatment may be one of the following:

For stage IIA cancer:

- Internal and external radiation therapy.
- Radical hysterectomy and lymph node dissection.
- Radical hysterectomy and lymph node dissection followed by radiation therapy plus chemotherapy.
- Radiation therapy plus chemotherapy.

For stage IIB cancer:

- Internal and external radiation therapy plus chemotherapy.

Stage III Cervical Cancer: Treatment may be one of the following:

- Internal and external radiation therapy plus chemotherapy.

Stage IV Cervical Cancer: Treatment may be one of the following:

For stage IVA cancer:

- Internal and external radiation therapy plus chemotherapy.

For stage IVB cancer:

- Radiation therapy to relieve symptoms caused by the cancer.
- Chemotherapy.

Recurrent Cervical Cancer: If the cancer has come back (recurred) in the pelvis, treatment may be one of the following:

- Radiation therapy combined with chemotherapy.
- Chemotherapy to relieve symptoms caused by the cancer.

If the cancer has come back outside of the pelvis, a patient may choose to go into a clinical trial of systemic chemotherapy.

Part Three

Endometrial Cancer

Chapter 11

Understanding Endometrial Cancer

What Is Endometrial Cancer?

Endometrial cancer is a cancer that develops from the endometrium, the inner lining of the *uterus* (womb).

About the Uterus and Endometrium

The uterus is a hollow organ, about the size and shape of a medium-sized pear. The uterus has two main parts. The lower end of the uterus, which extends into the vagina, is called the *cervix*. The upper part is the *body* of the uterus, also known as the *corpus*. (Corpus is the Latin word for body.) The body of the uterus has two layers. The inner layer is called the *endometrium*. (Endo is Latin for inside and metrium is Latin for uterus.) The outer is called the myometrium. (Myo is Latin for muscle.) The myometrium is the thick layer of muscle that expels the baby during delivery.

Hormonal changes during a woman's menstrual cycle cause the endometrium to continually change. During the early part of the menstrual cycle the endometrium changes and thickens in order to nourish an embryo in case a pregnancy occurs. After ovulation at the mid-point of the cycle, if pregnancy does not occur, the hormones change and the top layer of the lining begins to die. By the end of the

Excerpted from "Endometrial Cancer," © 2001 American Cancer Society; reprinted with permission. Full text available online at http://www.cancer.org/eprise/main/docroot/CRI/content/CRI_2_4_7x_CRC_Endometrial_Cancer_PDF.

cycle, the dead tissue is shed from the uterus (womb) and becomes the menstrual flow. This cycle repeats throughout a woman's life until menopause.

Cancers of the Uterus and Endometrium

Nearly all endometrial cancers are *adenocarcinomas* (cancers of glandular cells). More than 75% are *endometrioid adenocarcinomas*. Although endometrial and endometrioid are spelled somewhat alike, the words are not identical. Endometrioid cancers are a specific type of endometrial cancers. One-third to one-half of endometrioid cancers have glandular areas as well as areas formed by *squamous cells* (the type of cells found on the surface of the cervix and the skin). If the squamous cells look benign (noncancerous) under a microscope, and the glandular cells look cancerous these tumors are called *adenoacanthomas*. If the squamous areas and glandular areas both look malignant (cancerous), these tumors are called *adenosquamous carcinomas*. However, both adenoacanthomas and adenosquamous carcinomas are cancerous tumors. *Papillary serous adenocarcinomas* (about 10% of endometrial cancers) and *clear cell adenocarcinomas* (less than 5%) are less common types of endometrial cancer that often grow and spread rapidly. The above cancers of the endometrium develop from its glandular cells. Doctors call this layer of glandular cells the *endometrial epithelium.*

Three less common uterine cancers that do not come from glandular tissue of the endometrium are called *uterine sarcomas* and can involve the endometrium. These include (1) *stromal sarcomas* which develop in the stroma (supporting connective tissue) of the endometrium, (2) *malignant mixed mesodermal tumors* (MMMT, or carcinosarcomas) which may combine features of endometrial carcinoma and those of sarcomas, and (3) *leiomyosarcomas* which start in the myometrium or muscular wall of the uterus. These three types of cancer are not discussed in this document because their treatment and *prognosis* (the outlook for survival) are different from the most common cancers of the endometrium. A document on these three types of uterine cancer is available from the American Cancer Society upon request.

Cancers of the cervix are different from cancers of the body of the uterus and are described in another American Cancer Society document.

What Are the Key Statistics about Endometrial Cancer?

In the United States, cancer of the endometrium is the most common cancer of the female reproductive organs. The American Cancer

Society expects there will be 38,300 new cases of cancer of the uterine body, diagnosed in the United States during 2001. About more than 95% of these uterine body cancers are endometrial cancers. The American Cancer Society also estimates that about 6,600 women in the United States will die from cancers of the uterine body during 2001.

When all cases of endometrial cancer are considered together, the 5-year relative survival rate is 84%. However, the prognosis (the outlook for chances of survival) for any single woman depends on the stage of her cancer as well as several other factors.

The 5-year survival rate refers to the percentage of women who live at least 5 years after their cancer is diagnosed. Many of these women live much longer than 5 years after diagnosis, and 5-year rates are used to produce a standard way of discussing prognosis. Five-year *relative* survival rates exclude women dying of other diseases from the calculations, and are considered to be a more accurate way to describe the prognosis for women with a particular type and stage of cancer. Of course, 5-year survival rates are based on women diagnosed and initially treated more than 5 years ago. Improvements in treatment often result in a more favorable outlook for recently diagnosed patients.

Can Endometrial Cancer Be Found Early?

In most cases, being alert to any signs and symptoms (see "How is Endometrial Cancer Diagnosed?") of endometrial cancer and discussing them promptly with your health care team allows the disease to be diagnosed at an early stage. Early detection improves the chances that your endometrial cancer will be treated successfully. Unfortunately, some endometrial cancers may reach an advanced stage before recognizable signs and symptoms are present.

Signs and Symptoms of Endometrial Cancer

Unusual bleeding, spotting, or other discharge: If you have gone through menopause, it is especially important to report unusual bleeding or spotting to your health care team. About 90% of patients diagnosed with endometrial cancer have post-menopausal bleeding or irregular vaginal bleeding. Although this symptom also can occur with hyperplasia and some other noncancerous conditions, it is important to have immediate medical evaluation of irregular bleeding. Absence of visible blood in an abnormal vaginal discharge does not mean cancer is absent. In about 10% of cases, the discharge associated with endometrial cancer is white rather than blood-tinged. Any abnormal discharge should be investigated by your doctor.

Pelvic pain and/or mass and weight loss: These symptoms usually occur in later stages of the disease. Nonetheless, delays in seeking medical help may allow the disease to progress even further. This reduces the odds for successful treatment.

Early Detection Tests

Women at average endometrial cancer risk: Early detection refers to testing to find a disease such as cancer in people who do not have symptoms of that disease. At this time, there are no early detection tests or examinations recommended for women without symptoms who are at average endometrial cancer risk. Women over age 40 should have an annual pelvic exam by a health professional. Women who are between 18 and 39 years old should have a pelvic exam every 3 years. Although the pelvic exam can find some female reproductive system cancers, including some advanced uterine cancers, it is not very effective in finding early endometrial cancers. The Pap test can find some early endometrial cancers, but most cases are not detected by this test. In contrast, the Pap test is very effective in finding early cancers of the *cervix* (the lower part of the uterus). For this reason, the American Cancer Society recommends a yearly Pap test and pelvic exam starting at age 18 or when a woman first becomes sexually active, whichever is first. If Pap tests are negative three years in a row, the doctor or nurse may choose to do them less often, depending on a woman's risk factors. However, even if Pap tests are done less often, women over age 40 should continue to have annual pelvic exams.

The American Cancer Society recommends that, at the time of menopause, all women should be informed about the risks and symptoms of endometrial cancer, and strongly encouraged to report any vaginal bleeding or spotting to their doctor.

Women at increased endometrial cancer risk: The American Cancer Society recommends that women at increased risk (due to increasing age, history of unopposed estrogen therapy, late menopause, tamoxifen therapy, nulliparity, infertility or failure to ovulate, obesity, diabetes, or hypertension) should be informed about endometrial cancer early detection testing. Women with or at risk for hereditary nonpolyposis colon cancer (HNPCC) should be offered annual testing for endometrial cancer with endometrial biopsy beginning at age 35. This includes women known to carry HNPCC-associated gene mutations, women who are likely to carry such a mutation (those with a mutation known to be present in the family), and women from families with a predisposition to colon cancer where genetic testing has not been done.

How Is Endometrial Cancer Diagnosed?

History and Physical Examination

If a woman has any of the symptoms of endometrial cancer described in the section on "Can Endometrial Cancer Be Found Early?" she should visit her doctor. The doctor will ask her about her symptoms, risk factors, and family medical history. The doctor will also perform a general physical examination and an examination of the pelvis.

Consultation with a Specialist

If endometrial cancer is suspected, the woman should be examined by a doctor qualified to diagnose and treat diseases of the female reproductive system. Specialists in reproductive cancers are called *gynecologic oncologists.*

Sampling Endometrial Tissue

These procedures are usually done by a specialist such as a gynecologist. To determine if endometrial hyperplasia or endometrial cancer is present, the doctor must remove endometrial tissue so that it can be examined under the microscope. Endometrial tissue can be obtained by *endometrial biopsy* or by *dilation and curettage (D & C)* with or without a *hysteroscopy* (a test in which a gynecologist can view the inside of the uterus through a thin lighted tube).

Endometrial biopsy: An endometrial biopsy is an office procedure in which a sample of endometrial tissue is obtained through a very thin flexible tube inserted into the uterus through the cervix. The tube removes a small amount of endometrium using suction. The suctioning takes about a minute or less. The discomfort is similar to severe menstrual cramps and can be helped by taking a nonsteroidal anti-inflammatory drug such as ibuprofen an hour before the procedure.

91

Dilation and Curettage (D & C): If the endometrial biopsy sample doesn't provide an adequate amount of tissue or is suggestive of but not diagnostic for cancer, a D & C with or without a hysteroscopy must be done. In this outpatient procedure, the cervix is dilated and a special surgical instrument is used to scrape tissue from inside the uterus. The procedure takes about an hour and may require general anesthesia or *conscious sedation* (medication given into a vein to make the patient drowsy but still awake). A dilation and curettage is usually done in an outpatient surgery area of a clinic or hospital. Most women have little discomfort after this procedure.

Testing of Endometrial Tissue

Endometrial tissue samples removed by biopsy or D & C are examined under the microscope to determine whether cancer is present. If cancer is found, it will be characterized and graded. The lab report will state whether it is an endometrioid cancer or any of the other special types of endometrial cancer mentioned in the section "What Is Endometrial Cancer?" The grade of the endometrial cancer, which is based on examination under the microscope, is very important. If 95% or more of the cancer resembles glands of normal endometrial tissue, it is called grade 1. Cancers with less than half of the tissue forming glands are given a grade of 3. Grade 2 tumors have between 6% and 50% gland formation. Women with lower grade cancers are less likely to have advanced disease or recurrences.

The biopsy or D & C specimen can also be used for a test to see if the cancer cells contain *progesterone receptors*. Progesterone and estrogen are hormones that help regulate growth of normal endometrial cells and are produced by the ovaries. Having too much estrogen relative to progesterone increases endometrial cancer risk. In order for normal cells or endometrial cancer cells to respond to these hormones, the cells must contain special proteins that recognize estrogen and progesterone. These recognition proteins are called *receptors,* and can be identified by laboratory tests. Endometrial cancers that contain progesterone receptors tend to grow and spread more slowly. The presence or absence of these receptors can be used to predict prognosis.

Transvaginal Ultrasound or Sonography

A transvaginal sonogram uses sound waves to create images of the uterus. A probe inserted into the vagina releases sound waves that echo off tissue of the pelvic organs. The pattern of echoes is analyzed by a computer to create images on a video screen. These images often help determine if a tumor is present and if it extends into the myometrium.

Introducing saline (saltwater) into the uterus through a catheter before the transvaginal sonogram allows the doctor to see abnormalities of the uterine lining more clearly. This procedure is called a saline infusion sonogram or ultrahysterosonogram.

Tests to Detect Metastasis (Spread) of Endometrial Cancer

If the pathologist examining the endometrial biopsy or D & C specimen determines that cancer is present, the next step is surgery to remove the uterus. First, though, some tests are necessary to determine whether the cancer has spread to other organs. These tests typically include some routine blood tests and imaging tests.

CA 125 blood test: CA 125 is a substance released into the bloodstream by many but not all endometrial and ovarian cancers. Very high blood CA 125 levels suggest that an endometrial cancer has probably spread beyond the uterus. If CA 125 levels are elevated, some doctors use follow-up measurements to estimate the effectiveness of treatment (levels will drop if treatment is effective) and to identify cancer recurrence after initially successful treatment.

Cystoscopy and proctoscopy: If a woman has symptoms or signs that suggest the endometrial cancer has spread to the bladder or rectum, the inside of these organs can be viewed through a lighted tube. These examinations are called cystoscopy and proctoscopy, respectively. In cystoscopy the tube is placed into the bladder through the urethra. This allows the doctor to check the bladder and urethra for possible cancers. Small tissue samples can also be removed during cystoscopy for pathologic (microscopic) testing. This procedure can be done using a local anesthetic but some patients may require general anesthesia. Your doctor will let you know what to expect before and after the procedure.

Computed tomography (CT) scan: This test uses a special x-ray machine that rotates around the body, taking pictures from many angles. These pictures are combined by a computer to produce detailed cross-sectional images that are often helpful in determining if and where endometrial cancer has spread beyond the uterus (in the lower or lymph nodes, for example). This is most useful if the pelvic exam or CA 125 level indicates the cancer may have spread outside the uterus.

Magnetic resonance imaging (MRI): Like computed tomography, MRI displays a cross-section of the body. However, MRI uses powerful magnetic fields instead of x-rays. The procedure can present cross-sectional views from several angles. MRI may be done if the pelvic exam or CA 125 level indicates the cancer may have spread outside the uterus, but CT scans are used more often in this situation.

Chest x-ray: This can show if the cancer has spread to the lungs. It may also be used to determine if there are any serious lung or heart diseases.

Intravenous pyelogram (IVP): If it is suspected that the cancer has spread around the ureters (the tubes that connect the kidneys to the bladder), an IVP may be done. This is an x-ray test that outlines the urinary system. However, a computed tomography (CT) scan with contrast will provide the same information and is used more often than an IVP.

What Should You Ask Your Physician about Endometrial Cancer?

It is important for you to have honest, open discussions with your cancer care team. You should ask questions, no matter how trivial you may think they are. Some questions to consider:

- What type and grade of endometrial cancer do I have?

- Has my cancer spread beyond the uterus?

- What is the stage of my cancer and what does that mean in my case?

- What treatments are appropriate for me? What do you recommend? Why?

- What should I do to be ready for treatment?

- What risks or side effects should I expect?

- What are the chances of recurrence of my cancer with the treatment programs we have discussed?

- Should I follow a special diet?

- Will I be able to have children after my treatment?

- What is my expected prognosis, based on my cancer as you view it?

- Does this cancer prevent me from considering estrogen replacement therapy?

- How will I feel during treatment?

- When can I resume my usual activities at work and/or around the house?

In addition to these sample questions, be sure to write down some of your own. For instance, you may need specific information about anticipated recovery times so you can plan your work schedule. You may also want to ask about second opinions or about clinical trials for which you may qualify.

Chapter 12

Prevention of Endometrial Cancer

Prevention

Doctors can not always explain why one person gets cancer and another does not. However, scientists have studied general patterns of cancer in the population to learn what things around us and what things we do in our lives may increase our chance of developing cancer.

Anything that increases a person's chance of developing a disease is called a risk factor; anything that decreases a person's chance of developing a disease is called a protective factor. Some of the risk factors for cancer can be avoided, but many can not. For example, although you can choose to quit smoking, you can not choose which genes you have inherited from your parents. Both smoking and inheriting specific genes could be considered risk factors for certain kinds of cancer, but only smoking can be avoided. Prevention means avoiding the risk factors and increasing the protective factors that can be controlled so that the chance of developing cancer decreases.

Although many risk factors can be avoided, it is important to keep in mind that avoiding risk factors does not guarantee that you will not get cancer. Also, most people with a particular risk factor for cancer do not actually get the disease. Some people are more sensitive than others to factors that can cause cancer. Talk to your doctor about methods of preventing cancer that might be effective for you.

CancerNet, National Cancer Institute (www.nci.nih.gov), June 2000.

Purposes of This Summary

The purposes of this summary on endometrial cancer prevention are to:

- give information on endometrial cancer and how often it occurs

- describe endometrial cancer prevention methods

- give current facts about which women or groups of women would most likely be helped by following endometrial cancer prevention methods

You can talk to your doctor or health care professional about cancer prevention methods and whether these methods would be likely to help you.

Endometrial Cancer Prevention

The endometrium is the layer of tissue that lines the inside of the uterus. It is part of the female reproductive system.

Significance of Endometrial Cancer

In the United States, endometrial cancer is the most common cancer of the female reproductive system. The number of new cases of endometrial cancer has been decreasing, as has the number of deaths from this disease.

Endometrial Cancer Prevention

Endometrial cancer can sometimes be associated with known risk factors for the disease. Many risk factors are modifiable though not all can be avoided.

Age at onset of menstruation and menopause. Beginning menstruation at an early age and beginning menopause at a late age increase the risk of developing endometrial cancer.

Diet and lifestyle. The risk of developing endometrial cancer is increased in women who are obese. Eating a high fat diet is also associated with an increased risk of developing endometrial cancer.

Hereditary conditions. Women who carry the hereditary nonpolyposis colorectal cancer (HNPCC) genetic abnormality have an increased risk of developing endometrial cancer.

Hormone Therapy. The use of estrogens, a female hormone used to treat symptoms of menopause, is associated with an increased risk of endometrial cancer. The use of progestins in combination with estrogen replacement therapy decreases the risk of developing endometrial cancer or precancerous lesions, such as atypical hyperplasia. Using tamoxifen increases a woman's risk of developing endometrial cancer.

Number of children. Women who have never been pregnant have a greater risk of developing endometrial cancer than women who have had children.

Oral contraceptive use. The use of combination oral contraceptives by premenopausal women is associated with a decreased risk of developing endometrial cancer.

Chapter 13

Factors that Affect Your Risk of Developing Endometrial Cancer

Factors that Increase Your Risk

Seven factors that increase your risk of developing endometrial cancer are:

1. Age

You are at higher risk if you are post-menopausal and are over age 50.

2. Obesity

Women who weigh over 200 pounds have a seven-fold higher chance of getting endometrial cancer than women weighing less than 125 pounds. Excessive weight can put you at the highest risk of developing endometrial cancer.

3. Irregular Menstrual Periods

Obese women may not ovulate regularly during the reproductive years. This can upset the delicate balance between estrogenic hormones that encourage the development of cancer and the progestigenic hormones that protect against cancer.

Excerpted from "Endometrial Cancer," © 2000 Women's Cancer Network; reprinted with permission. Full text available at http://www.wcn.org.

4. Hypertension

Hypertension (high blood pressure) has been associated with uterine cancer, but not as strongly as some of the risk factors mentioned earlier. The relationship between hypertension and uterine cancer may be due to the fact that many women with hypertension are also obese, which is a very strong risk factor for uterine cancer.

5. Diabetes

Women with diabetes have twice the risk of uterine cancer as women who do not have diabetes. As is the case with hypertension, however, many women with diabetes are also obese. It is not entirely clear how much of the increased risk in women with diabetes is due to the diabetic condition as opposed to being overweight.

6. Estrogen Replacement Therapy

Estrogen replacement therapy after menopause has a number of beneficial effects including prevention of hot flashes and osteoporosis (thinning of the bones), and decreases the risk of heart disease. However, using estrogen replacement therapy without also taking progestins after menopause can cause a 2 to 12-fold increase in your risk of getting uterine cancer. The longer you take estrogens alone, the greater your risk of developing uterine cancer.

7. Late Menopause

Women who have a later menopause have a slightly increased risk of developing endometrial cancer.

Seven Factors that Can Decrease Your Risk

1. Age under 50

Uterine cancer before the age of 45 is unusual. Most young women who get the disease at an early age are obese.

2. Maintaining Normal Body Weight

Exercise and diet regimens that result in significant weight loss can markedly decrease your risk of developing uterine cancer and also can decrease the risk of a number of other illnesses including heart disease.

3. Regular Menstrual Cycles

Women who have regular menstrual periods have a somewhat lower risk of developing endometrial cancer.

4. Use of Birth Control Pills

Prescriptions that contain estrogens and/or progestins can have an impact on your risk of endometrial cancer. Taking birth control pills during child-bearing years can markedly decrease your risk of both uterine and ovarian cancer. Although it is not widely known, several studies have demonstrated that use of the pill for 5-10 years decreases the risk of this type of cancer by about 50%.

5. Smoking

Smoking increases the risk of lung cancer as well as many other types of cancer. Interestingly, however, if you smoke, you have approximately half the risk of developing uterine cancer than non-smokers. This may be explained by the fact that women who smoke have lower estrogen levels and tend to undergo menopause at an earlier age.

6. Estrogen Replacement Therapy

Taking estrogen later in life after the childbearing years can significantly reduce the risk of uterine cancer and offers additional benefits including prevention of hot flashes, thinning of the vagina, cardiovascular disease, and osteoporosis. If you use progestins with estrogen replacement, the risk of endometrial cancer is lowered to less than that of women who do not receive hormone replacement.

7. Early Menopause

Women who undergo menopause at an earlier age have a lower risk of getting endometrial cancer.

Additional Factors to Consider

Race

For reasons that are not entirely clear, uterine cancer is approximately twice as common in whites as it is in African Americans and other non-whites. On the other hand, African Americans who get this type of cancer are more likely to die of their disease.

Tamoxifen

Although several studies have shown that tamoxifen significantly increases the risk of uterine cancer, it is believed that the lowered incidence of breast cancer deaths when taking this drug outweighs the risk of developing uterine cancer. If you are receiving tamoxifen, you do not need routine x-rays or biopsies, but you should be examined by your gynecologist at least once a year or right away if irregular bleeding occurs.

Uterine Cancer before Age 45

Although this is relatively unusual, most young women who get the disease at a young age are obese.

Heavy Exercise

Some women who exercise a lot may not have menstrual periods because they are not ovulating, but this does not increase their risk of endometrial cancer.

Pregnancy

It is thought that pregnancy protects against endometrial cancer because, although menstrual cycles do not occur during pregnancy, high levels of progestins are produced.

Hereditary Predisposition

Unlike breast and ovarian cancers, which can run in some families, there is little evidence that this is the case for uterine cancer.

Childbearing

Although decisions regarding contraception and family planning are complex, you should be aware that bearing children decreases the risk of developing both uterine and ovarian cancer.

For More Information

Contact the Women's Cancer Network, c/o Gynecologic Cancer Foundation, 401 N. Michigan Avenue, Chicago, IL 60611. Toll Free: 800-444-4441 (for a referral to a gynecologic cancer specialist); Phone: 312-644-6610; Internet: www.wcn.org; E-mail: gcf@sba.com

Chapter 14

Treatment of Endometrial Cancer

What Is Cancer of the Endometrium?

Cancer of the endometrium, a common kind of cancer in women, is a disease in which cancer (malignant) cells are found in the lining of the uterus (endometrium). The uterus is the hollow, pear-shaped organ where a baby grows. Cancer of the endometrium is different from cancer of the muscle of the uterus, which is called sarcoma of the uterus.

A doctor should be seen if there are any of the following problems: bleeding or discharge not related to periods (menstruation), difficult or painful urination, pain during intercourse, and pain in the pelvic area.

Endometrial cancer has been found in a few breast cancer patients who have been treated with the hormone tamoxifen. If this hormone is being taken, a patient should go to a doctor for a pelvic examination every year and report any vaginal bleeding other than menstrual bleeding as soon as possible.

A doctor may use several tests to see if a person has cancer, usually beginning with an internal (pelvic) examination. During the examination, the doctor will feel for any lumps or changes in the shape of the uterus. The doctor will then do a Pap test, using a piece of cotton, a brush, or a small wooden stick to gently scrape the outside of the cervix (opening of the uterus) and vagina to pick up cells.

CancerNet, National Cancer Institute (www.nci.nih.gov), November 2000.

Because cancer of the endometrium begins inside the uterus, it does not usually show up on the Pap test. For this reason, a doctor may also do a dilation and curettage (D & C) or similar test to remove pieces of the lining of the uterus. During a D & C, the opening of the cervix is stretched with a spoon-shaped instrument and the walls of the uterus are scraped gently to remove any growths. This tissue is then checked for cancer cells.

The chance of recovery (prognosis) and choice of treatment depend on the stage of the cancer (whether it is just in the endometrium or has spread to other parts of the uterus or other parts of the body) and the patient's general health. The chance of recovery may also depend on how cells look under the microscope. If there is early-stage cancer, the prognosis may also depend on whether female hormones (progesterones) affect the growth of the cancer.

Stages of Cancer of the Endometrium

Once cancer of the endometrium has been found, more tests will be done to find out if the cancer has spread from the endometrium to other parts of the body (staging). To plan treatment, a doctor needs to know the stage of the disease. The following stages are used for cancer of the endometrium:

Stage I: Cancer is found only in the main part of the uterus (it is not found in the cervix).

Stage II: Cancer cells have spread to the cervix.

Stage III: Cancer cells have spread outside the uterus but have not spread outside the pelvis.

Stage IV: Cancer cells have spread beyond the pelvis, to other body parts, or into the lining of the bladder (the sac which holds urine) or rectum.

Recurrent: Recurrent disease means the cancer has come back (recurred) after it has been treated.

How Cancer of the Endometrium Is Treated

There are treatments for all patients with cancer of the endometrium. Four kinds of treatment are used:

- surgery (taking out the cancer in an operation)
- radiation therapy (using high-dose x-rays or other high-energy rays to kill cancer cells and shrink tumors)
- chemotherapy (using drugs to kill cancer cells)
- hormone therapy (using female hormones to kill cancer cells)

Surgery is the most common treatment of cancer of the endometrium. A doctor may take out the cancer using one of the following operations.

- Total abdominal hysterectomy and bilateral salpingo-oophorectomy: taking out the uterus, fallopian tubes, and ovaries through a cut in the abdomen. Lymph nodes in the pelvis may also be taken out (lymph node dissection). (The lymph nodes are small, bean-shaped structures that are found throughout the body. They produce and store infection-fighting cells, but may contain cancer cells.)
- Radical hysterectomy: taking out the cervix, uterus, fallopian tubes, ovaries, and part of the vagina. Lymph nodes in the area may also be taken out (lymph node dissection).

Radiation therapy is the use of high-dose x-rays to kill cancer cells and shrink tumors. Radiation may come from a machine outside the body (external radiation) or from putting materials that produce radiation (radioisotopes) through thin plastic tubes into the area where the cancer cells are found (internal radiation). Radiation may be used alone or before or after surgery.

Chemotherapy is the use of drugs to kill cancer cells. Chemotherapy may be taken by pill, or it may be put into the body by inserting a needle into a vein. Chemotherapy is called a systemic treatment because the drugs enter the bloodstream, travel through the body, and can kill cancer cells outside the uterus.

Hormone therapy is the use of hormones, usually taken by pill, to kill cancer cells.

Treatment by Stage

Treatment for cancer of the endometrium depends on the stage of the disease, the type of disease, and the patient's age and overall condition.

Standard treatment may be considered based on its effectiveness in patients in past studies, or participation in a clinical trial may be considered. Not all patients are cured with standard therapy and some standard treatments may have more side effects than are desired. For these reasons, clinical trials are designed to find better ways to treat cancer patients and are based on the most up-to-date information. Clinical trials are ongoing in most parts of the country for most stages of cancer of the endometrium. To learn more about clinical trials, call the National Cancer Institute's Cancer Information Service at 1-800-4-CANCER (1-800-422-6237); TTY at 1-800-332-8615.

Stage I endometrial cancer: Treatment may be one of the following:

- Surgery to remove the uterus and both ovaries and fallopian tubes (total abdominal hysterectomy and bilateral salpingo-oophorectomy) with removal of some of the lymph nodes in the pelvis and abdomen to see if they contain cancer.

- Total abdominal hysterectomy and bilateral salpingo-oophorectomy with removal of some of the lymph nodes in the pelvis and abdomen to see if they contain cancer, followed by radiation therapy to the pelvis.

- Clinical trials of radiation and/or chemotherapy following surgery.

- Radiation therapy alone for selected patients.

Stage II endometrial cancer: Treatment may be one of the following:

- Total abdominal hysterectomy, bilateral salpingo-oophorectomy, and removal of some of the lymph nodes in the pelvis and abdomen to see if they contain cancer, followed by radiation therapy.

- Internal and external-beam radiation therapy followed by surgery to remove the uterus and both ovaries and fallopian tubes (total abdominal hysterectomy and bilateral salpingo-oophorectomy). Some of the lymph nodes in the pelvis and abdomen are also removed to see if they contain cancer.

- Surgery to remove the cervix, uterus, fallopian tubes, ovaries, and part of the vagina (radical hysterectomy). Lymph nodes in the area may also be taken out (lymph node dissection).

Stage III endometrial cancer: Treatment may be one of the following:

- Surgery to remove the cervix, uterus, fallopian tubes, ovaries, and part of the vagina (radical hysterectomy). Lymph nodes in the area may also be taken out (lymph node dissection). Surgery is usually followed by radiation therapy.

- Internal and external-beam radiation therapy.

- Hormone therapy.

Stage IV endometrial cancer: Treatment may be one of the following:

- Internal and external-beam radiation therapy.

- Hormone therapy.

- Clinical trials of chemotherapy.

Recurrent endometrial cancer: If the cancer has come back, treatment may be one of the following:

- Radiation therapy to relieve symptoms, such as pain, nausea, and abnormal bowel functions.

- Hormone therapy.

- Clinical trials of chemotherapy.

Part Four

Ovarian Cancer

Chapter 15

Ovarian Cancer: An Overview

Introduction

The diagnosis of ovarian cancer brings with it many questions and a need for clear, understandable answers. We hope this National Cancer Institute (NCI) information will help. It describes the symptoms, detection, diagnosis, and treatment of this disease. Having this important information can make it easier for women and their families to handle the challenges they face.

Cancer researchers continue to study and learn more about ovarian cancer. The Cancer Information Service and the other sources of NCI information can provide the latest, most accurate information on ovarian cancer. Publications mentioned in this chapter and others are available from the Cancer Information Service at 1-800-4-CANCER. Also, many NCI publications may be viewed or ordered on the Internet at http://cancer.gov/publications/.

The Ovaries

The ovaries are a pair of organs in the female reproductive system. They are located in the pelvis, one on each side of the uterus (the hollow, pear-shaped organ where a baby grows). Each ovary is about the size and shape of an almond. The ovaries have two functions: they produce eggs and female hormones (chemicals that control the way certain cells or organs function).

National Cancer Institute, NIH Pub. No. 00-1561, June 2000.

Every month, during the menstrual cycle, an egg is released from one ovary in a process called ovulation. The egg travels from the ovary through the fallopian tube to the uterus.

The ovaries are also the main source of the female hormones estrogen and progesterone. These hormones influence the development of a woman's breasts, body shape, and body hair. They also regulate the menstrual cycle and pregnancy.

Understanding Ovarian Cancer

Cancer is a group of many related diseases that begin in cells, the body's basic unit of life. To understand cancer, it is helpful to know about normal cells and what happens when they become cancerous.

The body is made up of many types of cells. Normally, cells grow, divide, and produce more cells when the body needs them. This orderly process helps to keep the body healthy. Sometimes, however, cells keep dividing when new cells are not needed. These extra cells form a mass of tissue, called a growth or tumor. Tumors can be benign or malignant.

- **Benign tumors** are not cancer. They often can be removed and, in most cases, they do not come back. Cells in benign tumors do not spread to other parts of the body. Most important, benign tumors are rarely a threat to life.

- **Ovarian cysts** are a different type of growth. They are fluid-filled sacs that form on the surface of an ovary. They are not cancer. Cysts often go away without treatment. If a cyst does not go away, the doctor may suggest removing it, especially if it seems to be growing.

- **Malignant tumors** are cancer. Cells in these tumors are abnormal and divide without control or order. They can invade and damage nearby tissues and organs. Cancer cells can also spread (metastasize) from their original site to other parts of the body.

A malignant tumor that begins in the ovaries is called ovarian cancer. There are several types of ovarian cancer. Ovarian cancer that begins on the surface of the ovary (epithelial carcinoma) is the most common type. This is the type of cancer discussed in this chapter. Ovarian cancer that begins in the egg-producing cells (germ cell tumors) and cancer that begins in the supportive tissue surrounding the ovaries (stromal tumors) are rare and are not discussed in this text.

The National Cancer Institute's Cancer Information Service at 1-800-4-CANCER can provide information or suggest resources that deal with these types of ovarian cancer.

Ovarian cancer cells can break away from the ovary and spread to other tissues and organs in a process called shedding. When ovarian cancer sheds, it tends to seed (form new tumors) on the peritoneum (the large membrane that lines the abdomen) and on the diaphragm (the thin muscle that separates the chest from the abdomen). Fluid may collect in the abdomen. This condition is known as ascites. It may make a woman feel bloated, or her abdomen may look swollen.

Ovarian cancer cells can also enter the bloodstream or lymphatic system (the tissues and organs that produce and store cells that fight infection and disease). Once in the bloodstream or lymphatic system, the cancer cells can travel and form new tumors in other parts of the body.

Ovarian Cancer: Who's at Risk?

The exact causes of ovarian cancer are not known. However, studies show that the following factors may increase the chance of developing this disease:

Family history. First-degree relatives (mother, daughter, sister) of a woman who has had ovarian cancer are at increased risk of developing this type of cancer themselves. The likelihood is especially high if two or more first-degree relatives have had the disease. The risk is somewhat less, but still above average, if other relatives (grandmother, aunt, cousin) have had ovarian cancer. A family history of breast or colon cancer is also associated with an increased risk of developing ovarian cancer.

Age. The likelihood of developing ovarian cancer increases as a woman gets older. Most ovarian cancers occur in women over the age of 50, with the highest risk in women over 60.

Childbearing. Women who have never had children are more likely to develop ovarian cancer than women who have had children. In fact, the more children a woman has had, the less likely she is to develop ovarian cancer.

Personal history. Women who have had breast or colon cancer may have a greater chance of developing ovarian cancer than women who have not had breast or colon cancer.

Fertility drugs. Drugs that cause a woman to ovulate may slightly increase a woman's chance of developing ovarian cancer. Researchers are studying this possible association.

Talc. Some studies suggest that women who have used talc in the genital area for many years may be at increased risk of developing ovarian cancer.

Hormone replacement therapy (HRT). Some evidence suggests that women who use HRT after menopause may have a slightly increased risk of developing ovarian cancer.

About 1 in every 57 women in the United States will develop ovarian cancer. Most cases occur in women over the age of 50, but this disease can also affect younger women.

As we learn more about what causes ovarian cancer, we may also learn how to reduce the chance of getting this disease. Some studies have shown that breast feeding and taking birth control pills (oral contraceptives) may decrease a woman's likelihood of developing ovarian cancer. These factors decrease the number of times a woman ovulates, and studies suggest that reducing the number of ovulations during a woman's lifetime may lower the risk of ovarian cancer.

Women who have had an operation that prevents pregnancy (tubal ligation) or have had their uterus and cervix removed (hysterectomy) also have a lower risk of developing ovarian cancer. In addition, some evidence suggests that reducing the amount of fat in the diet may lower the risk of developing ovarian cancer.

Women who are at high risk for ovarian cancer due to a family history of the disease may consider having their ovaries removed before cancer develops (prophylactic oophorectomy). This procedure usually, but not always, protects women from developing ovarian cancer. The risks associated with this surgery and its side effects should be carefully considered. A woman should discuss the possible benefits and risks with her doctor based on her unique situation.

Having one or more of the risk factors mentioned here does not mean that a woman is sure to develop ovarian cancer, but the chance may be higher than average. Women who are concerned about ovarian cancer may want to talk with a doctor who specializes in treating women with cancer: a gynecologist, a gynecologic oncologist, or a medical oncologist. The doctor may be able to suggest ways to reduce the likelihood of developing ovarian cancer and can plan an appropriate schedule for checkups.

Detecting Ovarian Cancer

The sooner ovarian cancer is found and treated, the better a woman's chance for recovery. But ovarian cancer is hard to detect early. Many times, women with ovarian cancer have no symptoms or just mild symptoms until the disease is in an advanced stage. Scientists are studying ways to detect ovarian cancer before symptoms develop. They are exploring the usefulness of measuring the level of CA-125, a substance called a tumor marker, which is often found in higher-than-normal amounts in the blood of women with ovarian cancer. They also are evaluating transvaginal ultrasound, a test that may help detect the disease early. The Cancer Information Service can provide information about this research.

PLCO Screening Trial

A large-scale study, known as the PLCO (Prostate, Lung, Colorectal, and Ovarian) Cancer Screening Trial, is currently evaluating the usefulness of a blood test for the tumor marker known as CA-125 and a test called transvaginal ultrasound for ovarian cancer screening.

Recognizing Symptoms

Ovarian cancer often shows no obvious signs or symptoms until late in its development. Signs and symptoms of ovarian cancer may include:

- General abdominal discomfort and/or pain (gas, indigestion, pressure, swelling, bloating, cramps)
- Nausea, diarrhea, constipation, or frequent urination
- Loss of appetite
- Feeling of fullness even after a light meal
- Weight gain or loss with no known reason
- Abnormal bleeding from the vagina

These symptoms may be caused by ovarian cancer or by other, less serious conditions. It is important to check with a doctor about any of these symptoms.

Diagnosing Ovarian Cancer

To help find the cause of symptoms, a doctor evaluates a woman's medical history. The doctor also performs a physical exam and orders diagnostic tests. Some exams and tests that may be useful are described below:

Pelvic exam includes feeling the uterus, vagina, ovaries, fallopian tubes, bladder, and rectum to find any abnormality in their shape or size. (A Pap test, a good test for cancer of the cervix, is often done along with the pelvic exam, but it is not a reliable way to find or diagnose ovarian cancer.)

Ultrasound refers to the use of high-frequency sound waves. These waves, which cannot be heard by humans, are aimed at the ovaries. The pattern of the echoes they produce creates a picture called a sonogram. Healthy tissues, fluid-filled cysts, and tumors look different on this picture.

CA-125 assay is a blood test used to measure the level of CA-125, a tumor marker that is often found in higher-than-normal amounts in the blood of women with ovarian cancer.

Lower GI series, or **barium enema**, is a series of x-rays of the colon and rectum. The pictures are taken after the patient is given an enema with a white, chalky solution containing barium. The barium outlines the colon and rectum on the x-ray, making tumors or other abnormal areas easier to see.

CT (or CAT) scan is a series of detailed pictures of areas inside the body created by a computer linked to an x-ray machine.

Biopsy is the removal of tissue for examination under a microscope. A pathologist studies the tissue to make a diagnosis. To obtain the tissue, the surgeon performs a laparotomy (an operation to open the abdomen). If cancer is suspected, the surgeon performs an oophorectomy (removal of the entire ovary). This is important because, if cancer is present, removing just a sample of tissue by cutting through the outer layer of the ovary could allow cancer cells to escape and cause the disease to spread.

If the diagnosis is ovarian cancer, the doctor will want to learn the stage (or extent) of disease. Staging is a careful attempt to find out whether the cancer has spread and, if so, to what parts of the body. Staging may involve surgery, x-rays and other imaging procedures, and lab tests. Knowing the stage of the disease helps the doctor plan treatment.

Treatment for Ovarian Cancer

Treatment depends on a number of factors, including the stage of the disease and the general health of the patient. Patients are often treated by a team of specialists. The team may include a gynecologist, a gynecologic oncologist, a medical oncologist, and/or a radiation oncologist. Many different treatments and combinations of treatments are used to treat ovarian cancer.

Surgery is the usual initial treatment for women diagnosed with ovarian cancer. The ovaries, the fallopian tubes, the uterus, and the cervix are usually removed. This operation is called a hysterectomy with bilateral salpingo-oophorectomy. Often, the surgeon also removes the omentum (the thin tissue covering the stomach and large intestine) and lymph nodes (small organs located along the channels of the lymphatic system) in the abdomen.

Staging during surgery (to find out whether the cancer has spread) generally involves removing lymph nodes, samples of tissue from the diaphragm and other organs in the abdomen, and fluid from the abdomen. If the cancer has spread, the surgeon usually removes as much of the cancer as possible in a procedure called tumor debulking. Tumor debulking reduces the amount of cancer that will have to be treated later with chemotherapy or radiation therapy.

Chemotherapy is the use of drugs to kill cancer cells. Chemotherapy may be given to destroy any cancerous cells that may remain in the body after surgery, to control tumor growth, or to relieve symptoms of the disease.

Most drugs used to treat ovarian cancer are given by injection into a vein (intravenously, or IV). The drugs can be injected directly into a vein or given through a catheter, a thin tube. The catheter is placed into a large vein and remains there as long as it is needed. Some anticancer drugs are taken by mouth. Whether they are given intravenously or by mouth, the drugs enter the bloodstream and circulate throughout the body.

Another way to give chemotherapy is to put the drug directly into the abdomen through a catheter. With this method, called intraperitoneal chemotherapy, most of the drug remains in the abdomen.

After chemotherapy is completed, second-look surgery may be performed to examine the abdomen directly. The surgeon may remove fluid and tissue samples to see whether the anticancer drugs have been successful.

Radiation therapy, also called radiotherapy, involves the use of high-energy rays to kill cancer cells. Radiation therapy affects the cancer cells only in the treated area. The radiation may come from a machine (external radiation). Some women receive a treatment called intraperitoneal radiation therapy in which radioactive liquid is put directly into the abdomen through a catheter.

Clinical trials (research studies) to evaluate new ways to treat cancer are an important treatment option for many women with ovarian cancer. In some studies, all patients receive the new treatment. In others, doctors compare different therapies by giving the promising new treatment to one group of patients and the usual (standard) therapy to another group. Through research, doctors learn new, more effective ways to treat cancer. More information about treatment studies can be found in the NCI publication *Taking Part in Clinical Trials: What Cancer Patients Need To Know*. NCI also has a Web site at http://cancertrials.nci.nih.gov/ that provides detailed information about ongoing studies for ovarian cancer. Clinical trial information is also available from the Cancer Information Service by calling 1-800-4-CANCER (1-800-422-6237).

The NCI's CancerNet™ Web site provides information from numerous NCI sources, including PDQ®, NCI's cancer information database. PDQ contains information about ongoing clinical trials as well as current information on cancer prevention, screening, treatment, and supportive care. CancerNet also contains CANCERLIT®, a database of citations and abstracts on cancer topics from scientific literature. CancerNet can be accessed at http://cancernet.nci.nih.gov/ on the Internet.

Possible Side Effects of Treatment

The side effects of cancer treatment depend on the type of treatment and may be different for each woman. Doctors and nurses will explain the possible side effects of treatment, and they can suggest ways to help relieve problems that may occur during and after treatment.

Surgery causes short-term pain and tenderness in the area of the operation. Discomfort or pain after surgery can be controlled with medicine. Patients should feel free to discuss pain relief with their doctor. For several days after surgery, the patient may have difficulty emptying her bladder and having bowel movements.

When both ovaries are removed, a woman loses her ability to become pregnant. Some women may experience feelings of loss that may make intimacy difficult. Counseling or support for both the patient and her partner may be helpful.

Also, removing the ovaries means that the body's natural source of estrogen and progesterone is lost, and menopause occurs. Symptoms of menopause, such as hot flashes and vaginal dryness, are likely to appear soon after the surgery. Some form of hormone replacement therapy may be used to ease such symptoms. Deciding whether to use it is a personal choice; women with ovarian cancer should discuss with their doctors the possible risks and benefits of using hormone replacement therapy.

Chemotherapy affects normal as well as cancerous cells. Side effects depend largely on the specific drugs and the dose (amount of drug given). Common side effects of chemotherapy include nausea and vomiting, loss of appetite, diarrhea, fatigue, numbness and tingling in hands or feet, headaches, hair loss, and darkening of the skin and fingernails. Certain drugs used in the treatment of ovarian cancer can cause some hearing loss or kidney damage. To help protect the kidneys while taking these drugs, patients may receive extra fluid intravenously.

Radiation therapy, like chemotherapy, affects normal as well as cancerous cells. Side effects of radiation therapy depend mainly on the treatment dose and the part of the body that is treated. Common side effects of radiation therapy to the abdomen are fatigue, loss of appetite, nausea, vomiting, urinary discomfort, diarrhea, and skin changes on the abdomen. Intraperitoneal radiation therapy may cause abdominal pain and bowel obstruction (a blockage of the intestine).

Several NCI booklets, including *Chemotherapy and You*, *Radiation Therapy and You*, and *Eating Hints for Cancer Patients*, suggest ways for patients to cope with the side effects they experience during cancer treatment.

Doctors and nurses will explain the possible side effects of treatment, and they can suggest ways to help relieve problems that may occur during and after treatment.

The Importance of Followup Care

Followup care after treatment for ovarian cancer is important. Regular checkups generally include a physical exam, as well as a pelvic exam and Pap test. The doctor also may perform additional tests such as a chest x-ray, CT scan, urinalysis, complete blood count, and CA-125 assay.

In addition to having followup exams to check for the return of ovarian cancer, patients may also want to ask their doctor about checking them for other types of cancer. Women who have had ovarian cancer may be at increased risk of developing breast or colon cancer. In addition, treatment with certain anticancer drugs may increase the risk of second cancers, such as leukemia.

Emotional Support

Living with a serious disease is challenging. Apart from having to cope with the physical and medical challenges, people with cancer face many worries, feelings, and concerns that can make life difficult. They may need help coping with the emotional aspects of their disease.

In fact, attention to the emotional burden of having cancer is often a part of a patient's treatment plan. The support of the health care team (doctors, nurses, social workers), support groups, and patient-to-patient networks can help people feel less isolated and distressed and can improve the quality of their lives. Cancer support groups provide an environment where cancer patients can talk about living with cancer with others who may be having similar experiences. Patients may want to speak with their health care team about finding a support group. The Cancer Information Service and other NCI resources have helpful information about locating support groups. Also, useful information about coping with cancer is presented in many NCI fact sheets and booklets, including *Taking Time* and *Facing Forward*.

Ovarian Cancer: What the Future Holds

The National Cancer Institute is supporting and conducting research on the causes and prevention of ovarian cancer. Researchers have discovered that changes in certain genes (basic units of heredity) are responsible for an increased risk of developing ovarian and breast cancers. Members of families with many cases of these diseases may consider having a special blood test to see if they have a genetic change that increases the risk of these types of cancer. Although having such a genetic change does not mean that a woman is sure to develop ovarian or breast cancer, those who have the genetic change may want to discuss their options with a doctor. Information about gene testing is also available in the NCI publication *Understanding Gene*

Testing, which can be ordered from the CIS at 1-800-4-CANCER or on the Internet at http://cancer.gov/publications/.

Questions for Your Doctor

This information is designed to help you work with your doctor to get the information you need to make informed decisions about your health care. In addition, asking your doctor the following questions will help you further understand your condition. To help you remember what the doctor says, you may take notes or ask whether you may use a tape recorder. Some people also want to have a family member or friend with them when they talk to the doctor—to take part in the discussion, to take notes, or just to listen.

Diagnosis

- What tests can diagnose ovarian cancer?
- Are they painful? Do they carry any other risks to my health?
- How soon after the tests will I learn the results?
- What type of ovarian cancer do I have?

Treatment

- What treatments are recommended for me?
- What clinical trials are appropriate for my type of cancer?
- Will I need to be in the hospital to receive my treatment? For how long?
- How might my normal activities change during my treatment?

Side Effects

- What side effects should I expect? How long will they last?
- Whom should I call if I am concerned about a side effect?

Followup

- After treatment, how often do I need to be checked? What type of followup care should I have?
- Will I eventually be able to resume my normal activities?

The Health Care Team

- Who will be involved with my treatment and followup care? What is the role of each member of the health care team in my care?

- What has been your experience in caring for patients with ovarian cancer?

Resources

- Are there support groups in the area with people I can talk to?

- Are there organizations where I can get more information about ovarian cancer?

Chapter 16

Factors that Affect Your Risk of Developing Ovarian Cancer

Factors that Increase Your Risk

Family History

Family history is the most significant risk factor for ovarian cancer. Women should be encouraged to learn their family histories of breast, ovarian, uterine, colon, and prostate cancers on both the maternal and paternal family lineages. The genetic risk for ovarian cancer can be transmitted through either the mother or father and both of these family histories are of equal importance.

Other Genetic Factors

Recent advances in molecular biology have identified genes called BRCA-1 and BRCA-2 that appear to account for most of the genetic risk of ovarian cancer. Other genes associated with colon cancer in families and uterine cancers also lead to ovarian cancer. Only approximately 10% of the ovarian cancer cases are due to a familial risk. Approximately 15% of ovarian cancers in women 30-39 years old are associated with a genetic risk whereas the association is only 7% of the cases in women 50-59 years old.

Approximately 2 in 1000 women in the general population will carry a mutation in BRCA-1 and BRCA-2 genes associated with this increased risk of breast and ovarian cancers. In Jewish women of Ashkenazi heritage, however, approximately 2% or 2 in 100 women will harbor this altered gene. Women who have an altered BRCA-1 or BRCA-2 gene have approximately a 20% risk of developing ovarian cancer sometime in their life. Women should research their family tree and then discuss their genetic risk of ovarian cancer with their physicians.

Age

Epithelial ovarian cancer is rare among young women, but the incidence increases steeply around the time of the menopause and continues to increase into the older ages.

Risk Factors that Remain Controversial

Infertility

Infertility is a risk factor for ovarian cancer. It remains unclear whether all types of infertility have the same amount of risk. For example, a woman who has infertility due to male factor or low sperm count risk is likely different from a patient who has infertility due to an ovarian or hormonal factor. Nonetheless, never bearing children appears to place women at a slightly increased risk or ovarian cancer.

Use of Fertility Drugs

Fertility drugs also have been implicated as a risk factor for ovarian cancer. Whether or not this is just associated with the infertility also remains unclear. Women who use fertility drugs but later conceive and have a baby are not at an increased risk of ovarian cancer. Patients undergoing infertility treatment should discuss this possible association with their physicians.

Talcum Powder

Use of talcum powder on the perineum is also an equivocal risk factor. While some studies have noted that the use of talc on sanitary napkins and on the perineum have been found to be associated with an increased risk of ovarian cancer, other studies have not supported this and the risk appears to be equivocal.

Reproductive Factors

Age at the time menstruation begins, age at menopause, and breastfeeding are also of no significant effect on the incidence of ovarian cancer. The association of breastfeeding and ovarian cancer risk is also inconclusive, but if anything, there seems to be some level of protection associated with breastfeeding.

Weight and Diet

There appears to be no association between weight and ovarian cancer risk. While the risk factor associated with diet also remains unclear, it appears that a diet high in saturated fat and low in vegetables may be associated with an elevated ovarian cancer risk.

Smoking

Smoking has been associated with a slightly increased level of ovarian cancer, but this too remains controversial.

Factors that Decrease Your Risk of Ovarian Cancer

Childbearing

It is well established that ovarian cancer risk is reduced with each subsequent pregnancy. Results tend to show a 40% reduction in ovarian cancer risk associated with the first term pregnancy and a 10% to 15% reduction in risk with each additional term pregnancy.

Use of Birth Control Pills or Oral Contraceptives

Multiple studies have shown that the risk of ovarian cancer can be reduced 40% to 60% with the use of birth control pills. With each successive year of use between the beginning of menstruation and menopause, the risk of ovarian cancer continues to fall. For example, at the baseline, risk of ovarian cancer in the United States is 1 in 70. After accumulating 10 years of birth control pill use, a woman can reduce her risk to 1 in 350. Therefore, using birth control pills can provide benefits outside their normal use for contraception; most significantly, their ability to prevent and protect women against ovarian cancer.

Tubal Ligation

Tubal ligation is a sterilization procedure to prevent pregnancy. It appears that tubal ligation is associated with a significant reduction in ovarian cancer risk. Studies demonstrate that women who have undergone a tubal ligation reduce their risk of ovarian cancer by two-thirds or approximately 60%.

Hormone Replacement Therapy

While controversial in terms of its risk associated with breast cancer, hormone replacement therapy has not been associated with any significant alteration in ovarian cancer risk.

For More Information

Women's Cancer Network
c/o Gynecologic Cancer Foundation
401 N. Michigan Avenue
Chicago, IL 60611
Toll Free: 800-444-4441 (for a referral to a gynecologic cancer specialist)
Phone: 312-644-6610
Internet: www.wcn.org
E-mail: gcf@sba.com

Chapter 17

Do Infertility Drugs Increase the Risk of Ovarian Cancer?

Mary Kara Bucci, MD, OncoLink Editorial Assistant, responds to a question about whether infertility drugs increase the risk of ovarian cancer:

A report published in the September 22, 1994 issue of the *New England Journal of Medicine* implicates the long-term use (over twelve months) of an infertility drug, clomiphene, with an increased risk of ovarian cancer.

A previously published report (Whittemore et al, *American Journal of Epidemiology* 1992; 136:1184-203) implicated infertility drugs as a possible risk factor in the development of several different subtypes of ovarian cancer. To confirm these findings, doctors at the University of Washington in Seattle looked at 3,837 women evaluated for infertility over a ten-year period in Seattle. Of these women, eleven developed an ovarian cancer. This rate is 2.5 times the expected rate for women in the general population. The overall risk for any type of cancer was similar to the expected risk.

To determine if this increase was associated with infertility rather than an infertility drug, the study's authors compared the women who had taken clomiphene with those who were evaluated for infertility but had not taken the medication. They then compared the women who had taken clomiphene for twelve months or more with those who had taken it for fewer than twelve months or not at all. They found that women who had taken the drug at all were 3.1 times as likely to develop an ovarian cancer. Women who had taken the drug for twelve months or more were eleven times as likely as their comparison group to develop ovarian cancer, while women who were evaluated for infertility but had never taken the drug were not at increased risk. When they adjusted for obesity, a known risk factor for ovarian cancer, the authors found that women who had taken clomiphene for twelve months or more were eighteen times as likely to develop ovarian cancer.

The average elapsed time between seeking treatment for infertility and developing an ovarian cancer was almost 7 years. This is long enough to suggest that the ovarian cancer was not pre-existing (that is, it was not the cause of infertility and subsequent clomiphene use rather than the result).The presence of ovarian abnormalities, as opposed to the failure to conceive a child, was also assessed. The long-term use of clomiphene was associated with an increased risk of ovarian cancer in women both with and without ovarian abnormalities. This suggests that the higher rate of cancer seen in clomiphene users was not simply a reflection of underlying ovarian abnormalities.

The authors point out that they had a very small number of patients in their study, and a larger study would be needed to prove definitively that prolonged use of clomiphene may increase the risk of ovarian cancer.

Chapter 18

Accuracy of Screenings for Ovarian Cancer Is Still Inconsistent

Because screening for ovarian cancer is still in its infancy, women should educate themselves about symptoms and risk factors. There is no single, proven screening technique for ovarian cancer for the general population. However, there are recommendations for high-risk individuals and a combination of screening methods are being tested for the general population.

Genetic Predisposition

Women are at high risk of developing ovarian cancer if there is a strong family history of ovarian cancer or a combination of cancers linked to a family cancer syndrome, which may include breast, ovarian, uterine, and colorectal cancers. A genetic test is available to help determine if a women carries a mutated gene, known as BRCA1 or BRCA2, that makes her more likely to develop ovarian or related cancers. This test may be offered to women who appear to have a greater than 10% chance of getting such cancers.

The Froedtert and Medical College Cancer Genetics Screening Program includes a cancer geneticist/counselor and committee of doctors. After a review of family history and discussions with the patient, a blood test may be administered and analyzed for the mutated cancer genes. Typically, it will be offered to patients who have two or more first-degree relatives (mother or sisters) who developed ovarian cancer or family cancer syndrome cancers by the age of 50. An early onset or cluster of breast cancers, even in aunts and cousins, is of particular note. Patients with such a strong family history usually have a greater than 10% chance of getting ovarian and/or related cancers. If the test does not show a gene abnormality, it is most likely not a hereditary condition and the individual is not at high risk of developing the cancer.

If a gene abnormality is found, there are two approaches. In women who are older or who do not want more children, the ovaries are removed as a preventive measure. However, this is not 100% reliable, as primary peritoneal cancer, which mimics ovarian cancer, is still possible, although rare. In younger women who may want children, more screenings will be conducted. A blood test for CA125, the tumor marker for the most common form of ovarian cancer, will be administered every six months to a year thereafter. In addition, a transvaginal ultrasound, in which a probe is inserted into the vagina, will be administered on the same time schedule. A recto-vaginal pelvic exam will also be conducted every six months to a year thereafter.

Challenges

Unfortunately, the CA125 blood test is unreliable. Younger patients may have elevated tumor markers because of conditions unrelated to cancer, such as endometriosis or menstruation irregularities. Older, non-menstruating patients may show elevated CA125 markers if they have diverticulitis, for example. And individuals who have the initial, or Stage 1, ovarian cancer, display elevated CA125 markers only about half the time. It is far from a perfect test, and used alone, is not beneficial. An ongoing study is checking the efficacy of transvaginal ultrasound with the CA125 test.

Past studies of ovarian cancer screening tests typically found a small number of cancers, but usually in patients who had advanced symptoms already and who were beyond the curable stage. Some studies have found that false-positive screening results led to more women having unnecessary surgeries than the number of true-positive results detected by the test. Various blood tests are currently under study, and a screening for lysophosphitidic acid (LPA) shows promise in identifying early-stage ovarian cancer.

Stage 1 ovarian cancer is curable, but most ovarian cancer cases are discovered in Stage 3 in which the cancer has spread beyond the ovaries and pelvic area. Cure at an advanced stage is more elusive than in Stage 1. Stage 1 ovarian cancer symptoms are non-specific, making them difficult to identify. However, high-risk individuals and even the general population can benefit by knowing them. Symptoms include: an abdomen that is growing in size for no apparent reason; pelvic pain, pressure or bloating; heartburn; and a bladder that is not functioning well.

Until a better screening method is developed, women should learn the symptoms of ovarian cancer, determine if they are at high risk for the disease, and follow-up accordingly. If they are not at high risk, they should at least have an annual pelvic exam of the recto-vaginal areas.

— by Kenny Bozorgi, MD
Assistant Professor of Obstetrics and Gynecology
Medical College of Wisconsin and Froedtert Hospital

Chapter 19

Treating Ovarian Epithelial Cancer

What Is Cancer of the Ovary?

Cancer of the ovary is a disease in which cancer cells are found in the ovary. Approximately 25,000 women in the United States are diagnosed with this disease each year. The ovary is a small organ in the pelvis that makes female hormones and holds egg cells which, when fertilized, can develop into a baby. There are two ovaries: one located on the left side of the uterus (the hollow, pear-shaped organ where a baby grows) and one located on the right. This chapter has information on cancer that occurs in the lining (epithelium) of the ovary. Information on cancer that is found in the egg-making cells in the ovary, called a germ cell tumor of the ovary, is available from the Cancer Information Service at 1-800-4-CANCER. Also, many NCI publications may be viewed or ordered on the Internet at http://cancer.gov/publications.

Unfortunately, the vast majority of women with ovarian cancer are diagnosed with advanced disease. Although sometimes women with early ovarian cancer have symptoms, such as vague gastrointestinal discomfort, pelvic pressure, and pain, more often women with early ovarian cancer have no symptoms or very mild and nonspecific symptoms. By the time symptoms are present, women with ovarian cancer usually have advanced disease.

Because cancer of the ovary may spread to the peritoneum, the sac inside the abdomen that holds the intestines, uterus, and ovaries,

CancerNet, National Cancer Institute (www.nci.nih.gov), November 2000.

many women with cancer of the ovary may have fluid inside the peritoneum (called ascites), which causes swelling of the abdomen. If the cancer has spread to the muscle under the lung that controls breathing (the diaphragm), fluid may build up under the lungs and cause shortness of breath.

Some women are at higher risk of developing ovarian cancer because of a family history of ovarian cancer. Women with two or more close family members affected by ovarian cancer may be a part of a cancer family syndrome and should be counseled by a qualified specialist regarding their individual risk. A woman with one affected close relative (mother, sister, or daughter) has a 5.0% lifetime risk of ovarian cancer. This compares with a 1.5% lifetime risk of ovarian cancer in a woman with no affected relatives. At the present time, with current knowledge and technology, routine screening for ovarian cancer for women with one or no close relatives with ovarian cancer cannot be recommended.

The chance of recovery (prognosis) and choice of treatment depend on the patient's age and general state of health, the type and size of the tumor, and the stage of the cancer.

Stages of Cancer of the Ovary

Once cancer of the ovary has been found, more tests will be done to find out if the cancer has spread to other parts of the body (staging). An operation called a laparotomy is done for almost all patients to find out the stage of the disease. A doctor must cut into the abdomen and carefully look at all the organs to see if they contain cancer. During the operation the doctor will cut out small pieces of tissue (biopsy) so they can be looked at under a microscope to see whether they contain cancer. Usually the doctor will remove the cancer and other organs that contain cancer during the laparotomy (see section on how cancer of the ovary is treated). The doctor needs to know the stage of the disease to plan further treatment. The following stages are used for cancer of the ovary:

Stage I: Cancer is found only in one or both of the ovaries.

Stage II: Cancer is found in one or both ovaries and/or has spread to the uterus, and/or the fallopian tubes (the pathway used by the egg to get from the ovary to the uterus), and/or other body parts within the pelvis.

Stage III: Cancer is found in one or both ovaries and has spread to lymph nodes or to other body parts inside the abdomen, such as the surface of the liver or intestine. (Lymph nodes are small bean-shaped structures that are found throughout the body. They produce and store infection-fighting cells.)

Stage IV: Cancer is found in one or both ovaries and has spread outside the abdomen or has spread to the inside of the liver.

Recurrent or refractory: Recurrent disease means that the cancer has come back (recurred) after it has been treated. Refractory disease means the cancer is no longer responding to treatment.

How Cancer of the Ovary Is Treated

There are treatments for all patients with cancer of the ovary. Three kinds of treatments are used:

- surgery (taking out the cancer in an operation)
- radiation therapy (using high-energy x-rays to kill cancer cells)
- chemotherapy (using drugs to kill cancer cells)

Surgery: Adequate and complete surgical intervention is mandatory primary therapy for ovarian carcinoma, permitting precise staging, accurate diagnosis, and optimal debulking of the tumor (taking out as much of the cancer as possible). Such an operation generally involves total hysterectomy, bilateral salpingo-oophorectomy (removal of fallopian tubes and ovaries), omentectomy (removal of fatty tissue covering within the abdomen), and lymphadenectomy (sampling of lymph nodes). An aggressive approach to tumor debulking is important in ovarian cancer, since removal of the maximum amount of tumor is associated with improved survival. The procedure is best performed by a qualified gynecologic oncologist, who is a gynecologic surgeon with specialized training in pelvic cancers.

Radiation therapy is the use of high-energy x-rays to kill cancer cells and shrink tumors. Radiation may come from a machine outside the body (external-beam radiation therapy) or it may be put directly into the sac that lines the abdomen (peritoneum) in a liquid that is radioactive (intraperitoneal radiation).

Chemotherapy is the use of drugs to kill cancer cells. It may be taken by pill or put into the body by inserting a needle into a vein.

Chemotherapy is called a systemic treatment because the drugs enter the bloodstream, travel through the body, and kill cancer cells outside the ovaries. Chemotherapy can also be given by a needle put through the abdominal wall into the peritoneum.

Treatment by Stage

Treatment of cancer of the ovary depends on the stage of the disease, the type of disease, and the patient's age and overall condition.

Treatment may be received as part of an ongoing clinical trial for ovarian cancer. Clinical trials are designed to find better ways to treat cancer patients and are based on the most up-to-date information. Clinical trials are ongoing in most parts of the country for most stages of cancer of the ovary. If a clinical trial is not available, or the patient chooses not to participate, treatments are available that are considered standard based on their performance in prior clinical trials. To learn more about clinical trials, call the Cancer Information Service at 1-800-4-CANCER (1-800-422-6237); TTY at 1-800-332-8615.

Stage I ovarian epithelial cancer: All women who have ovarian cancer should have carefully performed surgical staging. Most women who have stage I ovarian cancer will have a total abdominal hysterectomy/bilateral salpingo-oophorectomy, omentectomy, and biopsy of lymph nodes and other tissues in the pelvis and abdomen. Depending on the pathologist's interpretation of the tumor cells, the specific cell type involved, and the grade of the tumor (how malignant it appears under a microscope), additional treatment may be recommended after surgery. Additional treatment may be one of the following:

- Radiation therapy, chemotherapy, or careful observation without immediate treatment (watchful waiting).

- Combination chemotherapy.

- A clinical trial evaluating new chemotherapy drugs or new combinations of drugs.

Stage II ovarian epithelial cancer: Treatment will include surgery to remove both ovaries, both fallopian tubes, the uterus, and as much of the cancer as possible (total abdominal hysterectomy and bilateral salpingo-oophorectomy with tumor debulking). During the surgery, samples of lymph nodes and other tissues in the pelvis and abdomen are cut out (biopsied) and checked for cancer. After the operation, treatment may be one of the following:

- Combination chemotherapy with or without radiation therapy.

- Combination chemotherapy.

- A clinical trial evaluating new chemotherapy drugs or new combinations of drugs.

Stage III ovarian epithelial cancer: Treatment will include surgery to remove both ovaries, both fallopian tubes, the uterus, and as much of the cancer as possible (total abdominal hysterectomy and bilateral salpingo-oophorectomy with tumor debulking). During the surgery, samples of lymph nodes and other tissues in the pelvis and abdomen are cut out (biopsied) and checked for cancer. After the operation, treatment may be one of the following:

- Combination chemotherapy.

- Combination chemotherapy possibly followed by surgery to find and remove any additional cancer.

Stage IV ovarian epithelial cancer: Treatment will probably be surgery to remove as much of the cancer as possible (tumor debulking), followed by combination chemotherapy.

Recurrent ovarian epithelial cancer: There is no standard treatment for cancer that recurs (comes back). Clinical trials are currently evaluating several treatment options. Treatment for recurrent cancer may be one of the following:

- Chemotherapy possibly followed by surgery.

- New chemotherapy drugs or new combinations of drugs.

- Surgery to ease the symptoms caused by the cancer.

- Combination chemotherapy.

Chapter 20

Treating Ovarian Low Malignant Potential Tumor

Description

Cancer of the ovary is a disease in which cancer cells are found in the ovary. The ovary is a small organ in the pelvis that makes female hormones and holds egg cells which, when fertilized, can develop into a baby. There are two ovaries: one located on the left side of the uterus (the hollow, pear-shaped organ where a baby grows) and one located on the right. This summary has information on cancer that occurs in the lining (epithelium) of the ovary.

Ovarian tumors of low malignant potential are considered border-line cancer. Approximately 15% of all cancers of the lining of the ovary (epithelial ovarian cancers) are low malignant potential tumors. These tumors are usually found early. Most women, however, survive even advanced stage ovarian low malignant potential tumors. Patients who do not survive usually die from complications of the disease (such as a small bowel obstruction) or the side effects of treatment, but rarely because the tumor has spread.

Treatment

There are treatments for all patients with cancer of the ovary. Three kinds of treatments are used:

- surgery (taking out the cancer in an operation)

PDQ Statement, National Cancer Institute (www.nci.nih.gov), January 2001.

- radiation therapy (using high-energy x-rays to kill cancer cells)
- chemotherapy (using drugs to kill cancer cells)

Surgery may be an unilateral salpingo-oophorectomy (surgery to remove one of the ovaries and the fallopian tube, the tube that connects the ovary to the uterus) or a combination of a hysterectomy (surgery to remove the uterus), a bilateral salpingo-oophorectomy (surgery remove both of the ovaries and fallopian tubes), and an omentectomy (partial removal of the lining of the abdominal cavity). The lymph nodes (small organs that fight infection and disease) may also be removed to check for signs of disease.

Radiation therapy is the use of high-energy x-rays to kill cancer cells and shrink tumors. Radiation may come from a machine outside the body (external-beam radiation therapy) or it may be put directly into the sac that lines the abdomen (peritoneum) in a liquid that is radioactive (intraperitoneal radiation).

Chemotherapy is the use of drugs to kill cancer cells. It may be taken by pill or put into the body by inserting a needle into a vein. Chemotherapy is called a systemic treatment because the drugs enter the bloodstream, travel through the body, and kill cancer cells outside the ovaries. Chemotherapy can also be given by a needle put through the abdominal wall into the peritoneum.

Treatment for early stage ovarian low malignant potential tumor (stage I/II disease) is complete removal of the tumor by surgery. If the patient plans to have children, only one ovary is removed. If both ovaries are affected, surgery to partially remove the ovaries may be possible. For women who do not wish to become pregnant, the uterus, cervix, and both ovaries are removed. To prevent a recurrence of borderline tumor or cancer, most physicians prefer to remove all ovarian tissue once a woman no longer intends to have children.

When disease is found in one ovary, the other ovary should also be checked carefully for signs of disease.

Patients who have advanced disease should undergo a hysterectomy, bilateral salpingo-oophorectomy, and omentectomy. The lymph nodes should also be checked for signs of disease.

If the tumor cannot be completely removed by surgery, patients may be treated with chemotherapy and/or radiation therapy. If the tumor continues to grow, patients may receive chemotherapy.

Chapter 21

New Treatment Approach to Ovarian Cancer Offers Promise

High-dose chemotherapy offers hope for some women with advanced ovarian cancer, according to researchers from the Autologous Blood and Marrow Transplant Registry (ABMTR) headquartered at the Medical College of Wisconsin. This is the largest study of its kind to date.

"We're not saying this is a miracle cure," says Mary Horowitz, MD, Professor of Medicine at the Medical College and Scientific Director of the International Bone Marrow Transplant Registry (IBMTR) and the ABMTR. "We're saying the results are encouraging enough or suggestively better than what is being reported as "salvage" or last-resort therapy to start more extensive clinical trials directly comparing this method with the conventional approach."

Patrick Stiff, MD, Ph.D., chairman of the ABMTR working committee for solid tumors and a faculty member at Loyola University Stritch School of Medicine in Chicago led the research, which is reported in the October 2000 issue of the *Annals of Internal Medicine*.

Ovarian cancer is the fifth leading cause of cancer deaths among women. According to the American Cancer Society, 23,100 new cases of ovarian cancer will be diagnosed in 2000 in the US. About 14,000 will die of the disease. Only 25% of ovarian cancers are found at an early stage before the cancer has spread beyond the ovaries.

The treatment studied involves high-dose chemotherapy combined with transplanting the woman's blood stem cells. Stem cells, which are removed prior to the chemotherapy, are primitive cells from which the body's various blood cells form. The study found that 39% of the women with chemotherapy-sensitive disease survived two years after treatment. Historically, only about 20% who get conventional treatment survive two years.

The study involved 421 women who were treated between 1989 and 1996 at 57 centers in North America. The results were reported to and analyzed at the ABMTR Statistical Center at the Medical College. "By putting together the experience of many centers, we've been able to identify the group of women in whom it's been more likely to work, and where we should be concentrating our efforts to determine if this adds to or is better than what we have available," says Dr. Horowitz.

The women who are the best candidates for this treatment are under 50 years of age, in good health aside from the cancer, and whose disease can respond to chemotherapy, according to Dr. Horowitz. Nevertheless, she says, these women had "very bad disease." The blood stem cells, which are found in the bone marrow, are removed to protect them (and thus the patient's blood cells) from the damage that chemotherapy can do to them.

"Doses of chemotherapy in ovarian cancer patients are limited because such drugs can destroy these vitally important stem cells," explains Dr. Horowitz. "Even for tumors that we believe can be cured with chemotherapy, we cannot give an unlimited amount. The other organs and tissues of the body tend to be more resistant to these chemotherapy agents than bone marrow stem cells. If you could ignore that toxicity, you can get an appreciable increase in the amount of drug that you can deliver," Dr. Horowitz says.

The stem cells are removed prior to the chemotherapy, frozen, and replaced after the chemotherapy. Though she finds the results of the study encouraging, Dr. Horowitz notes there are improvements that can be made in the treatment technique.

"There was still about a 10% mortality from the treatment. Part of that could be avoided by simply not treating patients who are too sick to withstand the treatment," she says. Because of the study's results, Horowitz argues, the time has come to seriously evaluate how good this treatment can really be. "We should be looking at this therapy in controlled, randomized trials," she says. Those trials would compare this therapy with existing forms of treatment.

Also involved in the study were Judith Veum-Stone, MS, Biostatistican, Medical College of Wisconsin; Dr. John Klein, Ph.D., Statistical Director of the IBMTR/ABMTR, Medical College of Wisconsin;

Hillard M. Lazarus, MD, Ireland Cancer Center at Case Western Reserve University; Lois Ayash, MD, University of Michigan Medical Center; John R. Edwards, MD, Walt Disney Memorial Cancer Institute at Florida Hospital in Orlando, Florida; Armand Keating, MD, Princess Margaret Hospital in Toronto, Ontario; David J. Oblon, MD, Sharp Health Care and the Sidney Kimmel Cancer Center, San Diego; Thomas C. Shea, MD, University of North Carolina; and Stephan Thomé, MD, Mayo Clinic.

Chapter 22

Fertility Sparing Surgery an Option for Some Ovarian Cancer Patients

An estimated 23,000 U.S. women will be diagnosed with ovarian cancer in 2000. While the disease strikes women over age 65 most frequently, many young women will also be diagnosed. Many of these patients will want to preserve their ability to have children after treatment.

Unfortunately, removal of both ovaries and the uterus is usually unavoidable for patients whose cancer has spread. But for women diagnosed with early-stage ovarian cancer (which includes about half of cases in women under 50) removal of one ovary has become a real option. This conservative surgery greatly increases the chances of preserving fertility.

"Certainly in older patients, for whom child bearing is no longer an issue, we tend to remove both ovaries. But in younger patients, we've learned that if one ovary is not involved in the cancer, it's not necessary to remove it," said Ted Trimble, M.D., a gynecologic surgeon at the National Cancer Institute.

The key to this approach is adequate information about how advanced the cancer is. Because the ovaries are so deep inside the body, the treating physician often will not know the extent of the cancer before surgery. The surgeon will sample tissue surrounding the ovaries and send it to the lab. With results in hand, the surgeon has to decide whether removing one ovary is safe.

Discussing the possible outcomes with the patient before the surgery and asking if she plans to have children is vital, says Trimble.

National Cancer Institute (http://cancertrials.nci.nih.gov), April 2000

147

"In many cases, we don't know when we're taking someone to surgery if they'll have cancer at all, or if they'll have cancer in one ovary or both ovaries. So we will work out a game plan with the patient, and tell them that we will try to remove the least amount of tissue possible. But you have to warn patients that there is a chance we might have to remove both ovaries or do a hysterectomy."

A recent study from Memorial Sloan-Kettering Cancer Center found that women with fertility-sparing surgery almost always resumed menstruation. The study looked at medical records for 92 patients who had both ovaries and the uterus removed and 16 patients who had fertility-sparing surgery.

Two of the 16 women (12 percent) had a recurrence in their remaining ovary and subsequently died. But twelve of the other fourteen either resumed normal menstruation or had a successful pregnancy.

In addition, fewer of the women who had fertility-sparing surgery had a cancer recurrence—12 percent compared to 15 percent in the radical surgery group. Survival times between the two groups were almost equal as well.

Another study from the University of Milan, Italy, found similar results. Of 56 women who had fertility-sparing surgery, 9 percent (5 patients) had their cancer return, while 12 percent (5 out of 43) who had the more radical surgery had a recurrence.

Summing up the trend toward fertility-sparing surgery whenever possible, the author of the Sloan-Kettering study, Carol Brown, M.D., said, "This is very reassuring news for young women with early-stage ovarian cancer."

References

"Preserving Fertility in Patients with Epithelial Ovarian Cancer: The Role of Conservative Surgery in Treatment of Early-Stage Disease," by C. Brown et al., presented at the 31st Annual Meeting of the Society of Gynecologic Oncologists, Feb. 2000.

"Conservative Surgery for Stage I Ovarian Carcinoma in Women of Childbearing Age," by G. Zanetta et al., *British Journal of Obstetrics and Gynecology*, Sept. 1997, pp. 1030-35.

Chapter 23

New Treatments in the Pipeline for Ovarian Cancer

The outlook for patients with advanced ovarian cancer brightened in the 1980s with the development of cisplatin and carboplatin and again in the 1990s, when paclitaxel, or Taxol®, emerged from clinical trials. But even with these advances, only a fraction of patients with stage III disease—by far the most common stage at diagnosis—survive five years.

Where the next advance will appear remains, therefore, an urgent question. What new strategy or strategies could be ready for large, randomized, studies? There is no overwhelming consensus on this issue, but in recent journal articles, experts propose several candidates for phase III trials.

Transplantation

Best known and perhaps most controversial of these candidates is high-dose chemotherapy with stem cell transplant. In this rigorous therapy, the transplant is used to restore bone marrow destroyed by the high doses of chemotherapy drugs.

High-dose chemotherapy and transplantation—first with bone marrow and later with stem cells—gained attention and supporters in the late 1980s and early 1990s, when it produced high response rates in early trials. The use of transplants began to grow, both outside of trials and in an ongoing stream of small, phase II studies. Many oncologists and patients became convinced of its benefits.

National Cancer Institute (http://cancertrials.nci.nih.gov), November 2000.

149

"People have very strong feelings about it, they believe in it," said Gisele Sarosy, M.D., an ovarian cancer researcher at the National Cancer Institute.

But skeptics point to problems with transplantation. They note the riskiness of high-dose chemotherapy plus the high cost of patient care and low quality of life during treatment. They also point out that transplantation has not so far been shown to prolong survival in a large, randomized trial.

Such a trial, comparing transplants to the best available standard therapy, is urgently needed, according to Patrick Stiff, M.D., and colleagues of Loyola University, Maywood, Ill. In a report in the Oct. 3, 2000 issue of the *Annals of Internal Medicine*, these longtime transplant researchers suggest a randomized trial in relapsed patients whose tumors are sensitive to the platinum-based drugs (cisplatin and carboplatin) and who have only very small tumors remaining after surgery.

This subgroup appears to have a good chance of benefiting from transplant, they say. That conclusion is based on an analysis of outcomes in 421 patients in the Autologous Blood and Marrow Transplant Registry. The analysis showed that 39 percent of a subset of transplant patients with relapsed, platinum-sensitive disease survived at least two years after diagnosis, results that the authors say "seem superior to those seen with conventional salvage chemotherapy."

One small phase III transplantation trial for ovarian cancer is currently under way in France and should be completed by the end of this year, but there is none in the United States. An NCI-sponsored trial closed recently, according to Edward Trimble, M.D., who coordinates gynecologic cancer trials and heads the surgery section in NCI's Cancer Therapy Evaluation Program. Trimble said that despite vigorous efforts to promote this trial, only 20 patients were enrolled in two and a half years.

"Without compelling data from phase III trials in other solid tumors, such as breast cancer," said Trimble, "I am pessimistic that we could successfully mount another phase III trial evaluating high-dose chemotherapy in women with ovarian cancer."

However, there are several other candidates for phase III trials. In an editorial that accompanies the Transplant Registry analysis, Sarosy and Eddie Reed, M.D., chief of the Medical Ovarian Cancer Section at NCI, propose several less toxic approaches that they consider at least as promising.

New Drug Strategies

One of these approaches, the use of newer drug combinations, has raised hopes because the drugs appear to overcome the platinum-drug resistance that develops in many ovarian cancers after initial treatment. In an article in the June 2000 issue of *Seminars in Oncology*, Trimble reviews the newer drugs—oxaliplatin, epirubicin, liposomal doxorubicin, topotecan, oral etoposide, gemcitabine, and vinorelbine—each of which has produced a response in ovarian cancer patients when used alone. They are now being tested in two-drug and three-drug combinations, said Trimble.

Also promising in early studies, say Sarosy and Reed, is the use of a second, or consolidation, round of standard-dose chemotherapy for patients whose tumors have responded well to the first round. They propose further study of consolidation with a combination of drugs that includes paclitaxel.

Intraperitoneal Therapy

Sarosy and Reed also suggest more phase III trials for intraperitoneal therapy, in which drugs are delivered directly to the abdominal cavity and its lining (peritoneum), the places where most ovarian cancers first spread. Like transplantation, this strategy has been used for some time without being fully studied.

Phase III intraperitoneal trials with various combinations of drugs have taken place, but the results have not shown clear-cut benefits over traditional chemotherapy, Trimble says. Currently, several studies of combination regimens are under way.

The Gynecologic Oncology Group, one of the NCI-sponsored Clinical Trials Cooperative Groups, has recently completed a phase III trial comparing standard intravenous carboplatin and paclitaxel to intravenous paclitaxel and to intraperitoneal cisplatin and paclitaxel. The results will be available in two to three years, Trimble said.

Other Treatments

Other innovative approaches to advanced ovarian cancer are in the pipeline. Trimble mentions several that are promising though not yet ready for phase III trials—therapeutic vaccines, gene therapy, and anti-angiogenic agents, which cut off the blood supply to tumors. To this list, Sarosy and Reed add graft-versus-tumor types of transplantation, in which the transplant may stimulate the patient's own immune system to fight the tumor.

The high number of investigational treatments is welcome in a disease in which current therapy is not curative, Trimble writes. "Based on this multitude of investigational questions and the low cure rates currently achieved, all women with advanced ovarian cancer should be offered participation in clinical trials."

Part Five

Other Gynecologic Cancers and Related Concerns

Chapter 24

Gestational Trophoblastic Tumor

What Is Gestational Trophoblastic Tumor?

Gestational trophoblastic tumor, a rare cancer in women, is a disease in which cancer (malignant) cells grow in the tissues that are formed following conception (the joining of sperm and egg). Gestational trophoblastic tumors start inside the uterus, the hollow, muscular, pear-shaped organ where a baby grows. This type of cancer occurs in women during the years when they are able to have children. There are two types of gestational trophoblastic tumors: hydatidiform mole and choriocarcinoma.

If a patient has a hydatidiform mole (also called a molar pregnancy), the sperm and egg cells have joined without the development of a baby in the uterus. Instead, the tissue that is formed resembles grape-like cysts. Hydatidiform mole does not spread outside of the uterus to other parts of the body.

If a patient has a choriocarcinoma, the tumor may have started from a hydatidiform mole or from tissue that remains in the uterus following an abortion or delivery of a baby. Choriocarcinoma can spread from the uterus to other parts of the body. A very rare type of gestational trophoblastic tumor starts in the uterus where the placenta was attached. This type of cancer is called placental-site trophoblastic disease.

Gestational trophoblastic tumor is not always easy to find. In its early stages, it may look like a normal pregnancy. A doctor should be

CancerNet, National Cancer Institute (www.nci.nih.gov), November 2000.

seen if the there is vaginal bleeding (not menstrual bleeding) and if a woman is pregnant and the baby hasn't moved at the expected time.

If there are symptoms, a doctor may use several tests to see if the patient has a gestational trophoblastic tumor. An internal (pelvic) examination is usually the first of these tests. The doctor will feel for any lumps or strange feeling in the shape or size of the uterus. The doctor may then do an ultrasound, a test that uses sound waves to find tumors. A blood test will also be done to look for high levels of a hormone called beta HCG (beta human chorionic gonadotropin) which is present during normal pregnancy. If a woman is not pregnant and HCG is in the blood, it can be a sign of gestational trophoblastic tumor.

The chance of recovery (prognosis) and choice of treatment depend on the type of gestational trophoblastic tumor, whether it has spread to other places, and the patient's general state of health.

Stages of Gestational Trophoblastic Tumor

Once gestational trophoblastic tumor has been found, more tests will be done to find out if the cancer has spread from inside the uterus to other parts of the body (staging). A doctor needs to know the stage of the disease to plan treatment. The following stages are used for gestational trophoblastic tumor:

Hydatidiform mole: Cancer is found only in the space inside the uterus. If the cancer is found in the muscle of the uterus, it is called an invasive mole (choriocarcinoma destruens).

Placental-site gestational trophoblastic tumor: Cancer is found in the place where the placenta was attached and in the muscle of the uterus.

Nonmetastatic: Cancer cells have grown inside the uterus from tissue remaining following treatment of a hydatidiform mole or following an abortion or delivery of a baby. Cancer has not spread outside the uterus.

Metastatic, good prognosis: Cancer cells have grown inside the uterus from tissue remaining following treatment of a hydatidiform mole or following an abortion or delivery of a baby. The cancer has spread from the uterus to other parts of the body. Metastatic gestational trophoblastic tumors are considered good prognosis or poor prognosis.

Metastatic gestational trophoblastic tumor is considered good prognosis if all of the following are true:

- The last pregnancy was less than 4 months ago.
- The level of beta HCG in the blood is low.
- Cancer has not spread to the liver or brain.
- The patient has not received chemotherapy earlier.

Metastatic, poor prognosis: Cancer cells have grown inside the uterus from tissue remaining following treatment of a hydatidiform mole or following an abortion or delivery of a baby. The cancer has spread from the uterus to other parts of the body. Metastatic gestational trophoblastic tumors are considered good prognosis or poor prognosis.

Metastatic gestational trophoblastic tumor is considered poor prognosis if any the following are true:

- The last pregnancy was more than 4 months ago.
- The level of beta HCG in the blood is high.
- Cancer has spread to the liver or brain.
- The patient received chemotherapy earlier and the cancer did not go away.
- The tumor began after the completion of a normal pregnancy.

Recurrent: Recurrent disease means that the cancer has come back (recurred) after it has been treated. It may come back in the uterus or in another part of the body.

How Gestational Trophoblastic Tumor Is Treated

There are treatments for all patients with gestational trophoblastic tumor. Two kinds of treatment are used: surgery (taking out the cancer) and chemotherapy (using drugs to kill cancer cells). Radiation therapy (using high-energy x-rays to kill cancer cells) may be used in certain cases to treat cancer that has spread to other parts of the body.

Surgery: The doctor may take out the cancer using one of the following operations:

- Dilation and curettage (D & C) with suction evacuation is stretching the opening of the uterus (the cervix) and removing the material inside the uterus with a small vacuum-like device. The walls of the uterus are then scraped gently to remove any material that may remain in the uterus. This is used only for molar pregnancies.

- Hysterectomy is an operation to take out the uterus. The ovaries usually are not removed in the treatment of this disease.

Chemotherapy uses drugs to kill cancer cells. It may be taken by pill or put into the body by a needle in a vein or muscle. It is called a systemic treatment because the drugs enter the bloodstream, travel through the body, and can kill cancer cells outside the uterus. Chemotherapy may be given before or after surgery or alone.

Radiation therapy uses high-energy x-rays to kill cancer cells and shrink tumors. Radiation may come from a machine outside the body (external beam radiation therapy) or from putting materials that produce radiation (radioisotopes) through thin plastic tubes into the area where the cancer cells are found (internal radiation).

Treatment by Stage

Treatment of gestational trophoblastic tumor depends on the stage of the disease, and the patient's age and overall condition.

Standard treatment may be considered because of its effectiveness in patients in past studies, or participation in a clinical trial may be considered. Not all patients are cured with standard therapy and some standard treatments may have more side effects than are desired. For these reasons, clinical trials are designed to find better ways to treat cancer patients and are based on the most up-to-date information. Clinical trials are ongoing in most parts of the country for most stages of gestational trophoblastic tumor. To learn more about clinical trials, call the Cancer Information Service at 1-800-4-CANCER (1-800-422-6237); TTY at 1-800-332-8615.

Hydatidiform mole: Treatment may be one of the following:

- Removal of the mole using dilation and curettage (D & C) and suction evacuation.

- Surgery to remove the uterus (hysterectomy).

Following surgery, the doctor will follow the patient closely with regular blood tests to make sure the level of beta HCG in the blood falls to normal levels. If the blood level of beta HCG increases or does not go down to normal, more tests will be done to see whether the tumor has spread. Treatment will then depend on whether the patient has nonmetastatic disease or metastatic disease (see the treatment sections on metastatic or nonmetastatic disease).

Placental-site gestational trophoblastic tumor: Treatment will probably be surgery to remove the uterus (hysterectomy).

Nonmetastatic gestational trophoblastic tumor: Treatment may be one of the following:

- Chemotherapy.
- Surgery to remove the uterus (hysterectomy) if the patient no longer wishes to have children.

Good prognosis metastatic gestational trophoblastic tumor: Treatment may be one of the following:

- Chemotherapy
- Surgery to remove the uterus (hysterectomy) followed by chemotherapy.
- Chemotherapy followed by hysterectomy if cancer remains following chemotherapy.

Poor prognosis metastatic gestational trophoblastic tumor: Treatment will probably be chemotherapy. Radiation therapy may also be given to places where the cancer has spread, such as the brain.

Recurrent gestational trophoblastic tumor: Treatment will probably be chemotherapy.

Chapter 25

Cancer of the Uterus

Introduction

Cancer of the uterus is the most common cancer of the female reproductive tract. The National Cancer Institute (NCI) has written this information to help women with cancer of the uterus and their families and friends better understand this disease. We hope others will read it as well to learn more about cancer of the uterus.

This chapter discusses symptoms, diagnosis, and treatment. It also has information about resources and sources of support to help women cope with cancer of the uterus.

Our knowledge of cancer of the uterus keeps increasing. For up-to-date information or to order publications, call the National Cancer Institute's Cancer Information Service (CIS). The toll-free number is 1-800-4-CANCER (1-800-422-6237). The number for callers with TTY equipment is 1-800-332-8615.

The CIS staff uses a National Cancer Institute cancer information database called PDQ and other NCI resources to answer callers' questions. Cancer Information Specialists can send callers information from PDQ and other NCI materials about cancer, its treatment, and living with the disease.

The Uterus

The uterus is a hollow, pear-shaped organ. It is located in a woman's lower abdomen between the bladder and the rectum. Attached to either

National Cancer Institute, NIH Pub. No. 98-1562, December 2000.

side of the top of the uterus are the fallopian tubes, which extend from the uterus to the ovaries.

The narrow, lower portion of the uterus is the cervix; the broad, middle part is the corpus; and the dome-shaped upper portion is the fundus. The walls of the uterus are made of two layers of tissue: the inner layer or lining (endometrium) and the outer layer or muscle (myometrium).

In women of childbearing age, the lining of the uterus grows and thickens each month so that it will be ready if pregnancy occurs. If a woman does not become pregnant, the thickened tissue and blood flow out of the body through the vagina; this flow is called menstruation.

What Is Cancer?

Cancer is a group of many different diseases that have some important things in common. They all affect cells, the body's basic unit of life. To understand cancer, it is helpful to know about normal cells and about what happens when cells become cancerous.

The body is made up of many types of cells. Normally, cells grow and divide to produce more cells only when the body needs them. This orderly process helps keep the body healthy. Sometimes cells keep dividing when new cells are not needed. A mass of extra tissue forms, and this mass is called a growth or tumor. Tumors can be benign or malignant.

Benign tumors are not cancer. They can usually be removed and, in most cases, they do not come back. Cells from benign tumors do not spread to other parts of the body. Most important, benign tumors are rarely a threat to life.

Fibroids are common benign tumors of the uterine muscle. These tumors do not develop into cancer. Fibroids are found mainly in women in their forties. Women may have many fibroid tumors at the same time. In most cases, fibroids cause no symptoms and require no treatment, although they should be checked by a doctor. Depending on the size and location of the tumors, however, symptoms sometimes occur. These symptoms may include irregular bleeding, vaginal discharge, and frequent urination. When fibroids cause heavy bleeding or press against nearby organs and cause pain, surgery or other treatment may be recommended. When a woman reaches menopause, fibroids are likely to become smaller, and sometimes disappear.

Endometriosis is another benign condition that affects the uterus. It does not develop into cancer. Endometriosis is seen mostly in women in their thirties and forties, particularly in women who have never been pregnant. It occurs when endometrial tissue begins to grow on the outside of the uterus and on nearby organs. This condition may cause painful menstrual periods, abnormal vaginal bleeding, and sometimes loss of fertility (ability to produce children). Treatment options generally include hormone therapy and surgery.

Endometrial hyperplasia, also a benign condition, is an increase in the number of cells lining the uterus. Although it is not cancer, endometrial hyperplasia is considered a precancerous condition; in some cases, it may develop into cancer. Heavy menstrual periods, bleeding between periods, and bleeding after menopause are common symptoms of hyperplasia. The treatment is usually hysterectomy or hormone therapy with progesterone, depending on the extent of the condition and whether a woman wants to have children.

Malignant tumors are cancer. Cancer cells can invade and damage tissues and organs near the tumor. Also, cancer cells can break away from a malignant tumor and enter the bloodstream or lymphatic system. This is how cancer spreads from the original (primary) tumor to form new tumors in other parts of the body. The spread of cancer is called metastasis.

Most cancers are named for the part of the body in which they begin. The most common type of cancer of the uterus begins in the endometrium. This type of cancer is called endometrial or uterine cancer. In this chapter, we will use the term uterine cancer to refer to cancer that begins in the endometrium. A different type of cancer, uterine sarcoma, develops in the uterine muscle. Cancer that begins in the cervix is also a different type of cancer. This text does not deal with uterine sarcoma or cancer of the cervix. The Cancer Information Service can provide information about uterine sarcoma and cancer of the cervix.

As uterine cancer grows, it may invade nearby organs. Uterine cancer cells also may break away from the tumor and spread to other parts of the body, such as the lungs, liver, and bones. When cancer spreads to another part of the body, the new cancer has the same kind of abnormal cells and the same name as the original (primary) cancer. For example, if uterine cancer spreads to the lungs, the cancer cells in the new tumor are uterine cancer cells. Cancer that has spread from the uterus to other parts of the body is called metastatic uterine cancer; it is not lung cancer.

Symptoms

Abnormal vaginal bleeding, especially after menopause, is the most common symptom of uterine cancer. Bleeding may start as a watery,

163

blood-streaked flow that gradually contains more blood. Although uterine cancer usually occurs after menopause, it sometimes occurs around the time that menopause begins. Abnormal bleeding should not be considered simply part of menopause; it should always be checked by a doctor.

A woman should see a doctor if she has any of the following symptoms:

- Unusual vaginal bleeding or discharge
- Difficult or painful urination
- Pain during intercourse
- Pain in the pelvic area

These symptoms can be caused by cancer or other less serious conditions. Most often, they are not cancer, but only a doctor can tell for sure.

Diagnosis

If a woman has symptoms, her doctor asks about her medical history and conducts a physical exam. In addition to checking general signs of health, the doctor usually performs blood and urine tests and one or more of the following procedures:

- The doctor performs a pelvic exam, checking the vagina, uterus, ovaries, bladder, and rectum. The doctor feels these organs for any lumps or changes in their shape or size. An instrument called a speculum is used to widen the vagina so the doctor can see the upper portion of the vagina and the cervix.

- The Pap test is often performed during a pelvic exam. The doctor uses a wooden scraper (spatula) or small brush to collect a sample of cells from the cervix and upper vagina. The cells are then sent to a medical laboratory to be checked for abnormal changes. Because uterine cancer begins inside the uterus, it may not show up on a Pap test, which examines cells from the cervix.

- A biopsy is necessary to help the doctor make a diagnosis. A biopsy can usually be done in the doctor's office. In a biopsy, the doctor removes a sample of tissue from the uterine lining. In some cases, a woman may require a dilation and curettage

(D&C), which is usually same-day surgery done in a hospital with anesthesia. During a D&C, the opening of the cervix is widened and the doctor scrapes tissue from the lining of the uterus. A pathologist examines the tissue to check for cancer cells, hyperplasia, or other conditions. After a D&C, women may have cramps and vaginal bleeding during healing.

A woman who needs a biopsy may want to ask the doctor some of the following questions:

- What type of biopsy will I have? Why?
- How long will it take? Will I be awake? Will it hurt?
- How soon will I know the results?
- If I do have cancer, who will talk with me about treatment? When?

Staging

Once uterine cancer is diagnosed, the doctor needs to know the stage, or extent, of the disease in order to plan the best treatment. Staging procedures help the doctor find out whether the cancer has spread and, if so, what parts of the body are affected. For most women, staging procedures include blood and urine tests and chest x-rays. Doctors may also order a CT scan, MRI, sigmoidoscopy, colonoscopy, ultrasonography, or other x-rays.

Treatment

After diagnosis and initial evaluation, the doctor considers treatment options that fit each woman's needs and discusses these options with her. The choice of treatment depends on the size of the tumor, the stage of the disease, whether female hormones affect tumor growth, and tumor grade. (The tumor grade tells how closely the cancer resembles normal cells and suggests how fast the cancer is likely to grow. Low-grade cancers are likely to grow and spread more slowly than high-grade cancers.) Other factors, including the woman's age and general health, are also considered when planning treatment. Women with uterine cancer may be treated by a team of specialists that may include a gynecologist, gynecologic oncologist (a doctor who specializes in treating cancer of the female reproductive tract), and a radiation oncologist.

Getting a Second Opinion

Before starting treatment, a woman may want a second specialist to confirm the diagnosis and review her treatment options. It may take a week or two to arrange for another opinion, but a short delay will not reduce the chance that treatment will be successful. Some insurance companies require a second opinion; many others cover a second opinion if the patient requests it. There are a number of ways to find a doctor who can give a second opinion:

- The woman's doctor may be able to suggest specialists to consult.

- The Cancer Information Service, at 1-800-4-CANCER, can tell callers about treatment facilities, including cancer centers and other programs supported by the National Cancer Institute.

- A woman can get the names of doctors from her local medical society, a nearby hospital, or a medical school.

- The *Official ABMS Directory of Board Certified Medical Specialists* lists doctors' names along with their specialty and their background. This resource is in most public libraries.

Preparing for Treatment

Many people with cancer want to learn all they can about their disease and their treatment choices so they can take an active part in decisions about their medical care. When a woman learns she has uterine cancer, shock and stress are natural reactions. These feelings may make it difficult for her to think of everything she may want to ask the doctor. Often, it helps to make a list of questions. To help remember what the doctor says, a woman may take notes or ask whether she may use a tape recorder. Some patients find it helpful to have a family member or friend with them when talking to the doctor to participate in the discussion, take notes, or just listen.

These are some questions a woman may want to ask the doctor:

- What kind of uterine cancer do I have?

- Is there any evidence the cancer has spread? What is the stage of the disease?

- What is the tumor grade?

- What are my treatment choices? Which do you recommend for me? Why?

- What are the expected benefits of each kind of treatment?
- What are the risks and possible side effects of each treatment?
- What is the treatment likely to cost?
- How will treatment affect my normal activities?
- How often should I have a checkup?
- Would a treatment study be appropriate for me?

Women do not need to ask all their questions or understand all the answers at once. They will have many chances to ask the doctor to explain things that are not clear and to ask for more information.

Methods of Treatment

Most women with uterine cancer are treated with surgery. Some have radiation therapy. A smaller number of women may be treated with hormone therapy or chemotherapy. Another treatment option for women with uterine cancer is to take part in treatment studies (clinical trials). Such studies are designed to improve cancer treatment. (See Treatment Studies for more information.) The following sections describe types of uterine cancer treatment.

Surgery to remove the uterus (hysterectomy) and the fallopian tubes and ovaries (bilateral salpingo-oophorectomy) is the treatment recommended for most women with uterine cancer. Lymph nodes near the tumor may also be removed during surgery to see if they contain cancer. If cancer cells have reached the lymph nodes, it may mean that the disease has spread to other parts of the body. If cancer cells have not spread beyond the endometrium, the disease can usually be cured with surgery alone.

These are some questions a woman may want to ask the doctor before having surgery:

- What kind of operation will it be?
- How will I feel after the operation?
- If I have pain, how will you help?
- How long will I have to stay in the hospital?
- Will I have any long-term effects because of this operation?
- When will I be able to resume my normal activities?
- Will follow-up visits be necessary?

In **radiation therapy** (also called radiotherapy), high-energy rays are used to kill cancer cells. The rays may come from a small container of radioactive material, called an implant, which is placed directly into or near the tumor site (internal radiation). It may also come from a large machine outside the body (external radiation). Some patients with uterine cancer need both internal and external radiation therapy. Like surgery, radiation therapy is a local therapy. It affects cancer cells only in the treated area. Radiation therapy may be used in addition to surgery to treat women with certain stages of uterine cancer. Radiation may be used before surgery to shrink the tumor or after surgery to destroy any cancer cells that remain in the area. Also, for a small number of women who cannot have surgery, radiation treatment is sometimes used instead.

In internal radiation therapy, tiny tubes containing a radioactive substance are inserted through the vagina and left in place for a few days. The patient is hospitalized during this treatment. Patients may not be able to have visitors or may have visitors only for a short period of time while the implant is in place. Once the implant is removed, there is no radioactivity in the body. External radiation therapy is usually given on an outpatient basis in a hospital or clinic 5 days a week for several weeks. This schedule helps protect healthy cells and tissue by spreading out the total dose of radiation.

These are some questions a woman may want to ask the doctor before having radiation therapy:

- What is the goal of treatment?
- How will the radiation be given?
- When will the treatments begin? When will they end?
- How will I feel during therapy? Are there side effects?
- What can I do to take care of myself during therapy?
- How will we know if the radiation therapy is working?
- Will I be able to continue my normal activities during treatment?

Hormone therapy is the use of drugs, such as progesterone, that prevent cancer cells from getting or using the hormones they may need to grow. Hormone treatment is a systemic therapy. The drugs, which are usually taken by mouth, enter the bloodstream, travel through the body, and control cancer cells outside the uterus. Women who are unable to have surgery are sometimes treated with hormone therapy.

Also, this form of treatment is often recommended for women who have metastatic or recurrent endometrial cancer.

These are some questions a woman may want to ask the doctor before having hormone therapy:

- Why do I need this treatment?
- What hormones will I be taking? What will they do?
- Will I have side effects? What can I do about them?
- How long will I be on this treatment?

Chemotherapy is the use of drugs to kill cancer cells. Anticancer drugs may be taken by mouth or given by injection into a blood vessel or a muscle. Like hormone therapy, chemotherapy is a systemic therapy; it can kill cancer cells throughout the body. Chemotherapy is being evaluated in treatment studies for patients with uterine cancer that has spread.

These are some questions a woman may want to ask the doctor before starting chemotherapy:

- What is the goal of this treatment?
- What drugs will I be taking?
- Will the drugs cause side effects? What can I do about them?
- How long will I need to take this treatment?
- How will we know if the drugs are working?

Treatment Studies

Doctors conduct treatment studies to learn about the effectiveness and side effects of new treatments. In some studies, all patients receive the new treatment. In other studies, doctors compare different therapies by giving the new treatment to one group of patients and the standard therapy to another group. Treatment studies are also designed to compare one standard treatment with another.

Women who take part in these studies have the first chance to benefit from treatments that have shown promise in earlier research. They also make an important contribution to medical science.

Doctors are studying new ways of giving radiation therapy and chemotherapy, new drugs and drug combinations, biological therapies, and new ways of combining various types of treatment. Some studies are designed to find ways to reduce the side effects of treatment and to improve the quality of women's lives.

Women who are interested in taking part in a study should talk with their doctor. They may want to read the National Cancer Institute booklet *Taking Part in Clinical Trials: What Cancer Patients Need to Know*, which explains the possible benefits and risks of treatment studies.

Another way to learn about treatment studies is through PDQ, a cancer information database developed by the National Cancer Institute. PDQ contains information about cancer treatment and about treatment studies in progress throughout the country. The Cancer Information Service can provide PDQ information to patients and the public.

Side Effects of Cancer Treatment

In treating cancer, it is hard to limit the effects of treatment so that only cancer cells are removed or destroyed. Because treatment also damages healthy cells and tissues, it often causes side effects.

The side effects of cancer treatment depend on a variety of factors, including the type and extent of the treatment. Side effects may not be the same for each person, and they may even change from one treatment to the next. Doctors and nurses can explain possible side effects, and they can help relieve symptoms that may occur during and after treatment.

Surgery

After a hysterectomy, women usually have some pain and general fatigue. In some cases, patients may have nausea and vomiting following surgery, and some women may have problems returning to normal bladder and bowel function. The effects of anesthesia and discomfort may also temporarily limit physical activity. Diet is usually restricted to liquids at first and gradually increases to regular meals. The length of the hospital stay may vary from several days to a week.

Women who have had a hysterectomy no longer have menstrual periods. When the ovaries are removed, menopause occurs immediately. Hot flashes and other symptoms of menopause caused by surgery may be more severe than those caused by natural menopause. In the general population, estrogen replacement therapy (ERT) is often prescribed to relieve these problems. However, ERT is not commonly used for women who have had endometrial cancer. Because estrogen has been linked to the development of uterine cancer (see Possible Causes and Prevention), many doctors are concerned that

ERT may cause uterine cancer to recur. Other doctors point out that there is no scientific evidence that ERT increases the risk of recurrence. A large research study is being conducted to determine whether women who have had early stage endometrial cancer can safely take estrogen.

After surgery, normal activities usually can be resumed in 4 to 8 weeks. Sexual desire and sexual intercourse are not usually affected by hysterectomy. However, some women may experience feelings of loss that may make intimacy difficult. Counseling or support for both the patient and her partner may be helpful.

Radiation Therapy

Radiation therapy destroys the ability of cells to grow and divide. Both normal and diseased cells are affected, but most normal cells are able to recover. With radiation therapy, the side effects depend largely on the treatment dose and the part of the body that is treated. During radiation therapy, people are likely to become very tired, especially in the later weeks of treatment. Resting is important, but doctors usually advise patients to try to stay as active as they can.

Patients receiving radiation for uterine cancer commonly have side effects that include dry, reddened skin and hair loss in the treated area, loss of appetite, and fatigue. Radiation therapy also may cause a decrease in the number of white blood cells that help protect the body against infection. Treatment may also cause diarrhea or frequent and uncomfortable urination. Some women have dryness, itching, tightening, and burning in the vagina. Women may be advised not to have intercourse during treatment; however, most can resume sexual activity within a few weeks after treatment ends. Women may be taught how to use a dilator, as well as a water-soluble lubricant to help minimize these problems.

The National Cancer Institute booklet *Radiation Therapy and You* has helpful information about radiation therapy and managing its side effects.

Hormone Therapy

Hormone therapy can cause a number of side effects. Women taking progesterone may experience fatigue and changes in appetite and weight, and they may retain fluid. Premenopausal women may have changes in their menstrual periods. Women may wish to discuss the side effects of hormone therapy with their doctor.

Chemotherapy

The side effects of chemotherapy depend mainly on the drugs and the doses received. In addition, as with other types of treatment, side effects vary for each individual. Generally, anticancer drugs affect cells that divide rapidly. These include blood cells, which fight infection, help the blood to clot, or carry oxygen to all parts of the body. When blood cells are affected by anticancer drugs, patients are more likely to get infections, may bruise or bleed easily, and may have less energy. Cells in hair roots and cells that line the digestive tract also divide rapidly. As a result, patients may lose their hair and may have other side effects, such as poor appetite, nausea and vomiting, or mouth sores. Usually, these side effects go away gradually during the recovery periods between treatments or after treatment is over.

The National Cancer Institute booklet *Chemotherapy and You* has helpful information about chemotherapy and coping with its side effects.

Nutrition for Cancer Patients

Good nutrition is important. Patients who eat well often feel better and have more energy. Eating well during cancer treatment means getting enough calories and protein to help prevent weight loss, regain strength, and rebuild normal tissues.

Some women find it hard to eat well during treatment. They may lose their appetite. In addition to loss of appetite, common side effects of treatment, such as nausea and vomiting, can make eating difficult. Also, women may not feel like eating when they are uncomfortable or tired.

Doctors, nurses, and dietitians can offer advice for healthy eating during cancer treatment. Patients and their families also may want to read the National Cancer Institute booklet *Eating Hints for Cancer Patients*, which contains many useful suggestions.

Follow-up Care

It is important for women who have had uterine cancer to have regular follow-up examinations after their treatment is over, in case the cancer comes back. Follow-up care is a part of the overall treatment plan, and women with cancer should not hesitate to discuss it with the doctor. Regular follow-up care ensures that any changes in health are discussed, and any recurrent cancer can be treated as soon as possible. Between follow-up appointments, women who have had uterine cancer should report any health problems as soon as they appear.

Checkups may include a physical exam, a pelvic exam, a chest x-ray, and laboratory tests.

Recovery and Outlook

People with cancer and their families are naturally concerned about their recovery from cancer. Sometimes people use statistics to try to figure out their chances of being cured. It is important to remember, however, that statistics are averages based on large numbers of patients. They cannot be used to predict what will happen to a particular patient because no two patients are alike; treatments and responses vary greatly. The patient's doctor is in the best position to discuss the issue of prognosis, or the probable outcome or course of the disease.

When doctors discuss a patient's prognosis, they may talk about surviving cancer rather than a cure. Although many patients with uterine cancer are actually cured, the disease can return. It is important to discuss the possibility of recurrence with the doctor.

Support for Cancer Patients

Living with a serious disease is not easy. People with cancer and those who care about them face many problems and challenges. Coping with these problems is often easier when people have helpful information and support services. Several useful National Cancer Institute booklets, including *Taking Time*, are available from the Cancer Information Service.

Friends and relatives can be very supportive. Also, it helps many patients to discuss their concerns with others who have cancer. Cancer patients often get together in support groups, where they can share what they have learned about coping with cancer and the effects of treatment. It is important to keep in mind, however, that each person is different. Treatments and ways of dealing with cancer that work for one person may not be right for another—even if they both have the same kind of cancer. It is always a good idea to discuss the advice of friends and family members with the doctor.

Cancer patients may worry about holding their jobs, caring for their families, keeping up with daily activities, or starting new relationships. Concerns about tests, treatments, hospital stays, and medical bills are common. Doctors, nurses, social workers, and other members of the health care team can answer questions about treatment, working, or other activities. They can also discuss outlook (prognosis) and the activity level people may be able to manage. Meeting with a social worker, counselor, or member of the clergy can be helpful to people who want to talk about their feelings or discuss their concerns.

It is natural for a woman to be worried about the effects of uterine cancer and its treatment on her sexuality. She may want to talk with the doctor about possible side effects and whether these side effects are likely to be temporary or permanent. Whatever the outlook, it may be helpful for women and their partners to talk about their feelings and help one another find ways to share intimacy during and after treatment.

Information about programs and local resources for women with uterine cancer and their families is available through the Cancer Information Service.

The Promise of Cancer Research

Over the last several decades, researchers have been unraveling the mysteries of cancer. As they learn more and more about cancer, they have begun to use this new knowledge to find better ways of preventing, detecting, and treating this disease. Opportunities exist as never before to build on this foundation and achieve new successes against cancer. Although there is much work to be done, there are many reasons to be optimistic about the future. Each achievement in laboratories and clinics brings researchers closer to the eventual control of cancer.

Possible Causes and Prevention

Scientists at hospitals and medical centers all across the country are studying uterine cancer. They are trying to learn more about what causes the disease and how to prevent it.

At this time, we do not know exactly what causes uterine cancer, and doctors can seldom explain why one woman gets this disease and another does not. It is clear, however, that uterine cancer is not caused by an injury, and is not contagious; no one can "catch" uterine cancer from another person.

By studying patterns of cancer in the population, researchers have found certain factors that are more common in women who get uterine cancer than in those who don't get this disease. It is important to know that most women with these risk factors do not get cancer, and many who do get uterine cancer have none of these factors.

The following are some of the known risk factors for this disease:

- **Age.** Cancer of the uterus is most common in women over age 50.

- **Endometrial hyperplasia.** Women who have endometrial hyperplasia have a higher risk of developing uterine cancer. This condition and its treatment are described in the What Is Cancer? section.

- **Estrogen replacement therapy.** Women who use estrogen replacement therapy to control symptoms associated with menopause, to prevent osteoporosis (thinning of the bones), or to reduce the risk of heart disease or stroke may have an increased risk of uterine cancer. Long-term treatment and large doses seem to increase this risk. Using a combination of estrogen and progesterone decreases the risk linked to the use of estrogen alone. The progesterone protects the endometrium from the cancer-causing effect of estrogen. A woman considering hormone replacement therapy should discuss the benefits and risks with her doctor. Regular follow-up visits with a health professional while taking estrogen replacement therapy may improve the chances of detecting and treating uterine cancer in the early stages should it develop.

- **Overweight.** Scientists believe that too much estrogen may be the reason why overweight women are more than twice as likely to develop uterine cancer as women of normal weight. Because fat converts certain hormones into a form of estrogen, women with excess fat produce higher levels of estrogen.

- **Diabetes and high blood pressure.** Some studies suggest that diabetes and high blood pressure increase the risk of uterine cancer. Because these conditions often occur in overweight people, researchers cannot be certain whether the conditions themselves or the relationship between body fat and estrogen levels increases uterine cancer risk.

- **Other cancers.** Women with a history of colon cancer, rectal cancer, or breast cancer have a slightly higher risk of developing uterine cancer than do most other women. Women who have had uterine cancer also have an increased risk of developing certain other cancers.

- **Tamoxifen.** An increased risk of developing uterine cancer has been found in women taking the drug tamoxifen for the treatment of breast cancer. This risk may be related to the estrogen-like effect of this drug on the uterus. Women taking tamoxifen should be closely monitored by the doctor for possible signs or symptoms of uterine cancer. Doctors emphasize that the benefits of tamoxifen as a treatment for breast cancer are firmly established and far outweigh the potential risk of other cancers.

- **Race.** White women have a greater chance of developing uterine cancer than black women.

Other risk factors for uterine cancer are also related to estrogen, including having few or no children or entering menopause late in life. Some studies of women who have used oral contraceptives that combine estrogen and progesterone show that these women have a lower than average risk of uterine cancer.

Women with known risk factors and those who are concerned about uterine cancer should talk with their doctor about the disease, the symptoms to watch for, and an appropriate schedule for checkups. The doctor's advice will be based on the woman's age, medical history, and other factors.

Chapter 26

Uterine Sarcoma

What is Sarcoma of the Uterus?

Sarcoma of the uterus, a very rare kind of cancer in women, is a disease in which cancer (malignant) cells start growing in the muscles or other supporting tissues of the uterus. The uterus is the hollow, pear-shaped organ where a baby grows. Sarcoma of the uterus is different from cancer of the endometrium, a disease in which cancer cells start growing in the lining of the uterus.

Women who have received therapy with high-dose x-rays (external beam radiation therapy) to their pelvis are at a higher risk to develop sarcoma of the uterus. These x-rays are sometimes given to women to stop bleeding from the uterus.

A doctor should be seen if there is bleeding after menopause (the time when a woman no longer has menstrual periods) or bleeding that is not part of menstrual periods. Sarcoma of the uterus usually begins after menopause.

If there are signs of cancer, a doctor will do certain tests to check for cancer, usually beginning with an internal (pelvic) examination. During the examination, the doctor will feel for any lumps or changes in the shapes of the pelvic organs. The doctor may then do a Pap test, using a piece of cotton, a small wooden stick, or brush to gently scrape the outside of the cervix (the opening of the uterus) and the vagina to pick up cells. Because sarcoma of the uterus begins inside, this cancer will not usually show up on the Pap test. The doctor may also

National Cancer Institute, Uterine Sarcoma (PDQ®), November 2000.

do a dilation and curettage (D & C) by stretching the cervix and inserting a small, spoon-shaped instrument into the uterus to remove pieces of the lining of the uterus. This tissue is then checked under a microscope for cancer cells.

The prognosis (chance of recovery) and choice of treatment depend on the stage of the sarcoma (whether it is just in the uterus or has spread to other places), how fast the tumor cells are growing, and the patient's general state of health.

Stages of Sarcoma of the Uterus

Once sarcoma of the uterus has been found, more tests will be done to find out if the cancer has spread from the uterus to other parts of the body (staging). A doctor needs to know the stage of the disease to plan treatment. The following stages are used for sarcoma of the uterus:

Stage I: Cancer is found only in the main part of the uterus (it is not found in the cervix).

Stage II: Cancer cells have spread to the cervix.

Stage III: Cancer cells have spread outside the uterus but have not spread outside the pelvis.

Stage IV: Cancer cells have spread beyond the pelvis, to other body parts, or into the lining of the bladder (the sac that holds urine) or rectum.

Recurrent: Recurrent disease means that the cancer has come back (recurred) after it has been treated.

How Sarcoma of the Uterus is Treated

There are treatments for all patients with sarcoma of the uterus. Four kinds of treatment are used:

- surgery (taking out the cancer in an operation)
- radiation therapy (using high-dose x-rays or other high-energy rays to kill cancer cells and shrink tumors)
- chemotherapy (using drugs to kill cancer cells)
- hormone therapy (using female hormones to kill cancer cells)

Surgery is the most common treatment of sarcoma of the uterus. A doctor may take out the cancer in an operation to remove the uterus, fallopian tubes and the ovaries, along with some lymph nodes in the pelvis and around the aorta (the main vessel in which blood passes away from the heart). The operation is called a total abdominal hysterectomy, bilateral salpingo-oophorectomy, and lymphadenectomy. (The lymph nodes are small bean-shaped structures that are found throughout the body. They produce and store infection-fighting cells, but may contain cancer cells.)

Radiation therapy uses x-rays or other high-energy rays to kill cancer cells and shrink tumors. Radiation therapy for sarcoma of the uterus usually comes from a machine outside the body (external radiation). Radiation may be used alone or in addition to surgery.

Chemotherapy uses drugs to kill cancer cells. Chemotherapy may be taken by pill, or it may be put into the body by a needle in a vein or a muscle. Chemotherapy is called a systemic treatment because the drugs enter the bloodstream, travel through the body, and can kill cancer cells outside the uterus.

Hormone therapy uses female hormones, usually taken by pill, to kill cancer cells.

Treatment by Stage

Treatment of sarcoma of the uterus depends on the stage and cell type of the disease, and the patient's age and overall condition.

Standard treatment may be considered because of its effectiveness in patients in past studies, or participation in a clinical trial may be considered. Not all patients are cured with standard therapy and some standard treatments may have more side effects than are desired. For these reasons, clinical trials are designed to find better ways to treat cancer patients and are based on the most up-to-date information. Clinical trials are ongoing in most parts of the country for most stages of sarcoma of the uterus. To learn more about clinical trials, call the Cancer Information Service at 1-800-4-CANCER (1-800-422-6237); TTY at 1-800-332-8615.

Stage I Uterine Sarcoma: Treatment may be one of the following:

- Surgery to remove the uterus, fallopian tubes and the ovaries, and some of the lymph nodes in the pelvis and abdomen (total abdominal hysterectomy, bilateral salpingo-oophorectomy, and lymph node dissection).

- Total abdominal hysterectomy, bilateral salpingo-oophorectomy, and lymph node dissection, followed by radiation therapy to the pelvis.
- Surgery followed by chemotherapy.
- Surgery followed by radiation therapy.

Stage II Uterine Sarcoma: Treatment may be one of the following:

- Surgery to remove the uterus, fallopian tubes and the ovaries, and some of the lymph nodes in the pelvis and abdomen (total abdominal hysterectomy, bilateral salpingo-oophorectomy, and lymph node dissection).
- Total abdominal hysterectomy, bilateral salpingo-oophorectomy, and lymph node dissection, followed by radiation therapy to the pelvis.
- Surgery followed by chemotherapy.
- Surgery followed by radiation therapy.

Stage III Uterine Sarcoma: Treatment may be one of the following:

- Surgery to remove the uterus, fallopian tubes and the ovaries, and some of the lymph nodes in the pelvis and abdomen (total abdominal hysterectomy bilateral salpingo-oophorectomy, and lymph node dissection). Doctors will also try to remove as much of the cancer that has spread to nearby tissues as possible.
- Total abdominal hysterectomy, bilateral salpingo-oophorectomy, and lymph node dissection, followed by radiation therapy to the pelvis.
- Surgery followed by chemotherapy.

Stage IV Uterine Sarcoma: Treatment will usually be a clinical trial using chemotherapy.

Recurrent Uterine Sarcoma: If the cancer has come back (recurred), treatment may be one of the following:

- Clinical trials of chemotherapy or hormone therapy.
- External radiation therapy to relieve symptoms such as pain, nausea, or abnormal bowel functions.

Chapter 27

Vaginal Cancer

What is Cancer of the Vagina?

Cancer of the vagina, a rare kind of cancer in women, is a disease in which cancer (malignant) cells are found in the tissues of the vagina. The vagina is the passageway through which fluid passes out of the body during menstrual periods and through which a woman has babies. It is also called the "birth canal." The vagina connects the cervix (the opening of the womb or uterus) and the vulva (the folds of skin around the opening to the vagina).

There are two types of cancer of the vagina: squamous cell cancer (squamous carcinoma) and adenocarcinoma. Squamous carcinoma is usually found in women between the ages of 60 and 80. Adenocarcinoma is more often found in women between the ages of 12 and 30.

Young women whose mothers took DES (diethylstilbestrol) are at risk for getting tumors in their vaginas. Some of them get a rare form of cancer called clear cell adenocarcinoma. The drug DES was given to pregnant women between 1945 and 1970 to keep them from losing their babies (miscarriage).

A doctor should be seen if there are any of the following: bleeding or discharge not related to menstrual periods, difficult or painful urination, and pain during intercourse or in the pelvic area. Also, there is still a chance of developing vaginal cancer in women who have had a hysterectomy.

National Cancer Institute, Vaginal Cancer (PDQ®), November 2000.

A doctor may use several tests to see if there is cancer. The doctor will usually begin by giving the patient an internal (pelvic) examination. The doctor will feel for lumps and will then do a Pap smear. Using a piece of cotton, a brush, or a small wooden stick, the doctor will gently scrape the outside of the cervix and vagina in order to pick up cells. Some pressure may be felt, but usually with no pain.

If cells that are not normal are found, the doctor will need to cut a small sample of tissue (called a biopsy) out of the vagina and look at it under a microscope to see if there are any cancer cells. The doctor should look not only at the vagina, but also at the other organs in the pelvis to see where the cancer started and where it may have spread. The doctor may take an x-ray of the chest to make sure the cancer has not spread to the lungs.

The chance of recovery (prognosis) and choice of treatment depend on the stage of the cancer (whether it is just in the vagina or has spread to other places) and the patient's general state of health.

Stages of Cancer of the Vagina

Once cancer of the vagina has been found (diagnosed), more tests will be done to find out if the cancer has spread from the vagina to other parts of the body (staging). A doctor needs to know the stage of the disease to plan treatment. The following stages are used for cancer of the vagina:

Stage 0 or carcinoma *in situ*: Stage 0 cancer of the vagina is a very early cancer. The cancer is found inside the vagina only and is in only a few layers of cells.

Stage I: Cancer is found in the vagina, but has not spread outside of it.

Stage II: Cancer has spread to the tissues just outside the vagina, but has not gone to the bones of the pelvis.

Stage III: Cancer has spread to the bones of the pelvis. Cancer cells may also have spread to other organs and the lymph nodes in the pelvis. (Lymph nodes are small bean-shaped structures that are found throughout the body. They produce and store cells that fight infection.)

Stage IVA: Cancer has spread into the bladder or rectum.

Stage IVB: Cancer has spread to other parts of the body, such as the lungs.

Recurrent: Recurrent disease means that the cancer has come back (recurred) after it has been treated. It may come back in the vagina or in another place.

How Cancer of the Vagina is Treated

Treatments are available for all patients with cancer of the vagina. There are three kinds of treatment:

- surgery (taking out the cancer in an operation)

- radiation therapy (using high-dose x-rays or other high-energy rays to kill cancer cells and shrink tumors)

- chemotherapy (using drugs to kill cancer cells)

Surgery is the most common treatment of all stages of cancer of the vagina. A doctor may take out the cancer using one of the following:

- Laser surgery uses a narrow beam of light to kill cancer cells and is useful for stage 0 cancer.

- Wide local excision takes out the cancer and some of the tissue around it. A patient may need to have skin taken from another part of the body (grafted) to repair the vagina after the cancer has been taken out.

- An operation in which the vagina is removed (vaginectomy) is sometimes done. When the cancer has spread outside the vagina, vaginectomy may be combined with surgery to take out the uterus, ovaries, and fallopian tubes (radical hysterectomy). During these operations, lymph nodes in the pelvis may also be removed (lymph node dissection).

- If the cancer has spread outside the vagina and the other female organs, the doctor may take out the lower colon, rectum, or bladder (depending on where the cancer has spread) along with the cervix, uterus, and vagina (exenteration).

- A patient may need skin grafts and plastic surgery to make an artificial vagina after these operations.

Radiation therapy uses x-rays or other high-energy rays to kill cancer cells and shrink tumors. Radiation may come from a machine outside the body (external radiation) or from putting materials that produce radiation (radioisotopes) through thin plastic tubes into the area where the cancer cells are found (internal radiation). Radiation may be used alone or after surgery.

Chemotherapy uses drugs to kill cancer cells. Chemotherapy may be taken by pill, or it may be put into the body by a needle in a vein. Chemotherapy is called a systemic treatment because the drugs enter the bloodstream, travel through the body, and can kill cancer cells outside the vagina. In treating vaginal cancer, chemotherapy may also be put directly into the vagina itself, which is called intravaginal chemotherapy.

Treatment by Stage

Treatment of cancer of the vagina depends on the stage of the disease, the type of disease, and the patient's age and overall condition.

Standard treatment may be considered because of its effectiveness in patients in past studies, or participation in a clinical trial may be considered. Not all patients are cured with standard therapy and some standard treatments may have more side effects than are desired. For these reasons, clinical trials are designed to find better ways to treat cancer patients and are based on the most up-to-date information. Clinical trials are ongoing in most parts of the country for most stages of cancer of the vagina. To learn more about clinical trials, call the Cancer Information Service at 1-800-4-CANCER (1-800-422-6237); TTY at 1-800-332-8615.

Stage 0 Vaginal Cancer: Treatment may be one of the following:

- Surgery to remove all or part of the vagina (vaginectomy). This may be followed by skin grafting to repair damage done to the vagina.

- Internal radiation therapy.

- Laser surgery.

- Intravaginal chemotherapy.

Stage I Vaginal Cancer: Treatment of stage I cancer of the vagina depends on whether a patient has squamous cell cancer or adenocarcinoma.

If squamous cancer is found, treatment may be one of the following:

- Internal radiation therapy with or without external beam radiation therapy.

- Wide local excision. This may be followed by the rebuilding of the vagina. Radiation therapy following surgery may also be performed in some cases.

- Surgery to remove the vagina with or without lymph nodes in the pelvic area (vaginectomy and lymph node dissection).

If adenocarcinoma is found, treatment may be one of the following:

- Surgery to remove the vagina (vaginectomy) and the uterus, ovaries, and fallopian tubes (hysterectomy). The lymph nodes in the pelvis are also removed (lymph node dissection). This may be followed by the rebuilding of the vagina. Radiation therapy following surgery may also be performed in some cases.

- Internal radiation therapy with or without external beam radiation therapy.

- In selected patients, wide local excision and removal of some of the lymph nodes in the pelvis followed by internal radiation.

Stage II Vaginal Cancer: Treatment of stage II cancer of the vagina is the same whether a patient has squamous cell cancer or adenocarcinoma.

Treatment may be one of the following:

- Combined internal and external radiation therapy.

- Surgery, which may be followed by radiation therapy.

Stage III Vaginal Cancer: Treatment of stage III cancer of the vagina is the same whether a patient has squamous cell cancer or adenocarcinoma.

Treatment may be one of the following:

- Combined internal and external radiation therapy.

- Surgery may sometimes be combined with radiation therapy.

Stage IVA Vaginal Cancer: Treatment of stage IVA cancer of the vagina is the same whether a patient has squamous cell cancer or adenocarcinoma.

Treatment may be one of the following:

- Combined internal and external radiation therapy.

- Surgery may sometimes be combined with radiation therapy.

Stage IVB Vaginal Cancer: If stage IVB cancer of the vagina is found, treatment may be radiation to relieve symptoms such as pain, nausea, vomiting, or abnormal bowel function. Chemotherapy may also be performed. A patient may also choose to participate in a clinical trial.

Recurrent Vaginal Cancer: If the cancer has come back (recurred) and spread past the female organs, a doctor may take out the cervix, uterus, lower colon, rectum, or bladder (exenteration), depending on where the cancer has spread. The doctor may give the patient radiation therapy or chemotherapy. A patient may also choose to participate in a clinical trial of chemotherapy or radiation therapy.

Chapter 28

Vulvar Cancer

What is Cancer of the Vulva?

Cancer of the vulva, a rare kind of cancer in women, is a disease in which cancer (malignant) cells are found in the vulva. The vulva is the outer part of a woman's vagina. The vagina is the passage between the uterus (the hollow, pear-shaped organ where a baby grows) and the outside of the body. It is also called the birth canal.

Most women with cancer of the vulva are over age 50. However, it is becoming more common in women under age 40. Women who have constant itching and changes in the color and the way the vulva looks are at a high risk to get cancer of the vulva. A doctor should be seen if there is bleeding or discharge not related to menstruation (periods), severe burning/itching or pain in the vulva, or if the skin of the vulva looks white and feels rough.

If there are symptoms, a doctor may do certain tests to see if there is cancer, usually beginning by looking at the vulva and feeling for any lumps. The doctor may then go on to cut out a small piece of tissue (called a biopsy) from the vulva and look at it under a microscope. A patient will be given some medicine to numb the area when the biopsy is done. Some pressure may be felt, but usually with no pain. This test is often done in a doctor's office.

The chance of recovery (prognosis) and choice of treatment depend on the stage of the cancer (whether it is just in the vulva or has spread to other places) and the patient's general state of health.

National Cancer Institute, Vulvar Cancer (PDQ®), November 2000.

187

Stages of Cancer of the Vulva

Once cancer of the vulva is diagnosed, more tests will be done to find out if the cancer has spread from the vulva to other parts of the body (staging). A doctor needs to know the stage of the disease to plan treatment. The following stages are used for cancer of the vulva:

Stage 0 or carcinoma *in situ:* Stage 0 cancer of the vulva is a very early cancer. The cancer is found in the vulva only and is only in the surface of the skin.

Stage I: Cancer is found only in the vulva and/or the space between the opening of the rectum and the vagina (perineum). The tumor is 2 centimeters (about 1 inch) or less in size.

Stage II: Cancer is found in the vulva and/or the space between the opening of the rectum and the vagina (perineum), and the tumor is larger than 2 centimeters (larger than 1 inch).

Stage III: Cancer is found in the vulva and/or perineum and has spread to nearby tissues such as the lower part of the urethra (the tube through which urine passes), the vagina, the anus (the opening of the rectum), and/or has spread to nearby lymph nodes. (Lymph nodes are small bean-shaped structures that are found throughout the body. They produce and store infection-fighting cells.)

Stage IV: Cancer has spread beyond the urethra, vagina, and anus into the lining of the bladder (the sac that holds urine) and the bowel (intestine); or, it may have spread to the lymph nodes in the pelvis or to other parts of the body.

Recurrent: Recurrent disease means that the cancer has come back (recurred) after it has been treated. It may come back in the vulva or another place.

How Cancer of the Vulva Is Treated

There are treatments for all patients with cancer of the vulva. Three kinds of treatment are used:

- surgery (taking out the cancer in an operation)
- radiation therapy (using high-dose x-rays or other high-energy rays to kill cancer cells)

- chemotherapy (using drugs to kill cancer cells)

Surgery is the most common treatment of cancer of the vulva. A doctor may take out the cancer using one of the following operations:

- Wide local excision takes out the cancer and some of the normal tissue around the cancer.

- Radical local excision takes out the cancer and a larger portion of normal tissue around the cancer. Lymph nodes may also be removed.

- Laser surgery uses a narrow beam of light to remove cancer cells.

- Skinning vulvectomy takes out only the skin of the vulva that contains the cancer.

- Simple vulvectomy takes out the entire vulva, but no lymph nodes.

- Partial vulvectomy takes out less than the entire vulva.

- Radical vulvectomy takes out the entire vulva. The lymph nodes around it are usually removed as well.

- If the cancer has spread outside the vulva and the other female organs, the doctor may take out the lower colon, rectum, or bladder (depending on where the cancer has spread) along with the cervix, uterus, and vagina (pelvic exenteration).

A patient may need to have skin from another part of the body added (grafted) and plastic surgery to make an artificial vulva or vagina after these operations.

Radiation therapy uses x-rays or other high-energy rays to kill cancer cells and shrink tumors. Radiation may come from a machine outside the body (external radiation) or from putting materials that contain radiation through thin plastic tubes into the area where the cancer cells are found (internal radiation). Radiation may be used alone or before or after surgery.

Chemotherapy uses drugs to kill cancer cells. Drugs may be given by mouth, or they may be put into the body by a needle in the vein or muscle. Chemotherapy is called systemic treatment because the drug enters the bloodstream, travels through the body, and can kill cancer cells throughout the body.

Treatment by Stage

Treatment of cancer of the vulva depends on the stage of the disease, the type of disease, and the patient's age and overall condition.

Standard treatment may be considered because of its effectiveness in patients in past studies, or participation in a clinical trial may be considered. Not all patients are cured with standard therapy and some standard treatments may have more side effects than are desired. For these reasons, clinical trials are designed to find better ways to treat cancer patients and are based on the most up-to-date information. Clinical trials are ongoing in most parts of the country for stages III and IV of cancer of the vulva. To learn more about clinical trials, call the Cancer Information Service at 1-800-4-CANCER (1-800-422-6237); TTY at 1-800-332-8615.

Stage 0 Vulvar Cancer: Treatment may be one of the following:

- Wide local excision or laser surgery or a combination of both.
- Skinning vulvectomy.
- Ointment containing a chemotherapy drug.

Stage I Vulvar Cancer: Treatment may be one of the following:

- Wide local excision.
- Radical local excision plus taking out all nearby lymph nodes in the groin and upper part of the thigh on the same side as the cancer.
- Radical vulvectomy and removal of the lymph nodes in the groin on one or both sides of the body.
- Radiation therapy alone (in selected patients).

Stage II Vulvar Cancer: Treatment may be one of the following:

- Radical vulvectomy and removal of the lymph nodes in the groin on both sides of the body. Radiation may be given to the pelvis following the operation if cancer cells are found in the lymph nodes.
- Radiation therapy alone (in selected patients).

Stage III Vulvar Cancer: Treatment may be one of the following:

- Radical vulvectomy and removal of the lymph nodes in the groin and upper part of the thigh on both sides of the body. Radiation may be given to the pelvis and groin following the operation if cancer cells are found in the lymph nodes or only to the vulva if the tumor is large but has not spread.

- Radiation therapy and chemotherapy followed by radical vulvectomy and removal of lymph nodes on both sides of the body.

- Radiation therapy (in selected patients) with or without chemotherapy.

Stage IV Vulvar Cancer: Treatment may be one of the following:

- Radical vulvectomy and removal of the lower colon, rectum, or bladder (depending on where the cancer has spread) along with the uterus, cervix, and vagina (pelvic exenteration).

- Radical vulvectomy followed by radiation therapy.

- Radiation therapy followed by radical vulvectomy.

- Radiation therapy (in selected patients) with or without chemotherapy, and possibly following surgery.

Recurrent Vulvar Cancer: If the cancer has come back, treatment may be one of the following:

- Wide local excision with or without radiation therapy.

- Radical vulvectomy and removal of the lower colon, rectum, or bladder (depending on where the cancer has spread) along with the uterus, cervix, and vagina (pelvic exenteration).

- Radiation therapy plus chemotherapy with or without surgery.

- Radiation therapy for local recurrences or to reduce symptoms such as pain, nausea, or abnormal body functions.

- Clinical trials of new forms of therapy.

Chapter 29

Questions and Answers about Metastatic Cancer

What is cancer?

Cancer is a group of many related diseases that begin in cells, the body's basic unit of life. The body is made up of many types of cells. Normally, cells grow and divide to produce more cells only when the body needs them. This orderly process helps keep the body healthy. Sometimes cells keep dividing when new cells are not needed. These extra cells may form a mass of tissue, called a growth or tumor. Tumors can be either benign (not cancerous) or malignant (cancerous).

Cancer can begin in any organ or tissue of the body. The original tumor is called the primary cancer or primary tumor and is usually named for the part of the body in which it begins.

What is metastasis?

Metastasis means the spread of cancer. Cancer cells can break away from a primary tumor and travel through the bloodstream or lymphatic system to other parts of the body.

Cancer cells may spread to lymph nodes near the primary tumor (regional lymph nodes). This is called nodal involvement, positive nodes, or regional disease. Cancer cells can also spread to other parts of the body, distant from the primary tumor. Doctors use the term metastatic disease or distant disease to describe cancer that spreads to other organs or to lymph nodes other than those near the primary tumor.

National Cancer Institute, CancerNet, August 2000.

When cancer cells spread and form a new tumor, the new tumor is called a secondary, or metastatic, tumor. The cancer cells that form the secondary tumor are like those in the original tumor. That means, for example, that if breast cancer spreads (metastasizes) to the lung, the secondary tumor is made up of abnormal breast cells (not abnormal lung cells). The disease in the lung is metastatic breast cancer (not lung cancer).

Is it possible to have a metastasis without having a primary cancer?

No. A metastasis is a tumor that started from a cancer cell or cells in another part of the body. Sometimes, however, a primary cancer is discovered only after a metastasis causes symptoms. For example, a man whose prostate cancer has spread to the bones in the pelvis may have lower back pain (caused by the cancer in his bones) before experiencing any symptoms from the prostate tumor itself.

How does a doctor know whether a cancer is a primary or a secondary tumor?

The cells in a metastatic tumor resemble those in the primary tumor. Once the cancerous tissue is examined under a microscope to determine the cell type, a doctor can usually tell whether that type of cell is normally found in the part of the body from which the tissue sample was taken.

For instance, breast cancer cells look the same whether they are found in the breast or have spread to another part of the body. So, if a tissue sample taken from a tumor in the lung contains cells that look like breast cells, the doctor determines that the lung tumor is a secondary tumor.

Metastatic cancers may be found at the same time as the primary tumor, or months or years later. When a second tumor is found in a patient who has been treated for cancer in the past, it is more often a metastasis than another primary tumor.

In a small number of cancer patients, a secondary tumor is diagnosed, but no primary cancer can be found, in spite of extensive tests. Doctors refer to the primary tumor as unknown or occult, and the patient is said to have cancer of unknown primary origin (CUP).

What treatments are used for metastatic cancer?

When cancer has metastasized, it may be treated with chemotherapy, radiation therapy, biological therapy, hormone therapy, surgery, or a combination of these. The choice of treatment generally depends on the type of primary cancer, the size and location of the metastasis, the patient's age and general health, and the types of treatments used previously. In patients diagnosed with CUP, it is still possible to treat the disease even when the primary tumor cannot be located.

New cancer treatments are currently under study. To develop new treatments, the National Cancer Institute (NCI) sponsors clinical trials (research studies) with cancer patients in many hospitals, universities, medical schools, and cancer centers around the country. Clinical trials are a critical step in the improvement of treatment. Before any new treatment can be recommended for general use, doctors conduct studies to find out whether the treatment is both safe for patients and effective against the disease. The results of such studies have led to progress not only in the treatment of cancer, but in the detection, diagnosis, and prevention of the disease as well. Patients interested in participating in research should ask their doctor to find out whether they are eligible for a clinical trial.

National Cancer Institute Information Resources

You may want more information for yourself, your family, and your doctor. The following National Cancer Institute (NCI) services are available to help you.

Telephone

Cancer Information Service (CIS) provides accurate, up-to-date information on cancer to patients and their families, health professionals, and the general public. Information specialists translate the latest scientific information into understandable language and respond in English, Spanish, or on TTY equipment.

Telephone 1-800-4-CANCER (1-800-422-6237)
TTY: 1-800-332-8615 (for deaf and hard of hearing callers)

Internet

These web sites may be useful:

http://www.nci.nih.gov

NCI's primary web site; contains information about the Institute and its programs.

http://cancernet.nci.nih.gov

CancerNet; contains material for health professionals, patients, and the public, including information from PDQ about cancer treatment, screening, prevention, genetics, supportive care, and clinical trials, and CANCERLIT, a bibliographic database.

http://cancertrials.nci.nih.gov

cancerTrials; NCI's comprehensive clinical trials information center for patients, health professionals, and the public. Includes information on understanding trials, deciding whether to participate in trials, finding specific trials, plus research news and other resources.

http://rex.nci.nih.gov

This site includes news, upcoming events, educational materials, and publications for patients, the public, and the mass media.

http://chid.nih.gov/ncichid

Cancer Patient Education Database; provides information on cancer patient education resources for patients, their families, and health professionals.

E-mail

CancerMail includes NCI information about cancer treatment, screening, prevention, genetics, and supportive care. To obtain a contents list, send e-mail to cancermail@icicc.nci.nih.gov with the word "help" in the body of the message.

Fax

CancerFax includes NCI information about cancer treatment, screening, prevention, genetics, and supportive care. To obtain a contents list, dial 301-402-5874 or 1-800-624-2511 from a touch-tone telephone or fax machine hand set and follow the recorded instructions.

Chapter 30

Hodgkin's Disease and Non-Hodgkin's Lymphoma during Pregnancy

Hodgkin's Disease During Pregnancy

This summary discusses the treatment of Hodgkin's disease during pregnancy.

What is Hodgkin's disease?

Hodgkin's disease is a type of lymphoma. Lymphomas are cancers that develop in the lymph system, part of the body's immune system.

The lymph system is made up of thin tubes that branch, like blood vessels, into all parts of the body. Lymph vessels carry lymph, a colorless, watery fluid that contains white blood cells called lymphocytes. Along the network of vessels are groups of small organs called lymph nodes. Clusters of lymph nodes are found in the underarm, pelvis, neck, and abdomen. The lymph nodes make and store infection-fighting cells. The spleen (an organ in the upper abdomen that makes lymphocytes and filters old blood cells from the blood), the thymus (a small organ beneath the breastbone), and the tonsils (an organ in the throat) are also part of the lymph system.

Because there is lymph tissue in many parts of the body, Hodgkin's disease can start to grow in almost any part of the body. The cancer can spread to almost any organ or tissue in the body, including the

National Cancer Institute, Hodgkin's Disease during Pregnancy (PDQ ®), January 2001, and Non-Hodgkin's Lymphoma during Pregnancy (PDQ ®), January 2001.

liver, bone marrow (the spongy tissue inside the large bones of the body that makes blood cells), and spleen.

Lymphomas are divided into two general types: Hodgkin's disease and non-Hodgkin's lymphomas. The cancer cells in Hodgkin's disease look a certain way under a microscope.

A doctor should be seen if any of the following symptoms persist for longer than two weeks: painless swelling of the lymph nodes in the neck, underarm, or groin; fever; night sweats; tiredness; weight loss without dieting; or itchy skin.

If symptoms are present, a doctor will carefully check for swelling or lumps in the neck, underarms, and groin. If the lymph nodes do not feel normal, a doctor may need to cut out a small piece and look at it under the microscope to see if there are any cancer cells. This procedure is called a biopsy.

The chance of recovery (prognosis) and choice of treatment depend on the stage of the cancer (whether it is in just one area or has spread throughout the body), the size of the swollen areas, the results of blood tests, the type of symptoms, and the patient's age, sex, and overall condition.

Description

Hodgkin's disease most commonly affects young adults and, therefore, young women may be diagnosed with the disease when they are pregnant. Treatment for Hodgkin's disease during pregnancy is chosen carefully so that the fetus is put in as little danger as possible. When treatment is being planned, the wishes of the patient, the seriousness and aggressiveness of the disease, and the number of months remaining in the pregnancy are also considered. The treatment plan may change as the symptoms, cancer, and pregnancy change.

Women who are in the first trimester of pregnancy are usually advised to end the pregnancy. Women who choose to continue pregnancy may delay treatment until the baby is delivered if the disease is slow growing and located above the diaphragm (above the stomach). If immediate treatment is needed for Hodgkin's disease, women may choose to receive radiation therapy or chemotherapy. Both radiation therapy and chemotherapy can cause harm to the fetus. In most cases, the fetus can be protected from exposure to radiation therapy with proper shielding. The fetus can not be protected against exposure to chemotherapy (using drugs to kill cancer cells), and some chemotherapy regimens may cause birth defects.

Most patients in the second half of pregnancy can delay treatment until the baby is induced at 32 to 36 weeks. Treatment for Hodgkin's disease can begin shortly after the baby is born. Patients with advanced Hodgkin's disease may require treatment before the baby is delivered. These patients may receive steroids (designed to fight tumor growth and help lung development in the fetus), radiation therapy, and/or chemotherapy. Because some chemotherapy regimens may cause birth defects, single-drug chemotherapy regimens are usually given. More extensive chemotherapy is usually given once the baby has been delivered. If the patient's breathing is being affected by a large tumor in the chest, a short course of radiation therapy can be given before delivery.

Women who have been treated for Hodgkin's disease during pregnancy appear to have survival rates similar to women who were treated while not pregnant. The long-term effects of anticancer treatment on the children of these women is not yet known; however, the risk does not appear to be significant.

Non-Hodgkin's Lymphoma During Pregnancy

This summary discusses the treatment of non-Hodgkin's lymphoma during pregnancy.

What is Non-Hodgkin's lymphoma?

Adult non-Hodgkin's lymphoma is a disease in which cancer (malignant) cells are found in the lymph system. The lymph system is made up of thin tubes that branch, like blood vessels, into all parts of the body. Lymph vessels carry lymph, a colorless, watery fluid that contains white blood cells called lymphocytes. Along the network of vessels are groups of small organs called lymph nodes. Clusters of lymph nodes are found in the underarm, pelvis, neck, and abdomen. The lymph nodes make and store infection-fighting cells. The spleen (an organ in the upper abdomen that makes lymphocytes and filters old blood cells from the blood), the thymus (a small organ beneath the breastbone), and the tonsils (an organ in the throat) are also part of the lymph system.

Because lymph tissue is found in many parts of the body, non-Hodgkin's lymphoma can start in almost any part of the body. The cancer can spread to almost any organ or tissue in the body, including the liver, bone marrow (the spongy tissue inside the large bones of the body that makes blood cells), spleen, and nose.

There are many types of non-Hodgkin's lymphomas. Some types spread more quickly than others. The type is determined by how the cancer cells look under a microscope. This determination is called the histology. The histologies for adult non-Hodgkin's lymphoma are divided into two groups: indolent lymphomas, which are slower growing and have fewer symptoms, and aggressive lymphomas, which grow more quickly.

- Indolent
  follicular small cleaved cell lymphoma
  follicular mixed cell lymphoma
  follicular large cell lymphoma
  adult diffuse small cleaved cell lymphoma
  small lymphocytic (marginal zone)

- Aggressive
  adult diffuse mixed cell lymphoma
  adult diffuse large cell lymphoma
  adult immunoblastic large cell lymphoma
  adult lymphoblastic lymphoma
  adult small noncleaved cell lymphoma

Other types of indolent non-Hodgkin's lymphoma are lymphoplasmacytoid lymphoma, monocytoid B-cell lymphoma, mucosa-associated lymphoid tissue (MALT) lymphoma, splenic marginal zone lymphoma, hairy cell leukemia, and cutaneous T-cell lymphoma (Mycosis fungoides/Sezary syndrome).

Other types of aggressive non-Hodgkin's lymphoma are anaplastic large-cell lymphoma, adult T-cell lymphoma/leukemia, mantle cell lymphoma, intravascular lymphomatosis, angioimmunoblastic T-cell lymphoma, angiocentric lymphoma, intestinal T-cell lymphoma, primary mediastinal B-cell lymphoma, peripheral T-cell lymphoma, lymphoblastic lymphoma, post-transplantation lymphoproliferative disorder, true histiocytic lymphoma, primary central nervous system lymphoma, and primary effusion lymphoma. Aggressive lymphomas are also seen more frequently in patients who are HIV-positive (AIDS-related lymphoma).

A doctor should be seen if any of the following symptoms persist: painless swelling in the lymph nodes in the neck, underarm, or groin; unexplained fever; drenching night sweats; tiredness; unexplained weight loss in the past 6 months; or itchy skin.

If these symptoms are present, a doctor will carefully check for swelling or lumps in the neck, underarms, and groin. If the lymph nodes don't feel normal, a doctor may need to surgically remove a small piece of tissue and look at it under a microscope to see if there are any cancer cells. This procedure is called a biopsy.

The chance of recovery (prognosis) and choice of treatment depend on the stage of the cancer (whether it is just in one area or has spread throughout the body), and the patient's age and overall condition.

Description

Non-Hodgkin's lymphoma (NHL) usually affects older adults and, therefore, women are seldom found to have NHL when they are pregnant. Most non-Hodgkin's lymphomas are aggressive and delaying treatment until after the baby has been delivered appears to lead to a poor outcome. Immediate treatment is often recommended, even during pregnancy. Children who were exposed to doxorubicin (a chemotherapy drug) before they were born have been monitored for up to 11 years, and they do not appear to suffer from side effects of the drug. Long-term studies have not been conducted to determine the effects of other chemotherapy drugs on children who were exposed to them before birth. Ending the pregnancy during the first trimester of pregnancy may also be an option for women who have aggressive NHL that must be treated immediately. Early delivery may reduce or avoid the fetus' exposure to chemotherapy drugs or radiation therapy. Women who have indolent (slow-growing) non-Hodgkin's lymphoma can usually delay treatment.

To Learn More

For more information, call the National Cancer Institute's Cancer Information Service at 1-800-4-CANCER (1-800-422-6237); TTY at 1-800-332-8615. The call is free and a trained information specialist is available to answer your questions.

The National Cancer Institute has booklets and other materials for patients, health professionals, and the public. These publications discuss types of cancer, methods of cancer treatment, coping with cancer, and clinical trials. Some publications provide information on tests for cancer, cancer causes and prevention, cancer statistics, and NCI research activities. NCI materials on these and other topics may be ordered online from the NCI Publications Locator Service at http://publications.nci.nih.gov/ or by telephone from the Cancer Information Service toll free at 1-800-4-CANCER.

There are many other places where people can get materials and information about cancer treatment and services. Local hospitals may have information on local and regional agencies that offer information about finances, getting to and from treatment, receiving care at home, and dealing with problems associated with cancer treatment. A list of organizations and websites that offer information and services for cancer patients and their families is available on CancerNet at http://cancernet.nci.nih.gov/cancerlinks.html.

For more information from the National Cancer Institute, please write to this address:

National Cancer Institute
Office of Communications
31 Center Drive, MSC 2580
Bethesda, MD 20892-2580

Chapter 31

Non-Cancerous Gynecologic Conditions

If you have a problem that affects your uterus or another part of your reproductive system, this information is for you. It explains most of the problems that can affect a woman's reproductive system and ways the problems can be treated, including medication, surgery, and other kinds of treatments.

About the Uterus

The uterus is located in the lower abdomen between the bladder and the rectum. The uterus is also called the womb. It is pear-shaped, and the lower, narrow end of the uterus is the cervix. When a woman is pregnant, the baby grows in the uterus until he or she is born.

On each side of the uterus at the top are the fallopian tubes and ovaries. Together, the uterus, vagina, ovaries, and fallopian tubes make up the reproductive system.

In women who have not gone through menopause ("the change" or "change of life"), the ovaries produce the hormone estrogen at the beginning of the menstrual cycle. Estrogen helps to prepare the lining of the uterus (called the endometrium) for possible pregnancy. When the uterus is ready, one of the ovaries releases an egg. The egg travels down the fallopian tube where it waits for possible fertilization.

"Common Uterine Conditions: Options for Treatment" U.S. Department of Health and Human Services, Agency for Health Care Policy and Research, AHCPR Pub. No. 98-0003, December 1997.

If the woman becomes pregnant, the fertilized egg travels to the uterus where it attaches to the endometrium. If she does not, the endometrium and the unfertilized egg are discharged through the vagina during the woman's next period (menstruation).

Some of the problems that can affect your uterus are:

- Noncancerous growths in the uterus, called fibroids, which can cause pain and bleeding.

- Endometriosis, a condition in which the tissue that forms the lining of the uterus grows outside the uterus.

- Heavy bleeding each time you have your period or between periods.

- Hormonal imbalances.

- Unexplained pelvic pain.

Treatment Options

Your doctor may have recommended that you have a hysterectomy or another kind of treatment. Before you decide what to do, it is important that you understand the problem and the different options you have for dealing with it.

The following information can help you think about your condition, learn about your treatment choices, and decide on some questions to ask your doctor.

Keep in mind that every woman is different and every situation is different. A good treatment choice for one woman may not be the best choice for another. That is why you should:

- Talk over your options carefully with your doctor.

- Ask questions until you understand what the doctor is telling you.

- Consider getting a second opinion.

- Work with your doctor to choose the treatment that is best for you.

You Are Not Alone

The first thing you need to know is that you are not alone. About 1 of every 10 women between the ages of 18 and 50 has this type of problem. Usually, the problem can be treated, and the symptoms can be relieved. Most women who have had treatment are satisfied with the results and are glad to be free of pain or other unpleasant symptoms.

The first step in getting relief is to find out what the problem is.

Finding Out about the Problem

There are several ways your doctor can find out (diagnose) what is causing your symptoms. The most common include:

A Medical History

The first step in diagnosing your problem is a medical history. The doctor—or sometimes the nurse—will ask you questions about your medical history. This will include questions about your symptoms and any serious illnesses you have had, as well as whether you have ever had surgery, been pregnant, or had children. You also may be asked about the medical history of close family members.

If you have been using herbs, acupuncture, or other "natural remedies," be sure to tell your doctor about them.

The doctor may ask about your sex life. You may be uncomfortable talking about such personal matters, but it is important for your doctor to know if something that is happening in your sex life might be related to your condition.

A Vaginal Exam

The doctor will use instruments to look inside your cervix and uterus. The doctor will use a speculum to keep the walls of the vagina apart during the exam. Sometimes this exam is uncomfortable. You may feel a slight cramp, but it usually is not painful. If you are able to relax, you will be more comfortable. The doctor may look inside the vagina and cervix with a lighted tube.

A Pap Test (or Pap Smear)

During the vaginal exam, the doctor usually takes a sample of cells from the cervix with a wooden scraper, cotton swab, or small brush. The test is quick and painless. The cells are placed on a glass slide, which is sent to a lab. A Pap test is one way that doctors can find cancer of the cervix or dysplasia, which is a condition that sometimes can turn into cancer.

All women over 18 years of age — and younger women who are sexually active — should have a Pap test done every 1 to 3 years.

Laboratory Tests

The doctor will take a sample of your blood and a urine specimen and send them to a lab to be examined. The results of these tests will tell the doctor a lot about your general health.

Imaging Tests

There are many ways to look inside the body without surgery. X-rays are the most well known. Your doctor may also suggest a sonogram, CAT scan, or MRI. These tests help the doctor to learn more about your body and what is causing your problem.

Depending on your symptoms, the doctor may suggest an endometrial biopsy, dilation and curettage (D&C), or other tests to help diagnose your problem.

Noncancerous Uterine Conditions

After your medical history, examination, and tests are done, your doctor will explain your condition to you and talk about your options for treatment. Later in this chapter you will find a list of questions you may want to ask your doctor.

Surgery, medicine (including hormones), a combination of the two, or "watchful waiting" are the most common choices for dealing with most noncancerous uterine conditions. Watchful waiting means having no treatment but seeing the doctor regularly to keep track of your condition and discuss symptoms. After a period of watchful waiting, if you are still having problems, you may decide with your doctor to consider one or more treatment options.

There are always new treatments in development. Be sure to ask your doctor if there are any new treatments for your condition that are not described in this chapter.

Your doctor may recommend that you have a hysterectomy. If so, you will want to see the section on hysterectomy.

Remember, all treatments — including medicine, surgery, other types of treatments, and even a decision to wait or not be treated — have risks and benefits. Be sure to ask your doctor about the risks and benefits of each treatment option you are offered. Then you can work with your doctor to weigh your options and make an informed choice.

Fibroids

What are fibroids?

Fibroids are growths in the walls of the uterus. Sometimes, a fibroid is attached to the outside of the uterus by a stalk. Fibroids can be as small as a seed or a pea or as large as an orange or small melon. Although fibroids are called "tumors," they are not cancer. They are smooth muscle growths.

About 2 of every 10 women who have not gone through menopause have fibroids. The technical term for a fibroid tumor is leiomyoma.

Fibroids may cause no symptoms at all, or they may cause pain or bleeding. Fibroids may make it hard to pass urine if they grow large enough to press on the bladder.

Fibroids also can make it hard for you to get pregnant. Sometimes fibroids can cause problems with pregnancy, labor, or delivery, including miscarriage and premature birth.

How are fibroids treated?

You may have several treatments to choose from if you have fibroids. It depends on how big the fibroids are, where they are, and whether you are pregnant or want to become pregnant.

Watchful waiting may be all the treatment you need if your fibroid is small and you do not have any symptoms. You will need regular visits to your doctor for a pelvic exam to monitor the growth of the fibroid.

Nonsurgical treatments for fibroids include hormones and pain relief medicines.

- Taking gonadotropin releasing hormone (GnRH) can cause fibroids to shrink. This may make surgery easier, or it may be used instead of an operation.

- Your doctor may prescribe ibuprofen (for example, Advil), acetaminophen (for example, Tylenol), or another medicine to relieve pain.

Surgical treatments for fibroids include hysterectomy and myomectomy.

- Hysterectomy is usually recommended when the fibroids are causing symptoms, when they have grown rapidly, or when the fibroids are large (as large as a grapefruit).

- Myomectomy is an operation to remove a fibroid tumor without taking out the uterus. This means that pregnancy is still possible, although a Cesarean section may be necessary.

  Recovery time after a myomectomy is about 3 to 4 weeks. About 20 percent of women who undergo myomectomy need a blood transfusion, about 30 percent have a fever after surgery, and many patients develop adhesions (scar tissue) in their pelvis in the months following surgery. These complications are more likely to occur when there is more than one fibroid and when the fibroids are large.

  The growths may come back after a myomectomy, and repeat surgery may be necessary. If you are considering a myomectomy, be sure to ask the doctor how likely it is that new fibroids might grow after the surgery.

  You also should ask your doctor how much experience he or she has in doing this procedure. Not all gynecologists have been trained to perform myomectomies.

- Another option is laser surgery, which usually is an outpatient procedure. With laser surgery, the doctor uses a high-intensity light to remove small fibroids.

- Depending on the location of the fibroid, it may be possible to remove it during a laparoscopy. Or, the doctor may put a thin tube (called a hysteroscope) with a laser through the vagina and into the uterus. The tube may have a small scraper to scrape away the fibroid from the wall of the uterus.

Endometriosis

What is endometriosis?

Endometrial tissue lines the uterus. Each month, in tune with the menstrual cycle, the endometrial tissue thickens and is shed during menstruation.

If you have endometriosis, it means that the same kind of tissue that lines your uterus is also growing in other parts of your body, usually in the abdomen. This can cause scar tissue to build up around your organs.

Endometriosis may cause severe pain and abnormal bleeding, usually around the time of your period. Pain during intercourse is another common symptom. However, it is possible to have endometriosis and not have any symptoms. Endometriosis is a leading cause of infertility (inability to get pregnant). Often it is not diagnosed until a woman has trouble getting pregnant.

Endometriosis will lessen after menopause and during pregnancy, since the growth of endometrial tissue depends on estrogen. If you have endometriosis and take estrogen-replacement therapy after menopause, the tissue may grow back.

The only way to be sure that you have endometriosis is through a surgical procedure, laparoscopy. Endometriosis can be a chronic condition and may return even after treatment with medicine or surgery.

How can endometriosis be treated?

There are several options for treating endometriosis. The best treatment for you may depend on whether you want to relieve pain, increase your chances of getting pregnant, or both. It is important to work with your doctor to weigh the benefits and risks of each treatment.

Nonsurgical treatments include:

- Medicine, including hormones. There are two types of hormone therapy: those that will make your body think it is pregnant and those that will make your body think it is in menopause. Both are meant to stop the body from producing the messages that cause the endometrial tissue to grow. Birth control pills may be used for a few months to try to shrink the adhesions in women who want to become pregnant. Other hormones—GnRH and danazol—also may help relieve the pain of endometriosis.

- Doctors sometimes prescribe pain relievers, such as ibuprofen (for example, Advil and Motrin) or, for severe pain, codeine.

- Other nonsurgical options include watchful waiting and changes in diet and exercise.

Several types of surgery are used to treat endometriosis, including:

- Laser laparoscopy, in which a cut is made in the abdomen and adhesions are removed, either by laser beams or electric cauterization.

- Hysterectomy, which may not cure endometriosis. Unless the ovaries are removed also, they will continue to produce estrogen. This may encourage endometrial tissue to grow in other areas of the body.

- Bowel resection, which means taking out a section of the bowel, if endometriosis is affecting the bowel.

- Cutting certain nerves, called the sacral nerves, in the lower back to relieve pain.

Endometrial Hyperplasia

What is hyperplasia?

Hyperplasia is a condition in which the lining of the uterus becomes too thick, which results in abnormal bleeding. Hyperplasia is thought to be caused by too much estrogen.

Depending on your age and how long you have had hyperplasia, your doctor may want to do a biopsy before beginning treatment to rule out cancer.

How is hyperplasia treated?

- Hormone treatment with birth control pills or progesterone helps some women who have hyperplasia.

- Hysterectomy is often recommended to treat hyperplasia. Because some types of hyperplasia can lead to cancer, your doctor will watch your condition carefully if you choose not to have a hysterectomy.

Uterine Prolapse

What is uterine prolapse?

If you have uterine prolapse, it means that your uterus has tilted or slipped. Sometimes it slips so far down that it reaches into the vagina. This happens when the ligaments that hold the uterus to the wall of the pelvis become too weak to hold the uterus in its place.

Uterine prolapse can cause feelings of pressure and discomfort. Urine may leak.

How is uterine prolapse treated?

Treatment choices depend on how weak the ligaments have become, your age, health, and whether you want to become pregnant. Options that do not involve an operation include:

- Exercises (called Kegel exercises) can help to strengthen the muscles of the pelvis. How to do Kegel exercises: Tighten your pelvic muscles as if you are trying to hold back urine. Hold the muscles tight for a few seconds and then release them. Repeat this exercise up to 10 times. Repeat the Kegel exercises up to four time each day.

- Taking estrogen to limit further weakening of the muscles and tissues that support the uterus.

- Inserting a pessary—which is a rubber, diaphragm-like device— around the cervix to help prop up the uterus. The pessary does have drawbacks. It may dislodge or cause irritation, it may interfere with intercourse, and it must be removed regularly for cleaning.

- Watchful waiting.

Surgical treatments include:

- Tightening the weakened muscles without taking out the uterus. This is usually done through the vagina, but it also can be done through the abdomen. Although this is a type of surgery, it is not as extensive as a hysterectomy.

- Hysterectomy. Doctors usually recommend this operation if symptoms are bothersome or if the uterus has dropped so far that it is coming through the vagina.

Ovarian Cysts

What are ovarian cysts?

Ovarian cysts are small, fluid-filled sacs that usually are not malignant. They may not cause any symptoms, or they may be quite painful. Sometimes, ovarian cysts appear in connection with the menstrual cycle, and they may go away on their own in a few months. When these cysts grow large, they may cause feelings of pressure or fullness.

Although most ovarian cysts are benign (not cancer), they must be taken very seriously. A sonogram will show whether a cyst is fluid-filled or has solid matter in it. If it is solid, it may be related to endometriosis, or it may be cancerous.

What are the treatments for ovarian cysts?

If you have not yet gone through menopause, you may not need any treatment, unless the cyst is very big or causing pain. Sometimes, taking birth control pills will make the cyst smaller. Surgery may be needed if the cyst is causing symptoms or is more than 2 inches across.

If surgery is needed, often the cyst can be removed without removing the ovary. Even if one ovary has to be removed, it is still possible to become pregnant as long as one ovary remains.

After menopause, the risk of ovarian cancer increases. Surgery to remove an ovarian cyst is usually recommended in this case. Your doctor will probably want to do a biopsy to see if cancer is present.

If you have gone through menopause and you have an ovarian cyst, talk with your doctor about what will be done during surgery. Make sure you understand whether he or she plans to remove just the cyst, the cyst and the ovary, or to do a hysterectomy. Talk over the options with your doctor and make your own wishes known.

Treatment options include:

- Watchful waiting.

- Hormone therapy to reduce the size of the cyst.

- Cystectomy to remove the cyst.

- Oophorectomy to remove the affected ovary.

- Hysterectomy. This usually is not necessary unless the cyst is cancerous.

Pelvic Inflammatory Disease

Pelvic inflammatory disease (PID) is caused by an infection that starts in the vagina. Most often, it is caused by a sexually transmitted disease (STD). The infection spreads upward into the uterus, fallopian tubes, and pelvis.

Women who use intrauterine devices (IUDs) are at increased risk for PID. Rarely, the bacteria that cause PID enter the body during childbirth or abortion.

PID can cause pelvic pain and fevers. It also may cause infertility (inability to get pregnant) because of damage to the fallopian tubes. Sacs of pus, called abscesses, may form in the pelvis. Sometimes the vagina will discharge a pus-like substance.

If PID is not treated, pain may be so intense that it is hard to walk. The infection may spread into the bloodstream and throughout the body, causing fever, chills, joint infections, and sometimes death.

How is PID treated?

- If you have PID and it is the result of an STD, you and your sexual partner will be given drugs called antibiotics to treat the infection.

- If an abscess has formed, it may need to be drained.

- Treatment may include hospitalization.

- An operation may be done to help heal scar tissue.

- If the disease cannot be stopped in any other way, you may need surgery to remove the infected organs.

Severe Menstrual Pain

What is severe menstrual pain?

Some women have extreme cramping just before and during their period. The technical term for this is dysmenorrhea. If you have this kind of pain, you should seek treatment. Severe menstrual pain may be a symptom of endometriosis.

What can be done about severe menstrual pain?

Several types of medicine are used to treat painful cramps. These include:

- Over-the-counter pain relievers, such as aspirin, ibuprofen, naproxen (for example, Aleve), or acetaminophen may be helpful.

- If over-the-counter medicines don't work, your doctor can give you a prescription for a stronger pain reliever, such as codeine.

- Birth control pills or other medicines may be used to reduce cramping.

- Surgery usually is not necessary if severe menstrual pain is the only problem.

Very Heavy Menstrual Bleeding

What is very heavy menstrual bleeding?

As you get closer to menopause, it may be hard to tell when your period is going to start. The time between your periods may be longer or shorter than usual. When it does start, bleeding may be very heavy and last for several weeks.

You may have dysfunctional uterine bleeding or DUB. DUB most often affects women over 45. Usually it is caused by an imbalance in the chemicals in the body (hormones) that control the menstrual cycle.

Younger women also may have heavy bleeding. Usually it is because of an irregular menstrual cycle. A woman may go for several months without a period, but the lining of her uterus continues to build up. When finally her body sheds the uterine lining, she may have very heavy bleeding.

The symptoms can be very upsetting and may make you feel limited in the things you can do. Sometimes, the symptoms are a sign of a more serious problem.

Your doctor will probably do a blood test. Depending on the results, your medical history, and your age, the doctor may recommend that you have a biopsy to rule out endometrial hyperplasia.

What treatments are used for very heavy menstrual bleeding?

• Birth control pills or other medicines may be helpful.

• Another choice is watchful waiting.

• A surgical procedure called endometrial ablation may help to relieve very heavy menstrual bleeding. Endometrial ablation causes sterility (inability to become pregnant), but it does not trigger menopause. The long-term effects of endometrial ablation are unknown.

Do you have a bleeding disorder?

If you have very heavy periods (lasting more than 7 days or soaking more than one pad or tampon every 2 to 3 hours), frequent or long-lasting nosebleeds, easy bruising, or prolonged oozing of blood after dental work, you may have a bleeding disorder such as von Willebrand Disease. This is not the same as very heavy menstrual bleeding, but it can be an underlying cause. It can be diagnosed at the Hemophilia Treatment Center, and it can be treated. Call the National Hemophilia

Foundation at 800-424-2634, extension 3051, to find the Hemophilia Treatment Center nearest you.

Chronic Pelvic Pain

What is chronic pelvic pain?

If you feel intense pain in your pelvis, but the doctor can find no cause, you may have chronic pelvic pain.

How is chronic pelvic pain treated?

Options that do not involve surgery include:

- Combination therapy—including anti-inflammatory medicines that contain ibuprofen, birth control pills, physical therapy, and nutritional and psychological counseling—may be helpful.

- Depending on the severity of the pain, watchful waiting may be another option.

Surgical options include:

- Surgery to take out scar tissue that may be causing pain. This is called adhesiolysis.

- Hysterectomy may be an option for women whose pelvic veins are persistently swollen or when all other measures have been tried without success. However, it does not always relieve the pain.

- Cutting certain nerves in the lower back to help relieve pain.

What You Should Know about Hysterectomy

Your doctor may have told you that you need a hysterectomy. This section describes the different kinds of hysterectomy and some of the things you will want to consider before you make a decision about surgery.

Make sure you understand all of your treatment options and the risks and benefits of each. Then you can work with your doctor to choose the best treatment for you.

A hysterectomy may be done to relieve symptoms caused by several conditions, including:

- Fibroids.

215

- Endometriosis.
- Hyperplasia.
- Uterine prolapse.
- Very heavy or irregular bleeding.

Like other operations, hysterectomy involves both risks and benefits. As with any surgery, there is some risk associated with the anesthesia and the operation itself.

After surgery, you will need to take it easy for several weeks. You will need help with household chores, shopping, and carrying things. If you have small children, you will need help caring for them.

Having a hysterectomy means that your periods will stop for good, and you will be unable to become pregnant. If your ovaries are removed, you may have symptoms associated with menopause.

If your doctor recommends that you have a hysterectomy, you will want to get as much information as possible before you make a decision. Be sure to ask the doctor about your other treatment options, including the benefits and risks of both surgical and nonsurgical alternatives to hysterectomy.

Here are some questions about hysterectomy. They can help you decide with your doctor whether a hysterectomy is the best choice for you.

What exactly is done during a hysterectomy?

The answer depends on which type of hysterectomy you have.

In a *subtotal* hysterectomy, the uterus is removed but the cervix, ovaries, and fallopian tubes are left in place.

In a *total* hysterectomy (also called a simple hysterectomy), the surgeon removes the uterus and cervix but leaves the ovaries and fallopian tubes.

In a hysterectomy with *bilateral salpingo-oophorectomy* (also called a radical hysterectomy), the uterus, cervix, ovaries, and fallopian tubes are removed.

Will I have a scar?

Whether or not you will have a scar and the kind of scar you will have depend on the kind of cut (incision) the doctor makes. The incision will depend on your condition and which method you choose.

In the first method, the surgeon cuts along the pubic hairline. Sometimes called a "bikini" cut, the scar may be harder to see after it heals.

Another method is to make a cut through the vagina. This method leaves no scar that can be seen. The surgeon may be able to use this method if your uterus is small or if it has slipped (prolapsed) into the vagina.

In the third method, the surgeon cuts downwards from just below the belly button to just above the pubic hairline. The cut is usually 4 to 6 inches long. This type of cut makes it easy for the surgeon to work inside the pelvis.

You should discuss these choices with your doctor and be sure that you understand them.

What about pain after the operation?

Your doctor can give you medicine to relieve the pain caused by surgery. Although you should rest as much as you need to, you will recover more quickly and feel better if you get a little bit of exercise each day.

What are the side effects of a hysterectomy?

Side effects depend on a number of things, including your age, condition, whether you are still having periods, and what type of hysterectomy you have. If you were still having periods before surgery, they will stop after the operation.

- If your ovaries are not removed, you will continue to have hormone changes like you did with your periods, but you will not have bleeding.

- If your ovaries are removed, you will go through changes like menopause. These might include hot flashes, vaginal dryness, night sweats, mood swings, or other symptoms.

Other side effects of hysterectomy are similar to the side effects for any type of surgery. If you work outside the home, you will need to be off for several weeks—how long depends on the type of hysterectomy you have and your doctor's orders. You will need help with routine activities such as child care, shopping, and housework. Additional side effects of surgery include:

Effects of anesthesia: The doctor will give you anesthesia so you will not feel pain during the operation. You may feel moody, tired, or weak for a few days after anesthesia. You also may feel a little sick to your stomach (nausea) after anesthesia. The doctor usually can give you something to help settle your stomach.

Infections: As with any type of operation, there is always a risk of infection. If you do get an infection, your doctor will give you medicine to treat it.

Too much bleeding: There is always a risk that you might bleed too much during an operation and need a transfusion. Ask your doctor if you should donate some of your own blood before the operation or if someone should give blood for you.

Damage to nearby organs: It is possible that during the operation a part of your body near the uterus might be damaged. Although this is unlikely, you should ask your doctor what might happen if an organ is damaged.

Studies have shown that for a small number of women, hysterectomy may be followed by one of more of the following problems: unwanted weight gain, constipation, fatigue, unexplained pelvic pain, and premature menopause, even when the ovaries are not removed.

If my ovaries are taken out during surgery, should I take medicine to replace the hormones the ovaries used to produce?

The ovaries produce the female hormone estrogen. Estrogen helps the body in a number of ways. For example, it helps to prevent heart disease and osteoporosis (a condition in which the bones become weak and can break easily). It also prevents vaginal dryness.

There is some concern that taking estrogen after your body stops producing it naturally might be harmful. Some research has shown that taking estrogen for many years may increase your risk for breast cancer. Also, if you had endometriosis before menopause, your endometriosis may come back if you start to take estrogen after menopause.

You should carefully consider the risks and benefits of estrogen replacement therapy. Ask your doctor to explain anything you don't understand.

How will I feel after a hysterectomy?

Of course, every woman has a different reaction to having this surgery. If your ovaries are removed along with your uterus, you may experience hot flashes or other menopause-like symptoms, as if you were going through "the change." Your doctor may recommend estrogen replacement therapy or other medicine to help relieve your symptoms.

You may be concerned that you won't enjoy sex after the surgery, or that your partner might not find you as appealing. Talk with other women who have had this surgery. You may be surprised to learn that they still enjoy an active and satisfying sex life after hysterectomy.

Age is an important factor in how a woman reacts emotionally to hysterectomy. This is especially true for younger women who have not started or completed their families. Sometimes doctors can find ways to help you manage your condition if you want to become pregnant before the surgery. Sometimes, a hysterectomy is needed to preserve a woman's health, and it may not be possible to delay the surgery.

If giving up the chance to become pregnant is a hard decision for you, you may want to talk with your doctor or a social worker about adoption, foster parenting, or other alternatives.

As a treatment for noncancerous uterine conditions, hysterectomy is more likely than not to improve a woman's life. In part because it means the end of painful symptoms. A few women, however, feel worse following surgery and regret their decision to have a hysterectomy.

Ask your doctor to help you sort out your options and weigh the pros and cons of this surgery as they relate to your situation. You also may want to talk this over carefully with your family or others who are close to you before making a decision.

You might want to ask your doctor or nurse about joining a support group before or after your surgery. Talking over your concerns with other women who have had this surgery can be helpful.

Should I get a second opinion?

Getting a second opinion from another doctor is a good way to make sure that hysterectomy is the right option for you. Don't be uncomfortable about telling your doctor you want a second opinion. Doctors expect their patients to ask for another opinion.

Many health insurance plans require that you get a second opinion before you have any surgery. Check with your insurance company to find out if they will pay for a second opinion.

If you go for a second opinion, be sure to bring your medical records from your first doctor so that the second doctor does not have to repeat tests. Be sure both doctors explain their opinions clearly to you.

In Conclusion

Living with a noncancerous uterine condition can be painful, embarrassing, frightening, exhausting, and sometimes dangerous. There is no need for you to suffer. Treatments are available, and in many cases you need not give up your ability to become pregnant. Hysterectomy is not always the only—or even the best—option.

Deciding on the treatment that is right for you should be done in partnership with your doctor and your family. It is always a good idea to discuss your options with more than one doctor. And, it is important to let those who care about you know that you will need support and help while you are being treated.

Facts about Hysterectomy

Did you know:

- Hysterectomy is the second most frequently performed operation for women, second only to Cesarean section.

- Hysterectomy rates are much higher in the United States than in Norway, Sweden, or England.

- By age 65, more than 37 percent of all women in the United States will have had a hysterectomy.

- About 583,000 hysterectomies were performed on U.S. women in 1995.

- U.S. women are more likely to have a hysterectomy if they live in the South or the Midwest.

- Recent studies suggest that about 15 percent of all hysterectomies may be unnecessary.

- Recently trained physicians are less likely to recommend a hysterectomy than ones trained earlier.

- Nearly three-quarters of all hysterectomies are done when women are between 30 and 54 years of age.

- Annual hospital costs for hysterectomy exceed $5 billion per year.

Questions to Ask Your Doctor

Here is a list of questions you might want to ask your doctor. Not every question will apply to you, but the questions may help you to organize your thoughts and concerns.

- What is the name of my condition?

- What do you think is causing my condition?

- Is my condition related to a disease that could be sexually transmitted? If so, what should I tell my partner? What can be done to protect me and my partner?

- Where can I get more information about my condition?

- What are my treatment options (hormone treatment, another kind of medicine, watchful waiting, surgery, or other alternative)?

- Which treatment would you recommend for me? Why?

- Is there anything I can do on my own to help lessen my symptoms?

- Are there ways to handle my problem without having surgery or taking medicines?

- If I need surgery, how long will it take me to recover from the operation? What limits might there be on my activities, including sex?

- What could happen if I decide not to have surgery or other treatment, or if I want to put off treatment for a while?

No matter which treatment your doctor recommends, you should get a second opinion and find out as much as you can about:

- How the procedure will be done or what medicines will be given.

- How pain can be handled.

- What the recovery period after surgery or other treatment will be like.

- What the common side effects of the treatment are and what can be done about them.

- Whether the treatment will affect your ability to become pregnant.

You may have thought of some other questions you want to ask. If so, you may want to make a list before you go to the doctor.

Chapter 32

Uterine Fibroids

Introduction

Uterine fibroids are nodules of smooth muscle cells and fibrous connective tissue that develop within the wall of the uterus (womb). Medically they are called uterine leiomyomata (singular: leiomyoma). Fibroids may grow as a single nodule or in clusters and may range in size from 1 mm to more than 20 cm (8 inches) in diameter. They may grow within the wall of the uterus or they may project into the interior cavity or toward the outer surface of the uterus. In rare cases, they may grow on stalks or peduncles projecting from the surface of the uterus.

The factors that initiate fibroid growth are not known. The vast majority of fibroids occur in women of reproductive age, and according to some estimates, they are diagnosed in black women two to three times more frequently than in white women. They are seldom seen in young women who have not begun menarche (menstruation) and they usually stabilize or regress in women who have passed menopause.

Fibroids are the most frequently diagnosed tumor of the female pelvis. It is important to know that these are benign tumors. They are not associated with cancer, they virtually never develop into cancer, and they do not increase a woman's risk for uterine cancer.

An undated publication produced by the National Institute of Child Health and Human Development, available online at www.nichd.nih.gov/publications/pubs/uterine.htm; accessed February 2001.

No one knows how many new cases of uterine fibroids occur within any given length of time nor how many women have fibroids at any time. It has been estimated that up to 20 to 30 percent of women of reproductive age have fibroids, though not all have been diagnosed. More careful studies, however, indicate that the prevalence may be much higher. A study of 100 uteri that had been removed in consecutive hysterectomies yielded the following results: 33 had been diagnosed as having fibroids prior to surgery; routine pathologic examination disclosed that 52 had fibroids. However, a surprising 77 specimens were found with fibroids upon very close examination. The majority of the tumors were less than 1 cm in diameter and were missed during routine pathologic examination. These results indicate that more than three-quarters of women have uterine fibroids.

This is a small study, however, and its results should not be interpreted as applying to the entire female population, but as an indicator that perhaps the prevalence of fibroids is much higher than has been believed.*

Who is at Risk for Uterine Fibroids?

No risk factors have been found for uterine fibroids other than being a female of reproductive age. However, some factors have been described that seem to be protective. In some studies, again of small numbers of women, investigators found that as a group, women who have had two liveborn children have one-half the risk of having uterine fibroids compared to women who have had no liveborn children. It could not be discerned whether having children actually protects a woman from developing fibroids or whether fibroids contributed to the infertility of women who had no children.

Obese women in some studies were at increased risk of having fibroids, but other studies failed to confirm this. A lower risk has been found in both smokers and users of oral contraceptives in some studies, but not in all. However, it is important to note that smoking poses far greater health hazards than do uterine fibroids. Athletic women also seem to have a lower prevalence compared with women who do not engage in any athletic activities.

In view of the lack of information on fibroids, the National Institute of Child Health and Human Development (NICHD) is conducting research on the scientific basis for better diagnosis and treatment of fibroid tumors. It is hoped that the results of this research will enable the medical community to better predict who is at risk for fibroids, what can be done to prevent their development, and/or how to provide the most effective treatment for them.

Symptoms of Uterine Fibroids

How do you know if you have uterine fibroids? Probably you do not know. Most fibroids do not cause any symptoms and do not require treatment other than regular observation by a physician. Fibroids may be discovered during routine gynecologic examination or during pre-natal care. Some women who have uterine fibroids may experience symptoms such as excessive or painful bleeding during menstruation, bleeding between periods, a feeling of fullness in the lower abdomen, frequent urination resulting from a fibroid that compresses the bladder, pain during sexual intercourse, or low back pain. Although reproductive symptoms such as infertility, recurrent spontaneous abortion, and early onset of labor during pregnancy have been attributed to fibroids [it is unknown whether fibroids cause] any of these symptoms. In rare cases, a fibroid can compress and block the fallopian tube, preventing fertilization and migration of the ovum (egg); after surgical removal of the fibroid, fertility is generally restored.

Treatment for Fibroids

Until very recently, a woman with growing uterine fibroids was considered a candidate for hysterectomy (removal of the uterus). However, treatment by hysterectomy in a woman of reproductive age means that she will no longer be able to bear children and hysterectomy may have other effects, both physical and psychological, as well. A woman considering hysterectomy should discuss the pros and cons thoroughly with her physicians.

Although the number of hysterectomies has been declining since 1987, this operation remains the second most frequently performed surgery in the U.S.; only cesarean section is performed more frequently. Fibroids remain the number one reason for hysterectomy with 150,000 to 175,000 operations carried out each year because of fibroids.

Hysterectomy for uterine fibroids historically has been based on uterine size. Once the uterus reached the size that it would be in the 12th week of pregnancy it was considered time to perform a hysterectomy. The decision was based mainly on the fact that fibroids of such volume could shield the presence of uterine cancer. Without effective diagnostic procedures the medical community considered it safer to remove the uterus than to possibly harbor a growing malignancy. Now, however, improved imaging procedures such as ultrasound and magnetic resonance imaging (MRI) can effectively determine whether or not a rapidly growing tumor is present, reducing the number of hysterectomies performed. Therapy for uterine fibroids should be based on symptoms and not the idea that uterine fibroids will continue to grow until it becomes necessary to perform a hysterectomy.

If a fibroid is particularly troublesome, the surgeon often can remove only the tumor, leaving the uterus intact (leiomyomectomy).

This may leave the wall of the uterus weakened, in which case any pregnancy that occurs later most likely will be delivered by cesarean section. Many women with fibroids have successful outcomes of pregnancy with no undue incidence of miscarriage or other unfavorable outcome.

More and more, physicians are beginning to realize that uterine fibroids may not require any intervention or, at most, limited treatment. For a woman with uterine fibroids that are not symptomatic the best therapy may be watchful waiting. Some women never exhibit any symptoms or have any problems associated with fibroids, in which case no treatment is necessary. For women who experience occasional pelvic pain or discomfort, a mild, over-the-counter anti-inflammatory or painkilling drug often will be effective. More bothersome cases may require stronger drugs available by prescription.

The fact that fibroids seemingly are estrogen-dependent has led to attempts to control them by reduction in available estrogen. Hormone-like agents that counter the action of gonadotropin-releasing hormone (GnRH) are being investigated as one such agent. The use of a GnRH agonist lowers blood levels of estrogen and reduces uterine volume by as much as 60 percent.

Of primary concern in the use of such agents is the possibility of increasing blood cholesterol levels and reducing bone density, which may lead to osteoporosis. Although only modest increases in blood cholesterol have been noted in women undergoing this treatment, the therapy itself was of short duration. Unfortunately, the uterus returned to its pre-treatment size within 3 to 6 months after GnRH agonists were stopped.

It would seem from these observations that the use of GnRH agonists is of limited application. But, in fact, defined protocols have been worked out for administration of these agents for use in women who have symptoms, are poor candidates for surgery, and are nearing menopause. Also, for patients needing a hysterectomy, the use of GnRH agonists can reduce uterine size considerably, making abdominal hysterectomy easier or even allowing a vaginal hysterectomy rather than an abdominal one.

Three GnRH agonists are currently available. Two must be given by injection and the third is administered by an inhaler. Side effects that have been found include hot flashes, depression, insomnia, decreased libido, and joint pain. Maximum uterine shrinkage is achieved after 3 months of therapy.

Studies have only just begun on the newest class of antihormonal agents, the antiprogestins, the best known of which is RU 486.* Even though fibroids appear primarily stimulated by estrogens, drugs in this class which oppose the other major female hormone, progesterone, also seem to be effective for treatment of uterine fibroids. Studies using these drugs are still in the early stages.**

* Cramer, DW. Epidemiology of Myomas. *Seminars in Reproductive Endocrinology* 10:320-324, 1992.

** Supported by San Diego Reproductive Medicine Educational and Research Foundation, and NIH Grant RR-00827.

*** Murphy, AA. et al. *Journal of Clinical Endocrinology and Metabolism.*

Chapter 33

Facts about Endometriosis

Endometriosis is a common yet poorly understood disease. It can strike women of any socioeconomic class, age, or race. It is estimated that between 10 and 20 percent of American women of childbearing age have endometriosis. While some women with endometriosis may have severe pelvic pain, others who have the condition have no symptoms. Nothing about endometriosis is simple, and there are no absolute cures. The disease can affect a woman's whole existence—her ability to work, her ability to reproduce, and her relationships with her mate, her child, and every one around her.

What Is Endometriosis?

The name endometriosis comes from the word "endometrium," the tissue that lines the inside of the uterus. If a woman is not pregnant this tissue builds up and is shed each month. It is discharged as menstrual flow at the end of each cycle. In endometriosis, tissue that looks and acts like endometrial tissue is found outside the uterus, usually inside the abdominal cavity.

Endometrial tissue residing outside the uterus responds to the menstrual cycle in a way that is similar to the way endometrium usually responds in the uterus. At the end of every cycle, when hormones cause the uterus to shed its endometrial lining, endometrial tissue

National Institute of Child Health and Human Development (NICHD), NIH Publication No. 91-2413; Reviewed and revised by David A. Cooke, M.D. March 11, 2001.

growing outside the uterus will break apart and bleed. However, un-like menstrual fluid from the uterus, which is discharged from the body during menstruation, blood from the misplaced tissue has no place to go. Tissues surrounding the area of endometriosis may be-come inflamed or swollen. The inflammation may produce scar tissue around the area of endometriosis. These endometrial tissue sites may develop into what are called "lesions," "implants," "nodules," or "growths." Although its tendency to spread in some ways resembles cancers, en-dometriosis is not considered a cancer, and is not malignant.

Endometriosis is most often found in the ovaries, on the fallopian tubes, and the ligaments supporting the uterus, in the internal area between the vagina and rectum, on the outer surface of the uterus, and on the lining of the pelvic cavity. Infrequently, endometrial growths are found on the intestines or in the rectum, on the bladder, vagina, cervix, and vulva (external genitals), or in abdominal surgery scars. Very rarely, endometrial growths have been found outside the abdomen, in the thigh, arm, or lung.

Physicians may use stages to describe the severity of endometrio-sis. Endometrial implants that are small and not widespread are con-sidered minimal or mild endometriosis. Moderate endometriosis means that larger implants or more extensive scar tissue is present. Severe endometriosis is used to describe large implants and exten-sive scar tissue.

What Are the Symptoms?

Most commonly, the symptoms of endometriosis start years after menstrual periods begin. Over the years, the symptoms tend to gradu-ally increase as the endometriosis areas increase in size. After meno-pause, the abnormal implants shrink away and the symptoms subside.

The most common symptom is pain, especially excessive menstrual cramps (dysmenorrhea) which may be felt in the abdomen or lower back or pain during or after sexual activity (dyspareunia). Infertility occurs in about 30 to 40 percent of women with endometriosis. Rarely, the irritation caused by endometrial implants may progress into in-fection or abscesses causing pain independent of the menstrual cycle. Endometrial patches may also be tender to touch or pressure, and intestinal pain may also result from endometrial patches on the walls of the colon or intestine.

The amount of pain is not always related to the severity of the dis-ease—some women with severe endometriosis have no pain; while others with just a few small growths have incapacitating pain.

Endometrial cancer is very rarely associated with endometriosis, occurring in less than 1 percent of women who have the disease. When it does occur, it is usually found in more advanced patches of endometriosis in older women and the long-term outlook in these unusual cases is reasonably good.

How Is Endometriosis Related to Fertility Problems?

Severe endometriosis with extensive scarring and organ damage may affect fertility. It is considered one of the three major causes of female infertility. However, unsuspected or mild endometriosis is a common finding among infertile women and how this type of endometriosis affects fertility is still not clear. While the pregnancy rates for patients with endometriosis remain lower than those of the general population, most patients with endometriosis do not experience fertility problems.

What Is the Cause of Endometriosis?

The cause of endometriosis is still unknown. One theory is that during menstruation some of the menstrual tissue backs up through the fallopian tubes into the abdomen, where it implants and grows. Another theory suggests that endometriosis may be a genetic process or that certain families may have predisposing factors to endometriosis. In the latter view, endometriosis is seen as the tissue development process gone awry.

Whatever the cause of endometriosis, its progression is influenced by various stimulating factors such as hormones or growth factors. In this regard, the National Institute of Child Health and Human Development (NICHD) investigators are studying the role of the immune system in activating cells that may secrete factors which, in turn, stimulate endometriosis.

In addition to these new hypotheses, investigators are continuing to look into previous theories that endometriosis is a disease influenced by delayed childbearing. Since the hormones made by the placenta during pregnancy prevent ovulation, the progress of endometriosis is slowed or stopped during pregnancy and the total number of lifetime cycles is reduced for a woman who had multiple pregnancies.

How Is Endometriosis Diagnosed?

Diagnosis of endometriosis begins with a gynecologist evaluating the patient's medical history. A complete physical exam, including a pelvic examination, is also necessary. However, diagnosis of endometriosis is only complete when proven by a laparoscopy. The woman is placed under anesthesia, and then her abdominal cavity is inflated with carbon dioxide gas. The laparoscope, which is a narrow rod containing a light and a camera lens is inserted into the abdomen through a very small incision. The laparoscope is moved around the abdomen. The surgeon can then check the condition of the abdominal organs and see the endometrial implants. Implants usually look like small, brown to blue spots on organs or the abdominal lining. The laparoscopy will show the locations, extent, and size of the growths and will help the patient and her doctor make better-informed decisions about treatment.

What Is the Treatment?

While the treatment for endometriosis has varied over the years, doctors now agree that if the symptoms are mild, no further treatment other than medication for pain may be needed. For women who are not interested in becoming pregnant, oral contraceptive pills are frequently prescribed. This tends to improve pain, and may halt progression of endometriosis. For those patients with mild or minimal endometriosis who wish to become pregnant, doctors are advising that, depending on the age of the patient and the amount of pain associated with the disease, the best course of action is to have a trial period of unprotected intercourse for 6 months to 1 year. If pregnancy does not occur within that time, then further treatment may be needed.

For patients with more serious disease who are not seeking a pregnancy and for whom a definitive diagnosis of endometriosis by laparoscopy has been made, a physician may suggest hormone suppression treatment. Since this therapy shuts off ovulation, women being treated for endometriosis will not get pregnant during such therapy, although some may elect to become pregnant shortly after therapy is stopped.

Hormone treatment is most effective when the implants are small. The doctor may prescribe a weak synthetic male hormone called Danazol, a synthetic progestin alone, or a combination of estrogen and progestin such as oral contraceptives.

Danazol has become a more common treatment choice than either progestin or the birth control pill. Disease symptoms are improved for 80 to 90 percent of the patients taking Danazol, and the size and the extent of implants are also reduced. While side effects with

Danazol treatment are not uncommon (e.g., acne, hot flashes, or fluid retention), most of them are relatively mild and stop when treatment is stopped. Overall, pregnancy rates following this therapy depend on the severity of the disease. However, some recent studies have shown that with mild to minimal endometriosis, Danazol alone does not improve pregnancy rates.

It is important to remember that Danazol treatment is unsafe if there is any chance that a woman is pregnant. A fetus accidentally exposed to this drug may develop abnormally. For this same reason, although pregnancy is not likely while a woman is taking this drug, careful use of a barrier birth control method such as a diaphragm or condom is essential during this treatment.

Another type of hormone treatment is a synthetic pituitary hormone blocker called gonadotropin-releasing hormone agonist, or GnRH agonist. This treatment stops ovarian hormone production by blocking pituitary gland hormones that normally stimulate ovarian cycles.

Several agents of this type have been developed over the past decade. Some names include leuprolide, nafarelin, and goserelin. Nafarelin is administered as a nasal spray, while leuprolide and goserelin are injections. All of these drugs are believed to improve endometriosis by reducing levels of hormones that stimulate endometrial implants to grow. The major side effects of these drugs are hot flashes, similar to those experienced by women undergoing menopause. There has also been concern about loss of bone mineral density that may occur with prolonged therapy. This may limit the duration and frequency of this type of treatment. As with Danazol, pregnancy cannot occur while taking these medications, but treatment for several months followed by discontinuation of the drug can improve fertility.

While pregnancy rates for women with fertility problems resulting from endometriosis are fairly good with no therapy and with only a trial waiting period, there may be women who need more aggressive treatment. Those women who are older and who feel the need to become pregnant more quickly or those women who have severe physical changes due to the disease, may consider surgical treatment. Also, women who are not interested in pregnancy, but who have severe, debilitating pain, may also consider surgery.

Surgical therapy of endometriosis is usually performed laparoscopically. In a procedure similar to that used to diagnose endometriosis, a laparoscope is inserted into the abdomen while the patient is under anesthesia. The endometrial implants are identified, and then destroyed using special tools attached to the laparoscope. Most often this is done using a laser, which vaporises the endometrial implants with minimal damage to healthy surrounding tissue. Other techniques include use of hot probes or cutting tools to remove the implants Less often, the surgery is done via laparotomy, which involves making a traditional surgical incision, and is performed in a hospital under anesthesia. Surgical removal of implants is moderately effective in reducing pain and improving fertility, although it does not succeed for all patients. Pregnancy rates are highest during the first year after surgery, as recurrences of endometriosis are fairly common. The specifics of the surgery should be discussed with a doctor.

Some women with endometriosis and infertility may benefit from In Vitro Fertilization (IVF) procedures, which are popularly known as "test-tube baby" methods. In IVF, the woman's eggs are directly harvested from her ovaries, then combined with the father's sperm in a laboratory. Fertilized eggs are then placed directly in the uterus. For women that have severe scarring of their ovaries and fallopian tubes, which interferes with her eggs reaching her uterus, this can be quite successful. However, it is expensive, and many health insurance plans do not cover it. It also increases the risk of multiple births.

Some patients may need more radical surgery to correct the damage caused by untreated endometriosis. Hysterectomy and removal of the ovaries may be the only treatment possible if the ovaries are badly damaged. In some cases, hysterectomy alone without the removal of the ovaries may be reasonable.

Where To Look For Answers

Because endometriosis affects each woman differently, it is essential that the patient maintains a good, clear, honest communication with her doctor. For the single truth about endometriosis is that there are no clear-cut, universal answers.

If pregnancy is an issue, then age may affect the treatment plan. If it is not an issue, then treatment decisions will depend primarily on the severity of symptoms.

A number of organizations provide information about the diagnosis and treatment of endometriosis and offer support to women affected by this disease and their families. Please note that while the groups listed below are valuable resources for information about endometriosis, they were not consulted in the writing of this publication.

The information presented here does not necessarily reflect the views of these organizations.

Endometriosis Association
8585 North 76th Place
Milwaukee, WI 53223
Phone: 414-355-2200

The American College of Obstetricians and Gynecologists
409 12th Street, SW
Washington, DC 20024-2188
Phone: 202-638-5577

American Fertility Society
2140-11th Avenue South, Suite 200
Birmingham, AL 35205-2800
Phone: 205-933-8494

Chapter 34

Ovarian Cysts

What is an ovarian cyst?

An ovarian cyst is a fluid-filled sac in the ovary. Many cysts are completely normal. These are called functional cysts. They occur as a result of ovulation (the release of an egg from the ovary). Functional cysts normally shrink over time, usually in about 1 to 3 months. If you have a functional cyst, your doctor may want to check you again in 1 to 3 months to make sure the cyst has gotten smaller. Or your doctor may want you to take birth control pills so you won't ovulate. If you don't ovulate, you won't form cysts.

If you are menopausal and are not having periods, you shouldn't form functional cysts. If you do have a cyst, your doctor will probably want you to have a sonogram so he or she can look at the cyst. What your doctor decides to do after that depends on your age, the way the cyst looks on the sonogram, and if you're having symptoms such as pain, bloating, feeling full after eating just a little, and constipation.

What is a sonogram?

A sonogram uses sound waves to make "pictures" of organs in the body. It's a good way to "look" at ovaries. This kind of sonogram can be done 2 ways, either through your abdomen or your vagina. Neither type is painful. The sonogram usually lasts about 30 minutes. It will give your doctor valuable information about the size and the appearance of your cyst.

Are there any other tests I might have?

Your doctor might test the level of a protein called CA-125 in your blood. This is a blood test that is often done in women with ovarian cancer. Sometimes this test is done in women with an ovarian cyst to see if their cyst could be cancerous. A normal CA-125 level is less than 35. However, this test is not always an accurate way to tell if a woman has cancer. For example, some women who do have ovarian cancer have a normal CA-125 level. Also, this level can sometimes be high in women who do not have cancer, particularly if they are in their childbearing years. For these reasons, the CA-125 blood test is usually only recommended for women who are at high risk for ovarian cancer.

Do I need surgery for an ovarian cyst?

The answer depends on several things, such as your age, whether you are having periods, the size of the cyst, its appearance, and your symptoms.

If you're having periods and the cyst is functional, you probably won't need to have surgery. If the cyst doesn't go away after several menstrual periods, if it gets larger, or if it doesn't look like a functional cyst on the sonogram, your doctor may want you to have an operation to remove it. There are many different types of ovarian cysts in women of childbearing age that do require surgery. Fortunately, cysts in women of this age are almost always benign (not cancer).

If you're past menopause and have an ovarian cyst, your doctor will probably want you to have surgery. Ovarian cancer is rare, but women 50 to 70 years of age are at greater risk. Women who are diagnosed at an early stage do much better than women who are diagnosed later.

What type of surgery would I need?

The type of surgery you need depends on several things, such as the size of the cyst, how the cyst looks on the sonogram, and if your doctor thinks it might be cancer. If the cyst is small (about the size of a plum) and if it looks benign on the sonogram, your doctor may decide to do a laparoscopy. This type of surgery is done with a lighted instrument called a laparoscope that's like a slender telescope. This is put into your abdomen through a small incision (cut) just above or just below your navel. With the laparoscope, your doctor can see your organs. Often the cyst can be removed with only small incisions in the pubic hair line. If the cyst looks too big to remove with the laparoscope or if it looks suspicious in any way, your doctor will probably do a laparotomy.

A laparotomy uses a bigger incision to remove the cyst or possibly the entire ovary. The cyst can be tested while you are under general anesthesia (puts you into a sleeplike state) to find out if it is cancer. If it is cancer, your doctor may need to remove both of the ovaries, the uterus, a fold of fatty tissue called the omentum, and some lymph nodes. It's very important that you talk to your doctor about all of this before the surgery. Your doctor will also talk to you about the risks of each kind of surgery, how long you are likely to be in the hospital and how long it will be before you can go back to your normal activities.

Chapter 35

Cervical Dysplasia and Human Papillomavirus (HPV)

What is cervical dysplasia?

When a female goes to a clinic or her health care provider for a Pap smear, they are screening the cells on her cervix to make sure that there are no abnormal or precancerous changes. If the Pap smear results show these cell changes, this is usually called cervical dysplasia. Other common terms the health care provider may use include:

- Abnormal cell changes
- Precancerous cells changes
- CIN (cervical intraepithelial neoplasia)
- SIL (squamous intraepithelial lesions)
- "Warts" on the cervix

All of these terms are equal—it simply means that abnormalities were found. Most of the time, these cell changes are due to human papillomavirus (HPV). There are many types of HPV that can cause cervical dysplasia. Most of these types are considered "high-risk" types, which means that they have been linked with cervical cancer.

- Just because a female has cervical dysplasia, it does not mean she will get cervical cancer. It means that her health care provider will want to monitor her closely every so often—and possibly do treatment—to prevent further cell changes that could become cancerous.

- HPV is a very common virus, and most females with HPV do not develop cervical cancer.

What about abnormal Pap smear results?

There term "abnormal Pap smear" is vague and not very specific. There are many different systems that health care providers use to classify a Pap smear. Within each system, there are different degrees of severity or abnormalities. Different classification systems and degrees of severity include:

- Descriptive System: mild, moderate, or severe dysplasia

- CIN System: CIN (cervical intraepithelial neoplasia) 1, 2, or 3

- Bethesda System: Low-Grade or High-Grade SIL (squamous intraepithelial lesion)

- Class System: Class 1 though Class 4.

Women with abnormal Pap smears are usually examined further for cervical problems. This may involve coming back for a colposcopy and biopsy, or coming back in a few months for another Pap smear.

It is important for a female to get a Pap smear at regular intervals by the time she reaches 18 years of age, or by the time she becomes sexually active—which ever comes first.

What's the difference between a Pap smear, a biopsy, and an HPV test?

A Pap smear is a screening to find abnormal cell changes on the cervix (cervical dysplasia) before they turn into cancer. These precancerous cervical changes are caused by HPV.

A biopsy is similar to a Pap smear, but a larger cluster of cells is removed from the cervix to see if there are abnormal cell changes. It is a good way to confirm the Pap smear and to rule out cancer.

An HPV test is different from a Pap smear or biopsy. This test checks directly for the genetic material (DNA) of HPV within cells. The only commercially available test for HPV is called Hybrid Capture II™, produced by Digene.

When is the HPV test used?

If a Pap smear result is borderline between "normal" and "abnormal." This is usually called "atypical cells" or "ASCUS." The HPV test is most commonly used to determine which women with a borderline result are likely to have precancerous changes on their cervix (HPV positive) and which are most likely to be normal cells (HPV negative). It helps to rule out whether HPV is causing the borderline abnormal cells.

When is the HPV test NOT used?

- If the Pap smear results show dysplasia or precancerous changes. This is because it is automatically assumed that the HPV is the cause.

- The HPV test can not be used on males.

- The HPV test is only FDA-approved to be used on the female's cervix.

Can a male find out if he has the cell-changing types of HPV?

Research has shown that the HPV test usually shows false negative results in men. This is because it is difficult to get a good cell sample to test from the thick skin on the penis.

Most people will not have visible symptoms if they are exposed to HPV. Therefore, for most, the virus is subclinical (invisible). This is especially true for males. If a male is exposed to the cell-changing types of HPV, he would be unlikely to have symptoms. If there are no symptoms for males, it is hard to test for it.

Most of the time, men will not have any health risks such as cancer with the "high-risk" types of HPV. It is the female's cervix that needs to be monitored.

How can a person get the types of HPV that cause cell changes?

- Any person who is sexually active can be exposed and get the cell-changing types of HPV.

- Most people are exposed to the cell-changing types of HPV at some point, but not everyone (especially males) will actually have abnormal cell changes (dysplasia).

- The types of HPV that cause abnormal cell changes are usually spread by direct skin-to-skin contact during vaginal, anal, or possibly through oral sex, with someone who has this infection.

- The cell-changing types of HPV are most likely to be given to a partner when dysplasia is actually present.

- Very little is known about passing subclinical (invisible) HPV to sex partners. Some experts think it may be less contagious than when the cell changes are present.

- The types of HPV that cause abnormal cell changes do not typically cause symptoms on other body parts such as the hands.

- Recent research studies have shown a relationship between a cell-changing type of HPV and some rare head and neck cancers, but there is not much evidence that oral sex definitely transmits these types of HPV.

How can someone reduce the risk of getting HPV?

Any one who is sexually active can come across this common virus. Ways to reduce the risk are:

- Not having sex with anyone.

- Having sex only with one partner who has sex only with you. People who have many sex partners are at higher risk of getting other STDs.

- If someone currently has abnormal cell changes, he or she should not have sexual activity until after the cells have been treated or have self resolved. This may help to lower the risk of transmission.

- Condoms (rubbers), used the right way from start to finish each time of having sex may help provide minimal protection—but only for the skin that is covered by the condom. Condoms do not cover all genital skin, so they don't give 100% protection.

- Spermicidal foams, creams, and jellies are not proven to act against HPV, but they work against some other STDs. These are best used along with condoms, not in place of condoms.

- If someone was exposed to the types of HPV that can cause abnormal cell changes, it would be unlikely that he or she will become re-infected with those same types since immunity will be set-up at some point.

- Realize that most people are exposed to one or more HPV types in their lifetime, and most will never even know it because they will not have visible symptoms.

- It is important for partners to understand the "entire picture" about HPV so that both people can make informed decisions based on facts, not fear or misconceptions.

How are abnormal cells treated?

- Currently, there is no treatment to cure HPV; there is no cure for any virus at this point. However, there are several treatment options available for treating the abnormal cells.

- Sometimes treatment may not even be necessary for mild cervical dysplasia. These cells can heal on their own and the health care provider will just want to monitor the cervix. HPV may then be in a latent (sleeping) state, but it is unknown if it totally gone or just not detectable.

- The goal of any treatment will be to get remove the abnormal cells. This may also end up removing most of the cells with the HPV in them.

- If the abnormal cells are treated, or if they have healed on their own, it may possibly help reduce the risk of transmission to a partner who may have never been exposed to the cell-changing types of HPV.

- When choosing what treatment to use, the health care provider will consider many things:
  - location of the abnormal cells
  - size of the lesions on the cervix
  - degree or severity of the Pap smear results
  - degree or severity of the colposcopy and biopsy results
  - HPV test results (if this test was needed)
  - age and pregnancy status
  - previous treatment history
  - patient and health care provider preferences

There are a variety of treatments for cervical dysplasia:

- Cryotherapy (freezing the cells with liquid nitrogen)

- LEEP (Loop Electrosurgical Excision Procedure)

- Conization (also called cone biopsy)

- Laser (not as widely used today due to high cost, lack of availability, and not all doctors are well-trained with using it. LEEP is more commonly used)

- No treatment at all; the health care provider will just monitor the cervix every three, four or six months until several Pap smear results in a row come back normal

What about pregnancy, HPV, and cervical dysplasia?

- For some pregnant women, cervical dysplasia may increase. This may be due to hormone changes during pregnancy, but this is not proven.

- If a woman has an abnormal Pap smear during pregnancy, even if it's severely abnormal, many health care providers will not do treatment. They will just monitor the cervix closely with a colposcope during the pregnancy.

- Sometime (a few weeks) after delivery of the baby, the provider will look at the cervix again and do another Pap smear or another biopsy. Many times after pregnancy, the cell changes will have spontaneously resolved—and no treatment will be necessary.

- The reason that many health care providers do not want to do treatment during pregnancy is because it may accidentally cause early labor.

- The types of HPV that can cause cell changes on the cervix and genital skin have not been found to cause problems for babies.

What about HPV and other cancers?

Anal dysplasia and anal cancer:

- Anal cancer is a rare occurrence that has been strongly linked to "high-risk" types of HPV.

- Abnormal cell changes in the anal area (anal dysplasia or anal neoplasia) are more common among individuals who engage in receiving anal sex.

- However, anal dysplasia has also been reported in some females who have a history of severe cervical dysplasia

- Treatment is available for anal dysplasia and anal cancer

Penile Intraepithelial Neoplasia (PIN) and penile cancer:

- Cancer of the penis is extremely rare in the United States, and HPV is not always the cause.

- There are some cases of cell changes (neoplasia) on the penis, which are caused by "high-risk" types of HPV.

- Most males do not ever experience symptoms or health risks if they get one or more "high-risk" types of HPV.

- Penile neoplasia can be treated.

- There is not a cancer screening for the penis because cancer of the penis is extremely rare, and because it is difficult to get a good cell sample from the penis.

Vaginal Intraepithelial Neoplasia (VAIN) and vaginal cancer:

- HPV has been linked with some, but not all, cases of cell changes in the vagina and with vaginal cancers.

- Various treatment options are available for vaginal neoplasia, depending on how mild or severe the cell changes are in this area.

Vulvar Intraepithelial Neoplasia (VIN) and vulvar cancer:

- HPV has been linked with some, but not all, cases of cell changes on the vulva (outside female genital area) and with vulvar cancers.

- Various treatment options are available for vulvar neoplasia, depending on how mild or severe the cell changes are in this area.

Is it normal to feel upset about HPV?

Yes, it is normal. Some people feel very upset. They feel ashamed, fearful, confused, less attractive or less interested in sex. They feel angry at their sex partner(s), even though it is usually not possible to know exactly when or from whom the virus was spread.

Some people are afraid that they will get cancer, or that they will never be able to find a sexual partner again. It is normal to have all, some, or none of these feelings. It may take some time, but it is important to know that it is still possible to have a normal, healthy life, even with HPV.

Ways to help cope with HPV emotionally:

• Talk to someone you can trust such as a friend or loved one

• Go to an HPV support group

• Get educated and learn the facts about HPV

For More Information

For more information about HPV and other sexually transmitted diseases, contact:

American Social Health Association
P.O. Box 13827
Research Triangle Park, NC 27709
Phone: (919) 361-8400
Fax: (919) 361-8425

Part Six

Cancer Screening and Prevention

Chapter 36

What You Need to Know about the Pap Examination

No cancer screening test in medical history is as effective for early detection of cancer as the Pap examination. Since the Pap examination was introduced after World War II, death rates from uterine cervical cancer have decreased 70 percent in the U.S. Unfortunately, thousands of women still fail to have annual Pap examinations. And sadly, of those women who do die of cervical cancer, 80 percent have not had a Pap examination in five years or more.

What is a Pap examination?

The Pap examination (sometimes called the Pap test or Pap smear) is named for George Papanicolaou, MD, a physician who pioneered this method of cancer detection in the 1930s.

A Pap examination is usually performed at the time of a pelvic examination, which can help detect signs of cancer in female organs other than the cervix. A Pap examination is a simple procedure in which your physician painlessly obtains cells from the surface of your cervix, often using a special brush to sample the area where most cancers begin to develop. The cells are placed on a glass slide, which is sent to a laboratory.

At the laboratory, the cells are stained and then examined under a microscope by specially trained cytotechnologists. If an abnormality is found, a pathologist, a physician who specializes in laboratory medicine, studies the cells and makes the final interpretation.

The results of your Pap examination are reported to your doctor within several weeks. Many doctors notify patients of their examination results in writing or by telephone. Others ask patients to call the office for their results. No matter what your doctor's preference, it's important that you find out the results of your Pap examination.

What can I learn from my Pap examination?

The Pap examination is a screening test for cervical cancer. Its primary purpose is to detect early cervical cancer and precancerous conditions. An abnormal Pap smear often means precancer, a change that can lead to cervical cancer if left untreated. If cancerous or precancerous cells are found, the next step is a more thorough examination of your cervix, during which your physician will obtain tissue biopsies for a pathologist to study. Sometimes, an abnormal Pap smear means there are uncertain cell changes that could be precancerous or could be entirely benign, needing no further investigation. Your physician may recommend repeat Pap smears or tissue biopsies to explain these uncertain changes.

A Pap examination also may detect infections such as bacteria, yeast, or viruses. One kind of sexually transmitted virus is important to detect because of its link to cervical cancer. This virus is human papillomavirus (HPV), sometimes called "condyloma," or genital warts.

Who should have a Pap examination?

Every woman should have an annual Pap examination when she becomes sexually active or turns 18 years old—whichever comes first. Regular Pap examinations should continue after menopause and after a hysterectomy (removal of the uterus).

When is the best time to get a Pap examination?

If you are having menstrual periods, the best time for a Pap examination is during the two weeks following the end of menstrual flow. If you've reached menopause, you can schedule your Pap examination anytime.

To ensure that the cells your physician obtains during the exam are adequate for evaluation, you should abstain from sexual activity and avoid using vaginal douches or lubricants for 48 hours before the examination.

How often should I have a Pap examination?

The College of American Pathologists recommends that you have yearly Pap and pelvic examinations. Cervical cancer takes time to develop into a deadly disease. With early detection by a Pap examination, cervical precancer or cancer can be treated with a high probability of cure. The pelvic exam is added insurance; it can help detect signs of cancer in female organs other than the cervix.

What does my doctor need to know about me?

Your physician and the pathologist who reviews your Pap examination need answers to the following questions:

- Have you ever had an abnormal Pap exam in the past?

- Are you or have you been sexually active? Have you been exposed to any sexually transmitted diseases?

- Have you had vaginal infections or abnormal vaginal discharge?

- When was your last menstrual period?

- Have you had any "spotting" or abnormal bleeding?

- Are you taking medications such as antibiotics, birth control pills, hormone pills or creams, or medication for heart disease?

- Have you had surgery, chemotherapy, or radiation treatment?

- Are you pregnant?

Are some women more at risk for cervical cancer than others?

Any woman can develop cancer of the cervix, but you are at a higher risk if:

- You have had multiple sex partners or a male partner who has had multiple female partners. If your partner has had sex with other women, you are at high risk even if you have had only one partner.

- You have had genital warts.

- You had sexual relations before the age of 18.

- You previously had an abnormal Pap examination.

Although not having a Pap examination doesn't cause cancer, you are at a greater risk if you have never had a Pap examination, or had your last one three or more years ago.

What are my responsibilities toward cancer detection?

If detected early, cervical cancer can be treated with a high rate of cure. Even better, most cases of cervical cancer can be prevented by detection and treatment of precancerous lesions. Do your part and make an annual Pap and pelvic examination part of your total health care program. It could save your life.

How reliable and accurate are Pap examinations?

No other screening procedure in medical history is as effective for detecting cancer. As effective as the Pap examination is, however, it is not perfect. A single Pap examination cannot be considered 100 percent reliable for several reasons:

- The cell-sample obtained might not include abnormal cells.

- Abnormal cells might have been washed away by douching, lubricants, or sexual activity.

- Abnormal cells may have escaped detection.

Your best assurance that cervical cancer will be detected early is to schedule a Pap examination once every year and to make sure that the sample is studied at an accredited laboratory.

What makes a laboratory accredited?

Find out if the laboratory evaluating your Pap examination is accredited by the College of American Pathologists or another recognized accrediting body. Accreditation guarantees that the laboratory has been inspected by outside professionals and that the personnel use quality control and quality assurance procedures daily. In an accredited laboratory, you can be sure that pathologists and cytotechnologists who analyze your Pap smear have the proper training and experience. To find out if the laboratory that evaluates your Pap examination is accredited, or for more information about women's health issues, call 800-LAB-5678.

Can I question my doctor about the quality of the laboratory that will examine my Pap smear?

Certainly! You can and should make sure your Pap examination will be evaluated by qualified personnel in an accredited laboratory. Some questions you might ask include:

- What is the name of the laboratory and where is it located?

- Is the laboratory accredited? Is it ever inspected?

- Do you (the physician) have good communication with the pathologist at the laboratory where my Pap examination will be evaluated?

- Can I see a copy of my Pap examination report? Will you explain the results to me?

- Will the laboratory inform you if my cell sample is not adequate for study so another sample can be taken?

If the laboratory that your doctor uses is not accredited, you can request that your Pap examination be sent to an accredited laboratory.

About the College of American Pathologists

The mission of the College of American Pathologists, the principal organization of board-certified pathologists, is to represent the interests of the public, patients, and pathologists by fostering excellence in the practice of pathology worldwide.

Please note the College of American Pathologists does not offer medical advice. This information is provided as a public service to help you better understand medical conditions. Consult your personal physician to seek medical advice.

Chapter 37

New Devices Aim at Improving Pap Test Accuracy

Early detection means everything with cervical cancer. There are no early-warning symptoms or physical changes that a woman can detect. The only defense is an accurate Pap test.

The Food and Drug Administration has recently approved three new automated systems that show promise of substantially improving the accuracy of Pap tests.

A Silent Cancer

Unlike many cancers that cause pain, noticeable lumps, or other early symptoms, cervical cancer has no telltale symptoms until it is so advanced that it is usually unresponsive to treatment. Symptoms may even be absent at that point, although they often include abnormal vaginal bleeding, such as following intercourse or douching, between menstrual periods, or after menopause. Only in its late stages does cervical cancer cause pain in the lower abdominal or back regions.

But because the cervix, or neck of the uterus, can be easily accessed through the vagina, doctors can test for cervical cancer as well as for precancerous changes in the cervix. Most cervical cancers grow slowly over several years and often are preceded by abnormal cells. Cervical cancer can often be prevented by the removal of these abnormal cells.

To detect abnormal or cancerous cervical cells, George Papanicolaou, M.D., Ph.D., of Cornell University developed in the 1940s what

This article originally appeared in the October 1996 *FDA Consumer*. This version contains revisions made in September 1997. Pub. No. (FDA) 97-4264.

is known today as the Pap test. In this test, a sample of cells is taken from in and around the cervix with a wooden scraper, cotton swab, or small cervical brush. The specimen is smeared on a glass slide, preserved with alcohol, and then sent to a laboratory. There cytotechnologists, specially trained in identifying abnormal cells, scrutinize the cervical cells under the microscope for any abnormal features associated with cancerous or precancerous cervical cells. These features include dark or irregularly shaped cell nuclei, or small or deformed cells.

The Pap test became a routine part of gynecological exams. As a result, there was a 70 percent drop in the number of women dying from cervical cancer between 1950 and 1970, according to the National Cancer Institute. But the problem of errors remained. Such errors are understandable when considering the magnitude of the task set before the cytotechnologist examining Pap slides. These standard-sized laboratory slides are lined with between 50,000 to 300,000 cervical cells. Lurking in these cells may be as few as a dozen abnormal cells. Finding such telltale cells is akin to finding a needle in a haystack, especially at the end of the day when cytotechnologists are likely to have examined nearly 100 Pap slides. In addition, abnormalities in cell shape may be slight and difficult for even the trained eye to detect, or may be masked by infection.

Improving Detection

A new slide preparation method may improve the accuracy of the initial screening.

The ThinPrep Processor Model 2000 is an automated slide preparation system for Pap smears that may make it easier to screen for atypical cells. Safety and effectiveness data submitted by the manufacturer to FDA demonstrated that slides prepared with the ThinPrep system are significantly more effective in a variety of patient populations for detecting low-grade squamous intraepithelial lesions (SILs) and some of the more severe lesions. In addition, the ThinPrep Processor is as safe and effective as the conventional method of preparing slides by hand for detecting all categories of atypical and diseased cervical cells.

In this system, improved quality comes from an automated process that concentrates the cellular material and filters out a lot of blood and other unneeded material.

The other new systems are computerized rescreening methods. In both systems, computers scan the slides for abnormal-looking cells.

One system, called PAPNET, uses neural net computer technology, which its manufacturer claims was originally created to detect flying missiles in what is known as the "Star Wars" defense strategy. PAPNET detects abnormal cervical cells with a computer system that essentially has learned by example. This system was created by feeding a series of digitized images of Pap slides to a computer. From these examples, the computer developed the guidelines for predicting abnormal cells.

PAPNET scans each Pap slide cytotechnologists have classified as normal and chooses the 128 cells or cell clusters that are most likely to be abnormal. Enlarged color images of these cells are then returned to the cytotechnologist for review.

Studies have used PAPNET rescreening to reexamine previous negative Pap smears taken from women with high-grade cervical cell abnormalities or cervical cancers. These studies found that in about one-third of these women, PAPNET testing detected abnormalities missed by manual screening on previous Pap smears.

The other Pap test rescreening system is called AutoPap 300 QC. This computerized system uses image interproduction and pattern recognition techniques to classify cells as abnormal. Hundreds of features—such as size, shape, density, and texture—are considered for each cell. Sophisticated statistical screens use this visual information to predict which cervical cells are abnormal. Following routine screening by a cytotechnologist, all "normal" slides are rescreened by AutoPap 300 QC, which selects 10 to 20 percent of slides with the highest probability of having abnormal cells. These are then rescreened manually by the cytotechnologist.

In one study, cytotechnologists randomly rescreening 10 percent of more than 4,000 Pap slides they originally classified as normal detected only about 1 of every 10 false negatives present. Cytotechnologists using AutoPap 300 QC to select the 10 percent of slides the system deemed as being most abnormal detected up to half of all the missed abnormals.

All three products are available for use by laboratories, but some labs may not yet be fully familiar with these new systems.

"Laboratories are starting to evaluate these devices and determine if and how they will use them," said Louise Magruder, of FDA's division of clinical laboratory devices.

Although use of ThinPrep, PAPNET and AutoPap 300 QC will considerably decrease the likelihood of missing a diagnosis of cervical cancer, none of these systems is perfect. Even if the rescreening systems could detect every abnormal cell on a Pap slide, some women with cervical cancer would still be told their Pap tests were normal because there were too few cells on the slide or the cell samples were not taken from both the inside and surface of the cervix. Douching or using vaginal spermicides or medicines a day or two before a Pap test can also wash away abnormal cells and thus reduce the test's accuracy.

Also, there is a small percentage of women who develop a rare form of aggressive cervical cancer that can develop to an advanced stage in less than a year. In addition, cervical cancer will continue to occur in women who don't receive regular gynecological exams and Pap tests. Most health professionals recommend that all women who are or have been sexually active or have reached age 18 have a Pap smear and gynecological exam as frequently as each year, but at least every three years, depending on their risk factors for cervical cancer.

There may be one exception to this recommendation: Researchers at Louisiana State University, writing in the Nov. 21, 1996, issue of the *New England Journal of Medicine,* found that the benefits of Pap tests for most women who have had hysterectomies are limited. The Pap test in such women is used to detect abnormal vaginal cells, and the researchers found the tests of little value for this use in women who had had hysterectomies for reasons other than cancer.

Risk Factors

Evidence collected over the past few decades suggests several risk factors for developing cervical cancer. These include having sexual intercourse before age 18, having several sexual partners, or having a sexual partner who previously had a long-term sexual relationship with a woman who had cervical cancer.

Scientists are closely scrutinizing the sexually transmitted human papillomaviruses (HPVs), some of which cause genital warts. Research strongly suggests some types of HPVs (there are more than 60 different types) can trigger the growth of abnormal cells in the cervix and are likely to play a key role in the development of cervical cancer. Women who have HPV or whose partners have HPV have an increased risk of developing cervical cancer.

However, many women infected with HPV do not develop cervical cancer, and not all women with cervical cancer harbor HPV. This suggests other factors act with HPV to cause cervical cancer. The genital herpes virus may play a role, as may the strength of a woman's immune system. Women infected with HIV, the virus that causes AIDS, are more likely to develop cervical cancer, as are female organ transplant patients who receive drugs that suppress the immune system to prevent rejection of the new organ.

Hormones may also influence the development of cervical cancer. The labeling of oral contraceptives states that some studies have found an increased incidence of cervical cancer in women taking birth control pills, but that this may be related to factors other than the pill. Women whose mothers took the estrogen-like drug diethylstilbestrol (DES) during pregnancy to prevent miscarriage are also more likely to develop cervical cancer. (DES was used to prevent miscarriages from about 1940 to 1970.)

Smoking also elevates the risk of cervical cancer, which rises with the number of cigarettes a woman smokes each day and with the number of years she has smoked. Women exposed to other people's tobacco smoke are also more likely to develop cervical cancer.

Research suggests women can reduce their risk of cervical cancer by using barrier methods of contraception, such as the diaphragm with spermicide and condoms, probably because such methods decrease the risk of being infected by a sexually transmitted disease.

At present, early detection of precancerous tissue remains the most effective way of preventing cervical cancer. When detected in its early stages nearly all cervical cancers can be cured with minor surgery or other practices.

In contrast, fewer than 20 percent of women with advanced cervical cancer survive more than five years, even with treatment, according to the National Cancer Institute. There are nearly 5,000 deaths due to cervical cancer each year in this country. Recent data from NCI reveal that the number of cases of cervical cancer in white women under the age of 50 in the United States has been increasing 3 percent each year since 1986. In contrast, incidence rates are declining in black women of all ages and in white women over age 50. According to the World Health Organization, cervical cancer is also the most common cancer among women in developing countries. New technologies available now may enhance the value of the Pap test, but for women the most important step is getting screened.

Early Detection Gives Time for Treatment

Most cervical cancers gradually progress over a period of years without immediately invading nearby tissue. Yet they leave telltale signposts along their way. Even the transition from a normal to a cancerous cervical cell is usually a gradual one, with several steps that can be seen with the aid of a microscope.

In what is thought to be one of the first steps in the development of cervical cancer, the nuclei of cervical cells enlarge and darken. A patch of these abnormal cells is termed a squamous intraepithelial lesion (SIL) because the abnormal cells are present only in the squamous epithelial cells which line the surface of the cervix. SILs are further classified as low-grade if the abnormal cells are of normal size, or high-grade if the cells are smaller than normal.

Low-grade SILs are common; most spontaneously revert to normal. But because some will progress to high-grade SILs and then to cervical cancer, most doctors ask women with this Pap diagnosis to have Pap tests every four to six months for about two years. After three consecutive Pap tests come back negative, women can return to a routine screening protocol.

If repeated Pap tests show persistent abnormalities, however, a woman's doctor may want to confirm the low-grade SIL diagnosis by further scrutinizing the cervix with other procedures.

Colposcopy is a widely used method to check the cervix for abnormal areas. The doctor applies special stains to the cervix and then uses an instrument much like a microscope (called a colposcope) to detect abnormal cells, which turn a different color than healthy cells.

The doctor also may want to remove a small amount of cervical tissue for examination with a biopsy. It also may be necessary to scrape more tissue from inside the cervical opening. These procedures can be done in the doctor's office under local anesthesia.

If the low-grade SIL diagnosis is confirmed, a doctor may ask the patient to continue to have frequent Pap tests. Alternatively, the doctor may prefer to destroy the abnormal area by freezing it (cryosurgery), burning it (cauterization), or by removing it with a laser or electrosurgical device. Such treatment may cause cramping or other pain, bleeding, or a watery discharge.

High-grade SILs rarely regress spontaneously. Most progress to cervical cancer over a period of 10 to 15 years, according to the National Cancer Institute. Women who have high-grade SIL Pap reports usually are asked to undergo a colposcopy or biopsy procedure to confirm diagnosis. Once the high-grade SIL diagnosis is certain, doctors usually destroy the lesion with one of the procedures described in the previous paragraph. Or, the lesion and adjacent tissue may be surgically removed.

If a high-grade SIL progresses to the point that the cell nuclei become jagged or irregular in shape, extremely dark, and enlarged, and the cells themselves are strangely shaped (tadpole- or spindle-shaped, for example, instead of round), the lesion is considered cancerous. If the cancer is limited in scope, it may be treated with some of the same methods used to destroy precancerous lesions. For more widespread cancers, more involved surgery is usually done, removing a larger portion of the cervix or the entire uterus, ovaries or fallopian tubes. Depending on the size and location of the tumor, radiation therapy or chemotherapy may also be necessary.

Chapter 38

Pap Smears:
When Yours Is Slightly
Abnormal

What Did My Pap Smear Show?

The Pap smear your family physician recently obtained from your cervix (the lower part of your womb) has shown some slightly abnormal changes. A Pap smear allows your doctor to look at cells from your cervix and see if there are any problems. Your Pap smear showed one or more of the following changes. Ask your doctor which of these changes you have.

ASCUS

ASCUS (pronounced "ask-us") stands for atypical squamous cells of undetermined significance. These changes in the squamous cells of your cervix mean that the cells on your Pap smear were slightly abnormal. ASCUS may be caused by a vaginal infection or an infection with a virus called HPV (human papillomavirus, or wart virus). Your doctor will talk with you about the options of looking at your cervix with a microscope (colposcopy) or repeating your Pap smear every 6 months for 2 years.

AGUS

AGUS stands for atypical glandular cells of undetermined significance. These changes in the cells of your cervix mean that these cells were slightly abnormal on your Pap smear. AGUS can occur with infections or with a change in the cells on the surface of your cervix or in the canal of your cervix. Your doctor will tell you how the abnormal results on your Pap smear need to be evaluated. Your doctor may recommend repeat Pap smears or colposcopy.

LSIL

LSIL stands for low-grade squamous intraepithelial lesion. This is a common condition of the cells of the cervix and often occurs when the HPV wart virus is present. These changes in the cervix can be present even if you and your sexual partner are monogamous and have never had visible warts. Changes due to LSIL often get better with time. Your doctor will talk with you about whether you need to have Pap smears every 6 months for 2 years or whether you should have colposcopy.

Inflammation

If inflammation is present in the cells on the Pap smear, it means that some white blood cells were seen on your Pap smear. Inflammation of the cervix is very common and usually does not mean there is a problem. If the Pap smear showed that the inflammation is severe, your doctor may want to find the cause, such as an infection. You may also need to have another Pap smear in 6 months to see if the inflammation has gone.

Hyperkeratosis

Hyperkeratosis is a finding of dried skin cells on your Pap smear. This change in the cells of the cervix often occurs from using a cervical cap or diaphragm or from having a cervical infection. Hyperkeratosis rarely needs any more evaluation than a repeat Pap smear in 6 months. If the hyperkeratosis is still present on the repeat Pap smear, your doctor may want to repeat your Pap smear in another 6 months or perform a colposcopy.

Stay in Touch with Your Doctor

Please be sure that you let your doctor's office know if you move or change your phone number so that you can be contacted with the results of your Pap smears or to arrange any other follow-up tests you may need.

The text in this chapter provides a general overview on this topic and may not apply to everyone. To find out if it applies to you and to get more information on this subject, talk to your family doctor.

Chapter 39

HPV Testing Shows Which Pap Abnormalities Need Attention

Testing for the human papillomavirus (HPV) may help doctors and patients decide what to do about the mildly abnormal and very common Pap test result known as ASCUS. Findings from a major, randomized, multicenter study by the National Cancer Institute (NCI) show that HPV testing is highly sensitive in identifying which Pap-detected abnormalities require immediate attention.

A report on the trial, which is known as the ASCUS/LSIL Triage Study or ALTS, appears Feb. 21, 2001 in the *Journal of the National Cancer Institute*. ASCUS and LSIL are acronyms for two mild abnormalities detected by Pap tests. One objective of ALTS was to determine whether HPV testing could sort out which women with ASCUS Pap test results need immediate attention and which do not.

What to do about ASCUS (short for atypical squamous cells of undetermined significance) has been a major issue in cervical cancer screening. Most of these mild abnormalities will go away without treatment. But physicians and patients have had no way to tell which will go away and which represent more serious conditions—precancer or cancer—that need to be treated.

In this study, HPV testing identified virtually all (96.3 percent) of the ASCUS abnormalities that needed treatment. "These results indicate that HPV testing is a viable option for women and their doctors to consider when deciding what to do about ASCUS," said NCI's Diane Solomon, M.D., principal investigator of ALTS.

National Cancer Institute, February 2001.

Although the HPV test proved highly sensitive, Solomon noted that the other two approaches to ASCUS remain options to consider. These are immediate colposcopy (examination with a magnifying instrument) with biopsy if indicated or follow-up by repeat Pap tests every six months. Patients and physicians may take several factors into account when deciding what to do about ASCUS, such as cost and patient preferences regarding follow-up appointments. The ALTS investigators plan to analyze the cost effectiveness of the three options when long-term data from the study become available.

Data from ALTS and other cervical screening studies will be evaluated by medical groups at two upcoming conferences, which are being convened to consider screening and management guidelines. NCI is convening the first of these, the Third Bethesda Workshop, April 30-May 2, 2001 in Bethesda, Md., to address the diagnosis and reporting of Pap test results. The second, led by the American Society for Colposcopy and Cervical Pathology, will develop evidence-based guidelines for clinical practice. It will take place in Bethesda, Md., Sept. 6-9, 2001.

ALTS included about 5,000 women with mildly abnormal Pap tests. About two-thirds had ASCUS and about one-third had the more definite abnormality called LSIL, or low-grade squamous intraepithelial lesion. Within each of these categories, women were assigned randomly to three different groups. One group had an immediate colposcopy—a procedure in which a physician examines the cervix through a magnifying instrument and biopsies any abnormal areas. A second group had repeat Pap tests. The third group was assigned to HPV triage. In this triage group, patients' Pap specimens were tested for HPV types associated with cervical cancer. Those who were HPV-positive had an immediate colposcopy and biopsy and those who were HPV-negative did not.

For the current study, the investigators analyzed the ALTS data from women who had been referred to colposcopy when they enrolled in the trial. The colposcopy results were compared to the results of HPV tests that patients also had on enrollment. The colposcopy results showed that about 5 percent to 10 percent of women with ASCUS had precancer or cancer and that, of these women, 96.3 percent had a positive HPV test. As a corollary, 99.5 percent of women with a negative HPV test did not have precancer or cancer.

The investigators conclude that HPV testing can help in deciding what to do about ASCUS. "A positive test suggests that precancer or, rarely, cancer may be present—we found precancers in 10 percent to 20 percent of ASCUS cases in which the HPV test was positive," said

NCI's co-principal investigator, Mark Schiffman, M.D. "A negative test provides strong reassurance that precancer or cancer is not present."

About 55 percent of women with ASCUS would have been referred to colposcopy if the HPV test had been used for triage in all cases. Thus, HPV testing reduced referrals to colposcopy by about a half compared to immediate colposcopy.

ALTS was conducted at four major medical centers: the University of Alabama at Birmingham; the University of Oklahoma in Oklahoma City; Magee-Womens Hospital of the University of Pittsburgh Medical Center in Pittsburgh, Pa.; and the University of Washington in Seattle. It was organized and funded by the NCI, which is the U.S. government's principal agency for cancer research.

For more information about cancer, visit NCI's Web site at: http://www.cancer.gov/

Chapter 40

Testing for Tumor Markers in Women

Tumor markers are substances that can often be detected in higher-than-normal amounts in the blood, urine, or body tissues of some patients with certain types of cancer. Tumor markers are produced either by the tumor itself or by the body in response to the presence of cancer or certain benign (noncancerous) conditions. This chapter describes some tumor markers found in the blood.

Measurements of tumor marker levels can be useful—when used along with x-rays or other tests—in the detection and diagnosis of some types of cancer. However, measurements of tumor marker levels alone are not sufficient to diagnose cancer for the following reasons:

- Tumor marker levels can be elevated in people with benign conditions.

- Tumor marker levels are not elevated in every person with cancer—especially in the early stages of the disease.

- Many tumor markers are not specific to a particular type of cancer; the level of a tumor marker can be raised by more than one type of cancer.

In addition to their role in cancer diagnosis, some tumor marker levels are measured before treatment to help doctors plan appropriate

Excerpted from "Tumor Markers," National Cancer Institute (NCI), April 1998; full text available at http://cis.nci.nih.gov/fact/5_18.htm.

therapy. In some types of cancer, tumor marker levels reflect the extent (stage) of the disease and can be useful in predicting how well the disease will respond to treatment. Tumor marker levels may also be measured during treatment to monitor a patient's response to treatment. A decrease or return to normal in the level of a tumor marker may indicate that the cancer has responded favorably to therapy. If the tumor marker level rises, it may indicate that the cancer is growing. Finally, measurements of tumor marker levels may be used after treatment has ended as a part of followup care to check for recurrence.

Currently, the main use of tumor markers is to assess a cancer's response to treatment and to check for recurrence. Scientists continue to study these uses of tumor markers as well as their potential role in the early detection and diagnosis of cancer. The patient's doctor can explain the role of tumor markers in detection, diagnosis, or treatment for that person. Described below are some of the most commonly measured tumor markers in women.

CA 125

CA 125 is produced by a variety of cells, but particularly by ovarian cancer cells. Studies have shown that many women with ovarian cancer have elevated CA 125 levels. CA 125 is used primarily in the management of treatment for ovarian cancer. In women with ovarian cancer being treated with chemotherapy, a falling CA 125 level generally indicates that the cancer is responding to treatment. Increasing CA 125 levels during or after treatment, on the other hand, may suggest that the cancer is not responding to therapy or that some cancer cells remain in the body. Doctors may also use CA 125 levels to monitor patients for recurrence of ovarian cancer.

Not all women with elevated CA 125 levels have ovarian cancer. CA 125 levels may also be elevated by cancers of the uterus, cervix, pancreas, liver, colon, breast, lung, and digestive tract. Noncancerous conditions that can cause elevated CA 125 levels include endometriosis, pelvic inflammatory disease, peritonitis, pancreatitis, liver disease, and any condition that inflames the pleura (the tissue that surrounds the lungs and lines the chest cavity). Menstruation and pregnancy can also cause an increase in CA 125.

Carcinoembryonic Antigen

Carcinoembryonic antigen (CEA) is normally found in small amounts in the blood of most healthy people, but may become elevated in people who have cancer or some benign conditions. The primary use of CEA is in monitoring colorectal cancer, especially when the disease has spread (metastasized). CEA is also used after treatment to check for recurrence of colorectal cancer. However, a wide variety of other cancers can produce elevated levels of this tumor marker, including melanoma; lymphoma; and cancers of the breast, lung, pancreas, stomach, cervix, bladder, kidney, thyroid, liver, and ovary.

Elevated CEA levels can also occur in patients with noncancerous conditions, including inflammatory bowel disease, pancreatitis, and liver disease. Tobacco use can also contribute to higher-than-normal levels of CEA.

Alpha-Fetoprotein

Alpha-fetoprotein (AFP) is normally produced by a developing fetus. AFP levels begin to decrease soon after birth and are usually undetectable in the blood of healthy adults (except during pregnancy). An elevated level of AFP strongly suggests the presence of either primary liver cancer or germ cell cancer (cancer that begins in the cells that give rise to eggs or sperm) of the ovary or testicle. Only rarely do patients with other types of cancer (such as stomach cancer) have elevated levels of AFP. Noncancerous conditions that can cause elevated AFP levels include benign liver conditions, such as cirrhosis or hepatitis; ataxia telangiectasia; Wiscott-Aldrich syndrome; and pregnancy.

Human Chorionic Gonadotropin

Human chorionic gonadotropin (HCG) is normally produced by the placenta during pregnancy. In fact, HCG is sometimes used as a pregnancy test because it increases early within the first trimester. It is also used to screen for choriocarcinoma (a rare cancer of the uterus) in women who are at high risk for the disease, and to monitor the treatment of trophoblastic disease (a rare cancer that develops from an abnormally fertilized egg). Elevated HCG levels may also indicate the presence of cancers of the testis, ovary, liver, stomach, pancreas, and lung. Pregnancy and marijuana use can also cause elevated HCG levels.

CA 19-9

Initially found in colorectal cancer patients, CA 19-9 has also been identified in patients with pancreatic, stomach, and bile duct cancer.

Researchers have discovered that, in those who have pancreatic cancer, higher levels of CA 19-9 tend to be associated with more advanced disease. Noncancerous conditions that may elevate CA 19-9 levels include gallstones, pancreatitis, cirrhosis of the liver, and cholecystitis.

CA 15-3

CA 15-3 levels are most useful in following the course of treatment in women diagnosed with breast cancer, especially advanced breast cancer. CA 15-3 levels are rarely elevated in women with early stage breast cancer.

Cancers of the ovary, lung, and prostate may also raise CA 15-3 levels. Elevated levels of CA 15-3 may be associated with noncancerous conditions, such as benign breast or ovarian disease, endometriosis, pelvic inflammatory disease, and hepatitis. Pregnancy and lactation can also cause CA 15-3 levels to rise.

CA 27-29

Similar to the CA 15-3 antigen, CA 27-29 is found in the blood of most breast cancer patients. CA 27-29 levels may be used in conjunction with other procedures (such as mammograms and measurements of other tumor marker levels) to check for recurrence in women previously treated for stage II and stage III breast cancer.

CA 27-29 levels can also be elevated by cancers of the colon, stomach, kidney, lung, ovary, pancreas, uterus, and liver. First trimester pregnancy, endometriosis, ovarian cysts, benign breast disease, kidney disease, and liver disease are noncancerous conditions that can also elevate CA 27-29 levels.

Chapter 41

The National Breast and Cervical Cancer Early Detection Program

A Decade of Progress

Recognizing the value of screening and early detection, Congress passed the Breast and Cervical Cancer Mortality Prevention Act of 1990. This act established Center for Disease Control and Prevention's (CDC) National Breast and Cervical Cancer Early Detection Program (NBCCEDP). Now in its tenth year, the NBCCEDP has provided more than 2 million screening exams to underserved women, including older women, women with low incomes, and women of racial and ethnic minority groups. The program has diagnosed over 5,800 breast cancers, over 31,000 precancerous cervical lesions, and over 500 cervical cancers. These numbers do not include the many women who, though screened outside the NBCCEDP, have benefited from its outreach programs.

The NBCCEDP operates in all 50 states, the District of Columbia, six U.S. territories, and 12 American Indian/Alaska Native organizations. Fiscal year 2000 appropriations of approximately $167 million enable CDC to increase education and outreach programs for women and health care providers, improve quality assurance measures for screening, and improve access to screening and follow-up services. Screening services provided by the NBCCEDP include clinical breast examinations, mammograms, pelvic examinations, and Pap tests. Postscreening diagnostic services, such as surgical consultation

The National Breast and Cervical Cancer Early Detection Program, Centers for Disease Control and Prevention (CDC), September 2000.

and biopsy, are also funded by the NBCCEDP to ensure that all women with abnormal screening results receive timely and adequate diagnostic evaluation and treatment referrals.

Preventing Deaths among Women

"Over 1.4 million women have taken advantage of services provided through CDC's National Breast and Cervical Cancer Early Detection Program. Now a decade old, this program operates in every state in the country, providing recommended screening to low-income women. Yet we are still able to reach only 15% of the eligible population. As a nation, we must step up our commitment to reaching all women."

— Jeffrey P. Koplan, MD, MPH, Director,
Centers for Disease Control and Prevention

Excluding skin cancer, breast cancer is the most common cancer among American women and is second only to lung cancer as a cause of cancer-related death. An estimated 182,800 new cases will be diagnosed among women in 2000, and 40,800 women will die of this disease. The incidence of invasive cervical cancer has decreased significantly over the last 40 years, in large part because of early detection efforts. Even so, an estimated 12,800 new cases will be diagnosed in 2000, and 4,600 women will die of this disease. Many of these deaths—which will occur disproportionately among women of racial and ethnic minority and low-income groups—could be avoided by making cancer screening services available to all women at risk.

Mammography is the best available method to detect breast cancer in its earliest, most treatable stage an average of 1.7 years before the woman can feel the lump. In most cases, the earlier breast cancer is detected, the better the survival rate. When breast cancer is diagnosed at a local stage, the 5-year survival rate is 96%; this rate decreases to 21% when the disease is diagnosed after spreading to other sites. Overall, timely mammography screening could prevent approximately 15%–30% of all deaths from breast cancer among women over the age of 40.

Cervical cancer screening, which is performed by using the Papanicolaou (Pap) test, detects not only cancer but also precancerous lesions. Detection and treatment of such lesions can actually prevent cervical cancer and thus can prevent virtually all deaths from this disease. Women whose cancer is detected in its earliest stage have a survival rate of almost 100% when they receive timely and appropriate treatment and follow-up.

Table 41.1. Percent Distribution of Screening Examinations among NBCCEDP Participants, by Race and Ethnicity, 1991–1998.

Race and Ethnicity	Mammograms	Papanicolaou Tests
White, non-Hispanic	53%	53%
Hispanic	19%	20%
Black, non-Hispanic	17%	15%
American Indian/Alaska Native	6%	7%
Asian	3%	3%
Other/Unknown	2%	2%

Table 41.2. Number of Screening Examinations among NBCCEDP Participants, Fiscal Years 1991–1998

Year	Mammograms	Papanicolaou Tests
1991–92	26,897	45,289
1993	65,713	109,994
1994	96,495	136,496
1995	136,139	170,717
1996	185,059	206,406
1997	225,088	223,305
1998	223,978	212,733
TOTAL	**959,369**	**1,104,940**

Public Education and Outreach: Eliminating Barriers to Screening

NBCCEDP programs work to reduce key barriers known to impede a woman's ability or decision to obtain screening. By promoting the life-saving benefits of early detection available through NBCCEDP-funded services, educational outreach programs help women overcome barriers such as the fear of learning that one has cancer, lack of transportation and child care, linguistic and cultural communication barriers, and lack of physician referral.

To address these barriers, CDC works with health care professionals and organizations, human services and voluntary organizations, academia, and health agencies to provide effective outreach programs.

State-Based Activities

With CDC's leadership, state-based programs have made significant progress in building state and community partnerships to reach women about the benefits of screening and early detection. For example:

* In Arizona, the Hopi Tribe has worked with physicians and staff from the Indian Health Service Unit in Keams Canyon, Arizona, to arrange home visits to Hopi women who have been referred for NBCCEDP funded screening. These one-on-one meetings, which occur in the native Hopi language, focus on the importance of women taking care of themselves—such as by keeping mammography or Pap test appointments—both for their own and for their families' sake.

* Arkansas' "Hats Off to Health" is a light-hearted but informative skit in which characters confront reasons women often give for not having breast cancer screening. Over 600 women have attended the program; surveys found that this nonthreatening approach to breast cancer screening education was effective in reducing self-perceived barriers to mammography.

* North Dakota's "Women's Way" program has set up 47 teams of volunteers statewide to employ diverse outreach strategies to educate and enroll local women in this breast and cervical cancer early detection program. Using either one-on-one or small group modes, these efforts use innovative methods (such as role model stories and program-related accessories) to convey their educational and motivational messages.

- A Minnesota Twin Cities community coalition has developed "Save Our Sisters," a screening campaign conducted at a popular eating and gathering place for the Minneapolis African American community. Sponsored by the Minnesota Department of Health and by local media, clinics, and churches, the campaign features free gospel music and food, local speakers who are breast cancer survivors, and opportunities to sign up for free mammograms.

- New Hampshire's "Let No Woman Be Overlooked" is an outreach strategy that uses public presentations, media advertising, and community networking to increase public knowledge that breast and cervical screening is free and accessible. Community out-reach workers enlist the support of local worksites, churches, and other community gathering places.

National Efforts

Examples of CDC collaboration with national organizations include the following:

- CDC collaborates with the American Cancer Society (ACS) to develop and disseminate comprehensive information on cancer prevention and early detection. Through CDC, ACS divisions have formed partnerships with state health departments to increase screening services to medically underserved women. CDC and ACS collaborate in many program areas, including establishing infrastructure and public and professional education activities.

- A unique public-private partnership was established among CDC, Avon Products Inc., and the National Cancer Institute. Avon's Breast Cancer Awareness Crusade has raised more than $37 million for breast cancer programs nationwide through the sale of its Breast Cancer Awareness pink ribbon products.

Enhanced Professional Services for Effective Screening and Follow-Up

Successful detection and treatment of breast and cervical cancer depends on the quality of diagnostic services and on appropriate medical and technical training. Improved screening techniques and diagnostic skills translate to more cancers diagnosed early and more lives saved. The NBCCEDP provides national guidance and support to ensure that screening-related professional and medical services incorporate current techniques and best practices.

Quality Assurance for Screening and Follow-Up

All health agencies participating in the NBCCEDP use mammography facilities certified by the American College of Radiology and laboratories that follow the Clinical Laboratory Improvement Amendments of 1988. CDC provides screening and diagnostic guidelines to all state-based programs and assists states in evaluating their clinical services. As more women are screened by the NBCCEDP, participating health agencies and providers will experience greater challenges in obtaining sufficient resources for treating women with breast and cervical cancer. To help women overcome financial, logistical, and other barriers to these follow-up services, the NBCCEDP has distributed case management procedures and policies to all participating programs.

Professional Education: Enhancing Health Care at the Source

Through professional education services, the NBCCEDP has helped a wide range of health care professionals—including physicians, nurses, radiology technologists, and cytologists—better understand and perform their key roles in the early detection of breast and cervical cancer.

- CDC's national training center for cancer detection and prevention has recently developed a self-study packet with a videotape to help providers—particularly those in rural areas—improve follow-up of women who have abnormal screening results from clinical breast examinations and mammograms. The training center also offers Native American nurses "Native Web" training to enhance their clinical breast examination skills.

- Professional education opportunities are also offered through the NBCCEDP's state, tribal, and territorial programs. For example, the Kentucky Cancer Program offers a self-study kit to help primary care physicians increase and improve routine breast and cervical cancer screenings. The program features a videotape discussing communication strategies, physical examination recommendations and techniques, risk management, and office reminder systems.

NBCCEDP Accomplishments

- Almost 1 million mammograms provided.
- About 1.1 million Pap tests provided.
- Over 5,800 breast cancers diagnosed.
- Over 31,000 precancerous cervical lesions diagnosed.
- Over 500 cervical cancers diagnosed.

Partnerships for Cancer Control in Populations at Higher Risk

Partnerships that focus their prevention efforts on populations at greater risk are essential for understanding and alleviating disparities. Both mammograms and Pap tests are underused by women who are members of racial and ethnic minority groups, have less than a high school education, are older, or live below the poverty level.

CDC funds a strong and effective network of partners who are well positioned in communities at risk. These partners have developed projects that are focused on underserved populations and cover a wide range of public and professional education interventions. For example, many projects are involved with developing low-literacy, bilingual, and culturally appropriate educational materials that are used in diverse training and outreach programs and educational campaigns. The various interventions used by the different projects contribute to the common goal of increasing access to and use of screening services among priority populations.

CDC funds the following partners to promote screening among populations at higher risk:

- American Social Health Association
- Association of Asian Pacific Community Health Organizations
- Baylor College of Medicine, Salud en Accion Program
- Institute for the Advancement of Social Work Research
- Mautner Project for Lesbians with Cancer
- National Asian Women's Health Organization
- National Association of Community Health Centers
- National Caucus and Center on Black Aged, Inc.
- National Center for Farmworkers Health, Inc.

- National Education Association Health Information Network
- National Hispanic Council on Aging
- U.S. Conference of Mayors' Research and Education Foundation
- The Witness Project
- World Education

For More Information

For more information, or to obtain copies of the document from which the text in this chapter was taken, please contact:

Centers for Disease Control and Prevention
National Center for Chronic Disease Prevention and
Health Promotion
Mail Stop K-64
4770 Buford Highway NE
Atlanta, GA 30341-3717
Phone: 770-488-4751
Toll Free Voice Information System: 888-842-6355
Fax: 770-488-4760
Website: http://www.cdc.gov/cancer

Chapter 42

Human Papillomaviruses (HPV) and Cancer Risk

Human Papillomaviruses

Human papillomaviruses (HPVs) are a group of more than 100 types of viruses. They are called papillomaviruses because certain types may cause warts, or papillomas, which are benign (noncancerous) tumors. The HPVs that cause the common warts which grow on hands and feet are different from those that cause growths in the mouth and genital area. Some types of HPVs are associated with certain types of cancer.

Of the more than 100 types of HPVs, over 30 types can be passed from one person to another through sexual contact. HPV infection is one of the most common sexually transmitted diseases (STDs). Some types of HPVs may cause warts to appear on or around the genitals or anus. Genital warts (technically known as condylomata acuminatum) are most commonly associated with two HPV types, numbers 6 and 11. Warts may appear within several weeks after sexual contact with a person who has HPV, or they may take months or years to appear; or they may never appear. HPVs may also cause flat, abnormal growths in the genital area and on the cervix (the lower part of the uterus that extends into the vagina). HPV infections often do not cause any symptoms.

HPVs and Cancer Risk

HPVs are now recognized as the major cause of cervical cancer. Studies also suggest that HPVs may play a role in cancers of the anus,

Fact Sheet 3.20, Cancer Info. Service (CIS), Nat'l Cancer Institute, 8/01.

vulva, vagina, and penis, and some cancers of the oropharynx (the middle part of the throat that includes the soft palate, the base of the tongue, and the tonsils).

Some types of HPVs are referred to as "low-risk" viruses because they rarely develop into cancer; these include HPV-6 and HPV-11. HPV viruses that can lead to the development of cancer are referred to as "high-risk." Both high-risk and low-risk types of HPVs can cause the growth of abnormal cells, but generally only the high-risk types of HPVs may lead to cancer. Sexually transmitted, high-risk HPVs have been linked with cancer in both men and women; they include HPV types 16, 18, 31, 33, 35, 39, 45, 51, 52, 56, 58, 59, 68, and 69. These high-risk types of HPVs cause growths that are usually flat and nearly invisible, as compared with the warts caused by HPV-6 and HPV-11. It is important to note, however, that the majority of HPV infections go away on their own and do not cause any abnormal growths.

Precancerous Cervical Conditions

Abnormal cervical cells can be detected when a Pap test is done during a gynecologic exam. Various terms have been used to describe the abnormal cells that may be seen in Pap tests. In the Bethesda system (the major system used to report the results of Pap tests in the United States), precancerous conditions are divided into low-grade and high-grade squamous intraepithelial lesions (SILs). Squamous cells are thin, flat cells that cover internal and external surfaces of the body, including the tissue that forms the surface of the skin, the lining of the hollow organs of the body, and the passages of the genital, respiratory, and digestive tracts. Other terms sometimes used to describe these abnormal cells are cervical intraepithelial neoplasia (CIN) and dysplasia. Low-grade SILs (mild dysplasias) are a common condition, especially in young women. The majority of low-grade SILs return to normal over months to a few years. Sometimes, low-grade SILs can progress to high-grade SILs. High-grade SILs are not cancer, but they may eventually lead to cancer and should be treated by a doctor.

Risk Factors for HPV and Cervical Cancer

Behaviors such as beginning sexual intercourse at an early age (before age 16) and having many sexual partners increase the chance that a woman will develop an HPV infection in the cervix. Most HPV infections go away on their own without causing any type of abnormality. It is important to note that infection with high-risk HPV types may increase the chance that mild abnormalities will progress to more severe abnormalities or cervical cancer. Still, of the women who do develop abnormal cell changes with high-risk types of HPV, only a small percentage will develop cervical cancer if the abnormal cells are not removed. Studies suggest that whether a woman develops cervical cancer depends on a variety of factors acting together with high-risk HPVs. The factors that may increase the risk of cancer in women with HPV infection include smoking, having many children, and human immunodeficiency virus (HIV) infection.

Screening and Followup for Precancerous Cervical Conditions

Screening for cervical cancer consists of regular Pap tests for women who are sexually active or who have reached 18 years of age. If high-grade abnormal cell changes are found on a Pap test, colposcopy and biopsy of any abnormal areas are recommended. (Colposcopy is a procedure in which a lighted magnifying instrument called a colposcope is used to examine the vagina and cervix. Biopsy is the removal of a small piece of tissue for diagnosis.) If low-grade changes are found, repeat Pap tests or colposcopy may be recommended.

Treatment of HPV Infection

Although there is currently no medical cure to eliminate a papillomavirus infection, the SILs and warts these viruses cause can be treated. Methods used to treat SILs include cryosurgery (freezing that destroys tissue), laser treatment (surgery using a high-intensity light), LEEP (loop electrosurgical excision procedure, the removal of tissue using a hot wire loop), as well as conventional surgery. Similar treatments may be used for external genital warts. In addition, three powerful chemicals (podophyllin, bichloroacetic acid, and trichloroacetic acid) will destroy external genital warts when applied directly to them. Podofilox (podophyllotoxin) can be applied topically either as a liquid or a gel to external genital warts. Imiquimod cream has also been approved to treat external warts. Also, fluorouracil cream (sometimes called 5-FU) may be used to treat the warts. Some doctors use interferon alpha to treat warts that have recurred after being removed by traditional means. Imiquimod and interferon alpha work by stimulating the immune (defense) system to fight the virus.

Current Research

The ASCUS/LSIL Triage Study (ALTS), a major study organized and funded by the National Cancer Institute (NCI), is currently evaluating different management approaches for women with mildly abnormal Pap test results. (ASCUS and LSIL are acronyms for the two mild abnormalities detected by Pap tests. ASCUS stands for atypical squamous cells of undetermined significance and LSIL for low-grade squamous intraepithelial lesions.) Preliminary findings from the ALTS study suggest that testing cervical samples for HPV is an excellent option to help direct followup for women with an ASCUS Pap test result. Repeat Pap tests or direct referral to colposcopy remain options for the followup of ASCUS results. The final study results, which are expected to be published in about 3 years, will help women and their doctors decide what course of action to take when mild abnormalities show up on Pap tests.

Researchers at NCI and elsewhere are studying how HPVs cause precancerous changes in normal cells and how these changes can be prevented. They are using HPVs grown in the laboratory to find ways to prevent the infection and its associated disease and to create vaccines against the viruses. Vaccines for certain papillomaviruses, such as HPV-16 and HPV-18, are being studied in clinical trials (research studies with people) for cervical cancer; similar trials for other types of cancer are planned. Information about clinical trials is available from the Cancer Information Service (CIS) (see below) or on the NCI's cancerTrials-R Web site at http://cancertrials.nci.nih.gov/ on the Internet.

Laboratory research has indicated that HPVs produce proteins known as E5, E6, and E7. These proteins interfere with the cell functions that normally prevent excessive growth. For example, HPV E6 interferes with the human protein p53. p53 is present in all people and acts to keep tumors from growing. This research is being used to develop ways to interrupt the process by which HPV infection can lead to growth of abnormal cells and, eventually, cancer.

Resources

The following Federal Government agencies and other organizations can provide more information about HPVs and their link to cancer:

National Cancer Institutes' Cancer Information Service
Telephone: 1-800-4-CANCER (1-800-422-6237)
TTY (for deaf and hard of hearing callers): 1-800-332-8615

National Institute of Allergy and Infectious Disease (NIAID)
Office of Communications and Public Liaison
Building 31, Room 7A-50
31 Center Drive MSC 2520
Bethesda, MD 20892-2520
Telephone: 301-496-5717
Internet website: http://www.niaid.nih.gov

The NIAID conducts research on HPVs and offers printed materials.

Centers for Disease Control and Prevention (CDC)
National STD Hotline 1-800-227-8922

The toll-free CDC National STD Hotline provides anonymous, confidential information on sexually transmitted diseases (STD) and how to prevent them. Staff provide referrals to free or low-cost clinics nationwide. Free educational literature about a wide variety of STDs and prevention methods is also available. The hotline is open Monday through Friday, 8 a.m.-11 p.m. EST.

More information about STDs, including HPV, is available on the CDC National STD Hotline's website at: http://www.ashastd.org/std/stdhotln.html

The CDC's Division of Sexually Transmitted Diseases Prevention website also has information about HPV, including treatment guidelines and surveillance statistics. It can be found at: http://www.cdc.gov/nchstp/dstd/dstdp.html

Chapter 43

Oral Contraceptives and Cancer Risk

Oral contraceptives (OCs) first became available to American women in the early 1960s. The convenience, effectiveness, and reversibility of action of birth control pills (which are popularly known as "the pill") has made them the most popular form of birth control in the United States. However, a correlation between estrogen and increased risk of breast cancer has led to continuing controversy about a possible link between OCs and cancer.

This chapter addresses only what is known about OC use and the risk of developing cancer. It does not deal with the most serious side effect of OC use—the increased risk of cardiovascular disease for certain groups of women.

Oral Contraceptives

Currently, two types of OCs are available in the United States. The most commonly prescribed OC contains two synthetic versions of natural female hormones (estrogen and progesterone) that are similar to the hormones the ovaries normally produce. Estrogen stimulates the growth and development of the uterus at puberty, thickens the endometrium (the inner lining of the uterus) during the first half of the menstrual cycle, and stimulates changes in breast tissue at puberty and childbirth. Two types of synthetic estrogens are used in OCs, ethinyl estradiol and mestranol.

CancerNet, National Cancer Institute (www.nci.nih.gov), February 2000.

Progesterone, which is produced during the last half of the menstrual cycle, prepares the endometrium to receive the egg. If the egg is fertilized, progesterone secretion continues, preventing release of additional eggs from the ovaries. For this reason, progesterone is called the "pregnancy-supporting" hormone, and scientists believe it to have valuable contraceptive effects. The synthetic progesterone used in OCs is called progestogen or progestin. Norethindrone and levonorgestrel are examples of synthetic progesterones used in OCs.

The second type of OC available in the United States is called the minipill and contains only a progestogen. The minipill is less effective in preventing pregnancy than the combination pill, so it is prescribed less often.

Because medical research suggests that cancers of the female reproductive organs sometimes depend on naturally occurring sex hormones for their development and growth, scientists have been investigating a possible link between OC use and cancer risk. Medical researchers have focused a great deal of attention on OC users over the past 30 years. This scrutiny has produced a wealth of data on OC use and the development of certain cancers, although results of these studies have not always been consistent.

Breast Cancer

A woman's risk of developing breast cancer depends on several factors, some of which are related to her natural hormones. Hormonal factors that increase the risk of breast cancer include conditions that allow high levels of estrogen to persist for long periods of time, such as early age at first menstruation (before age 12), late age at menopause (after age 55), having children after age 30, and not having children at all. A woman's risk of breast cancer increases with the amount of time she is exposed to estrogen.

Because many of the risk factors for breast cancer are related to natural hormones, and because OCs work by manipulating these hormones, there has been some concern about the possible effects of medicines such as OCs on breast cancer risk, especially if women take them for many years. Sufficient time has elapsed since the introduction of OCs to allow investigators to study large numbers of women who took birth control pills for many years beginning at a young age and to follow them as they became older.

However, studies examining the use of OCs as a risk factor for breast cancer have produced inconsistent results. Most studies have not found an overall increased risk for breast cancer associated with

OC use. In June 1995, however, investigators at the National Cancer Institute (NCI) reported an increased risk of developing breast cancer among women under age 35 who had used birth control pills for at least 6 months, compared with those who had never used OCs. They also saw a slightly lower, but still elevated, risk among women ages 35 to 44. In addition, their research showed a higher risk among long-term OC users, especially those who had started to take the pill before age 18.

A 1996 analysis of worldwide epidemiologic data, which included information from the 1995 study, found that women who were current or recent users of birth control pills had a slightly elevated risk of developing breast cancer. However, 10 years or more after they stopped using OCs, their risk of developing breast cancer returned to the same level as if they had never used birth control pills.

To conduct this analysis, the researchers examined the results of 54 studies conducted in 25 countries that involved 53,297 women with breast cancer and 100,239 women without breast cancer. More than 200 researchers participated in this combined exhaustive analysis of their original studies, which represented about 90 percent of the epidemiological studies throughout the world that had investigated the possible relationship between OCs and breast cancer.

The return of risk to normal levels after 10 years or more of not taking OCs was consistent regardless of family history of breast cancer, reproductive history, geographic area of residence, ethnic background, differences in study designs, dose and type of hormone, and duration of use. The change in risk also generally held true for age at first use; however, for reasons that were not fully understood, there was a continued elevated risk among women who had started to use OCs before age 20.

One encouraging aspect of the study is that the slightly elevated risk seen in both current OC users and those who had stopped use less than 10 years previously may not be due to the contraceptive itself. The slightly elevated risk may result from the potential of estrogen to promote the growth of breast cancer cells that are already present, rather than its potential to initiate changes in normal cells leading to the development of cancer.

Furthermore, the observation that the slightly elevated risk of developing breast cancer that was seen in this study peaked during use, declined gradually after OC use had stopped, then returned to normal risk levels 10 years or more after stopping, is not consistent with the usual process of carcinogenesis. It is more typical for cancer risk to peak decades after exposure, not immediately afterward. Cancer usually is more likely to occur with increased duration and/or degree of exposure to a carcinogen. In this analytical study, neither the dose and type of hormone nor the duration of use affected the risk of developing breast cancer.

Ovarian and Endometrial Cancers

Many studies have found that using OCs reduces a woman's risk of ovarian cancer by 40 to 50 percent compared with women who have not used OCs. The Centers for Disease Control and Prevention's (CDC) Cancer and Steroid Hormone Study (CASH), along with other research conducted over the past 20 years, shows that the longer a woman uses OCs, the lower her risk of ovarian cancer. Moreover, this lowered risk persists long after OC use ceases. The CASH study found that the reduced risk of ovarian cancer is seen in women who have used OCs for as little as 3 to 6 months, and that it continues for 15 years after use ends. Other studies have confirmed that the reduced risk of ovarian cancer continues for at least 10 to 15 years after a woman has stopped taking OCs. Several hypotheses have been offered to explain how oral contraceptives might protect against ovarian cancer, such as a reduction in the number of ovulations a woman has during her lifetime, but the exact mechanism is still not known.

Researchers have also found that OC use may reduce the risk of endometrial cancer. Findings from the CASH study and other reports show that combination OC use can protect against the development of endometrial cancer. The CASH study found that using combination OCs for at least 1 year reduced the risk of developing endometrial cancer to women who never took birth control pills. In addition, the beneficial effect of OC use persisted for at least 15 years after OC users stopped taking birth control pills. Some researchers have found that the protective effect of OCs against endometrial cancer increases with the length of time combination OCs are used, but results have not been consistent.

The reduction in risk of ovarian and endometrial cancers from OC use does not apply to the sequential type of pill, in which each monthly cycle contains 16 estrogen pills followed by 5 estrogen-plus-progesterone pills. (Sequential OCs were taken off the market in 1976, so few women have been exposed to them.) Researchers believe OCs reduce cancer risk only when the estrogen content of birth control pills is balanced by progestogen in the same pill.

Cancer of the Cervix

There is some evidence that long-term use of OCs may increase the risk of cancer of the cervix (the narrow, lower portion of the uterus). The results of studies conducted by NCI scientists and other researchers support a relationship between extended use of the pill (5 or more years) and a slightly increased risk of cervical cancer. However, the exact nature of the association between OC use and risk of cervical cancer remains unclear.

One reason that the association is unclear is that two of the major risk factors for cervical cancer (early age at first intercourse and a history of multiple sex partners) are related to sexual behavior. Because these risk factors may be different between women who use OCs and those who have never used them, it is difficult for researchers to determine the exact role that OCs may play in the development of cervical cancer.

Also, many studies on OCs and cervical cancer have not accounted for the influence of human papillomaviruses (HPVs) on cervical cancer risk. HPVs are a group of more than 70 types of viruses, some of which are known to increase the risk of cervical cancer. Compared to non-OC users, women who use OCs may be less likely to use barrier methods of contraception (such as condoms). Since condoms can prevent the transmission of HPVs, OC users who do not use them may be at increased risk of becoming infected with HPVs. Therefore, the increased risk of cervical cancer that some studies found to be caused by prolonged OC use may actually be the result of HPV infection.

There is evidence that pill users who never use a barrier method of contraception or who have a history of genital infections are at a higher risk for developing cervical cancer. This association supports the theory that OCs may act together with sexually transmitted agents (such as HPVs) in the development of cervical cancer. Researchers continue to investigate the exact nature of the relationship between OC use and cancer of the cervix.

OC product labels have been revised to inform women of the possible risk of cervical cancer. The product labels also warn that birth control pills do not protect against human immunodeficiency virus (HIV) and other sexually transmitted diseases such as HPV, chlamydia, and genital herpes.

Liver Tumors

There is some evidence that OCs may increase the risk of certain malignant (cancerous) liver tumors. However, the risk is difficult to evaluate because of different patterns of OC use and because these tumors are rare in American women (the incidence is approximately 2 cases per 100,000 women). A benign (noncancerous) tumor of the liver called hepatic adenoma has also been found to occur, although rarely, among OC users. These tumors do not spread, but they may rupture and cause internal bleeding.

Reducing Risks

After many years on the U.S. market, the overall health effects of OCs are still mixed. The most serious side effect of the pill continues to be an increased risk of cardiovascular disease in certain groups, such as women who smoke; women over age 35; obese women; and those with a history of high blood pressure, diabetes, or elevated serum cholesterol levels. Information about the increased risk of cardiovascular disease is available from the National Heart, Lung, and Blood Institute (NHLBI). The NHLBI Information Center can be reached at:

Post Office Box 30105
Bethesda, MD 20824-0105
Telephone: 301-592-8573
Fax: 301-592-8563
E-mail: NHLBIinfo@rover.nhlbi.nih.gov
Internet Web site: http://www.nhlbi.nih.gov

The NCI recommends that women in their forties or older get screening mammograms on a regular basis, every 1 to 2 years. Women who are at increased risk for breast cancer should seek medical advice about when to begin having mammograms and how often to be screened. A high-quality mammogram, with a clinical breast exam (an exam done by a professional health care provider), is the most effective way to detect breast cancer early.

Women who are or have been sexually active or are in their late teens or older can reduce their risk for cervical cancer by having regular Pap tests. Research has shown that women who have never had a Pap test or who have not had one for several years have a higher-than-average risk of developing cervical cancer.

Women who are concerned about their risk for cancer are encouraged to talk with their doctor. More information is also available from the Cancer Information Service.

Cancer Information Service
1-800-4-CANCER (1-800-422-6237)
TTY: 1-800-332-8615

References

Breast Cancer

Brinton LA, Daling JR, Liff JM, et al. Oral contraceptives and breast cancer risk among younger women. *Journal of the National Cancer Institute* 1995; 87(13):827-835.

The Centers for Disease Control and the National Institute of Child Health and Human Development. Oral contraceptive use and the risk of breast cancer: The Centers for Disease Control and the National Institute of Child Health and Human Development Cancer and Steroid Hormone Study. *New England Journal of Medicine* 1986; 315:405-411.

Chilvers C, McPherson K, Pike MC, et al. Oral contraceptive use and breast cancer risk in young women. *Lancet* 1989; 1:973-982.

McPherson K, Vessey MP, Neil A, et al. Early oral contraceptive use and breast cancer: results of another case-control study. *British Journal of Cancer* 1987; 56:653-660.

Meirik O, Lund E, Adami HO, et al. Oral Contraceptive use and breast cancer in young women: a joint national study in Sweden and Norway. *Lancet* 1986; 2:650-654.

Miller DR, Rosenberg L, Kaufman DW, et al. Breast cancer before age 45 and oral contraceptive use: new findings. *American Journal of Epidemiology* 1989; 129:269-280.

Olsson H, Olsson ML, Moeller TR, et al. Oral contraceptive use and breast cancer in young women in Sweden. *Lancet* 1985; 1:748-749.

Paul C, Skegg DCG, Spears GFS. Oral contraceptives and risk of breast cancer. *International Journal of Cancer* 1990; 46:366-373.

Pike MC, Henderson BE, Krailo MD, et al. Breast cancer in young women and use of oral contraceptives: possible modifying effect of formulation and age at use. *Lancet* 1983; 2:926-930.

Romiu I, Berlin JA, Colditz G. Oral contraceptives and breast cancer: review and meta-analysis. *Cancer* 1990; 66:2253-2263.

Rookus MA, Van Leeuwen FE. Oral contraceptives and risk of breast cancer in women aged 25-54 years: The Netherlands Oral Contraceptives and Breast Cancer Study Group. *Lancet* 1994; 344:844-851.

Thomas DB. Oral contraceptives and breast cancer: review of the epidemiologic literature. *Contraception* 1991; 43(6):597-642.

White E, Malone KE, Weiss NS, et al. Breast cancer among young U.S. women in relation to oral contraceptive use. *Journal of the National Cancer Institute* 1994; 86: 505-514.

Wingo PA, Lee NC, Ory HW, et al. Age-specific differences in the relationship between oral contraceptive use and breast cancer. *Cancer* Supplement 1993; 71(4):1506-1517.

Ovarian and Endometrial Cancers

Brinton LA, Huggins GR, Lehman HF, et al. Long-term use of oral contraceptives and risk of invasive cervical cancer. *International Journal of Cancer* 1986; 38:339-344.

The Centers for Disease Control. Oral contraceptive use and the risk of ovarian cancer: The Centers for Disease Control Cancer and Steroid Hormone Study. *Journal of the American Medical Association* 1983; 249:1596-1599.

The Centers for Disease Control. Combination oral contraceptive use and the risk of endometrial cancer: The Cancer and Steroid Hormone Study of the Centers for Disease Control and the National Institute of Child Health and Human Development. *Journal of the American Medical Association* 1987; 257(6):796-800.

The Centers for Disease Control and the National Institute of Child Health and Human Development. The reduction in risk of ovarian cancer associated with oral contraceptive use: The Cancer and Steroid Hormone Study of the Centers for Disease Control and the National Institute of Child Health and Human Development. *New England Journal of Medicine* 1987; 316:650-655.

Stanford JL, Brinton LA, Berman ML, et al. Oral contraceptives and endometrial cancer: do other risk factors modify the association? *International Journal of Cancer* 1993; 54(2):243-248.

Cervix

Brinton LA. Epidemiology of cervical cancer—overview. *IARC Scientific Publications* 1992; 119:3-23.

Brinton LA. Oral contraceptives and cervical neoplasia. *Contraception* 1991; 43(6):581-595.

Brinton LA, Huggins GR, Lehman HF, et al. Long-term use of oral contraceptives and risk of invasive cervical cancer. *International Journal of Cancer* 1986; 38(3):399-444.

Daling JR, Madeleine MM, McKnight B, et al. The relationship of human papillomavirus-related cervical tumors to cigarette smoking, oral contraceptive use, and prior herpes simplex virus type 2 infection. *Cancer Epidemiology, Biomarkers, and Prevention* 1996; 5(7):541-548.

Gram IT, Macaluso M, Stalsberg H. Oral contraceptive use and the incidence of cervical intraepithelial neoplasia. *American Journal of Obstetrics and Gynecology* 1992; 167(1):40-44.

Munoz N, Bosch FX, de Sanjose S, et al. The causal link between human papillomavirus and invasive cervical cancer: a population-based case-control study in Colombia and Spain. *International Journal of Cancer* 1992; 52(5):743-749.

Liver

Rooks JB, Ory HW, Ishak KG, et al. Epidemiology of hepatocellular adenoma: the role of oral contraceptive use. *Journal of the American Medical Association* 1979; 242:644-648.

Tao, LC. Oral contraceptive-associated liver cell adenoma and hepatocellular carcinoma. *Cancer* 1991; 68:341-347.

Palmer J, Rosenberg L, Kaufman DW, et al. Oral contraceptive use and liver cancer. *American Journal of Epidemiology* 1989; 130:878-882.

Chapter 44

Menopausal Hormone Replacement Therapy: Evaluating Cancer Risks

Menopause

Menopause is the time in a woman's life when hormonal changes cause menstruation to stop permanently. For most women, menopause is the last stage of a gradual biological process that actually begins during their mid-thirties.

Menopause is considered complete when a woman has stopped menstruating, or having her period, for 1 year. This usually occurs between ages 45 and 55, with variations in timing from woman to woman. By the time natural menopause is complete, hormone output has decreased significantly, but does not completely stop. Women who have surgery to remove both of their ovaries (an operation called bilateral oophorectomy) experience "surgical menopause," the immediate cessation of ovarian hormone production and menstruation. Doctors may recommend hormone replacement therapy (HRT), using either estrogen alone or estrogen in combination with progestin (a form of progesterone) to counter some of the possible effects of natural or surgical menopause on a woman's health and quality of life.

Because of advances in medical care and fewer deaths during childbirth, the average life expectancy for women in the United States increased from 51 years in 1900 to 79 years in 1990. A 50-year-old woman today can expect to live at least one-third of her life after menopause. An estimated 40 million women will go through menopause

CancerNet, National Cancer Institute (www.nci.nih.gov), April 2000.

in the next 20 years. Thus, an increasing number of women will need to weigh the benefits and risks of HRT.

Although menopause is defined by many people as simply the end of a woman's menstrual cycles and her ability to bear children, it is also the beginning of a new and distinct phase of her life, with its own special health issues.

Symptoms of Menopause

Each woman experiences menopause differently. Some women have minimal discomfort, while others have moderate or even severe problems. Hot flashes, the most common symptom, occur in more than 60 percent of menopausal women. Hot flashes often begin several years before other symptoms of menopause occur.

Other changes involve the vagina and urinary tract. Declining estrogen levels can make vaginal tissue drier, thinner, and less elastic, which can make sexual intercourse painful. Urinary tract tissue also becomes less elastic, sometimes leading to involuntary loss of urine upon coughing, laughing, sneezing, exercising, or sudden exertion (stress incontinence). Urinary tract infections tend to occur more frequently. Other possible effects of menopause include sleep disturbances, mood swings, depression, and anxiety.

Health Effects of Menopause

In addition to producing some potentially uncomfortable symptoms, menopause can have more serious, long-term effects on a woman's overall health and potential years of life. For example, the drop in estrogen that occurs at menopause is thought to cause adverse changes in levels of cholesterol and other blood lipids (fats), and in levels of fibrinogen (a substance that affects blood clotting). These changes may increase the risk of heart disease (the leading cause of death among American women) and stroke. More than 370,000 women in this country die each year from heart disease, and about 93,000 die from stroke.

Osteoporosis (thinning of the bones), another serious concern during later life, is aggravated by menopause. Menopause speeds up the bone depletion that occurs during normal aging processes. About 20 percent of women over age 50 have or are at risk for bone fragility and fractures as their estrogen levels decline. Fractures, which often require a long recovery period, are a common injury in women with osteoporosis. Fractures of the vertebrae can cause curvature of the spine (also called kyphosis), loss of height, and pain.

Hormone Replacement Therapy

Most women will eventually need to make decisions about whether to take HRT and, if so, for how long. Hormone replacement therapy can have beneficial effects, but there are also some concerns associated with it. Each woman should consider both risks and benefits when making her decisions.

Benefits of HRT

It has been well documented for several decades that HRT is the most effective remedy for the hot flashes and sleep disturbances that often accompany menopause. Hormone replacement therapy has also consistently been shown to decrease vaginal discomfort by increasing the thickness, elasticity, and lubricating ability of vaginal tissue. Urinary tract tissue also becomes thicker and more elastic, reducing the incidence of stress incontinence and urinary tract infections.

Some women and their doctors report that HRT can be helpful in relieving the depression and mood swings that may occur during menopause and can produce a general sense of well-being and increased energy. Also, some find that HRT increases skin thickness and elasticity, decreasing the appearance of wrinkles.

Although HRT was used initially to reduce the discomfort from short-term menopausal symptoms, studies have provided evidence that it may prevent or reduce some of the negative long-term health effects of menopause. Scientists continue to gather information to define the potential benefits from HRT and to identify the women for whom it may be most useful. Further research is also needed to determine when HRT should be started and how long it should be continued to achieve the greatest benefits.

Hormone replacement therapy plays a significant role in building and maintaining bone, thus helping to prevent osteoporosis. HRT is also sometimes used to treat bone loss that has already begun. HRT can prevent the decline of bone density and may reduce the incidence of fractures. It has been shown, however, that bone loss resumes upon discontinuation of HRT.

Research shows that HRT improves blood lipids and lowers fibrinogen levels. Some studies suggest that HRT may reduce the risk of heart disease and stroke. However, scientists are concerned that some of the apparent benefits of HRT in these studies may be due to the fact that healthier or more health-conscious women may be more likely to take replacement hormones. In one study of postmenopausal women with heart disease, the use of HRT did not prevent further heart attacks or death from heart disease. Additional research is in progress to clarify this issue.

Some studies suggest that taking estrogen may reduce the risk of developing Alzheimer's disease. However, scientists caution that additional research is needed to explore this possibility.

Concerns about HRT

Although HRT has potential benefits for many menopausal and postmenopausal women, it can also have drawbacks. Concerns about HRT center on the risk of endometrial cancer and breast cancer, especially after long-term use (more than 10 years).

Endometrial Cancer (Cancer of the Uterus)

When estrogen replacement became available for menopausal women in the 1940s, it was administered in high doses without progestin. As it became more popular in the 1960s, it was given to increasing numbers of women. In the 1970s, however, it became clear that women who received estrogen alone had a six- to eight-fold increased risk of developing cancer of the endometrium (lining of the uterus).

Now, most doctors prescribe HRT that includes progestin, along with much lower doses of estrogen, for women who have not had a hysterectomy (surgery to remove the uterus). Progestin counteracts estrogen's negative effect on the uterus by preventing the overgrowth of the endometrial lining. Adding progestin to HRT substantially reduces the increased risk of endometrial cancer associated with taking estrogen alone. (A woman who has had a hysterectomy does not need progestin and can receive HRT with estrogen alone.)

Because reports have shown that estrogen increases the risk of developing endometrial cancer, many women and their doctors are also concerned that HRT may increase the risk of recurrence in women with a history of endometrial cancer. At present, however, there is no scientific evidence that taking estrogen increases this risk. To help resolve this issue, the National Cancer Institute is sponsoring a clinical trial to determine the effects of estrogen in women treated for early stage endometrial cancer. The study will compare recurrence rates between women who are given estrogen and those who are not given estrogen.

Breast Cancer

The relationship between HRT and breast cancer is not clear. The possible increased risk of developing breast cancer is consistently cited by menopausal and postmenopausal women as the main reason they are reluctant to use HRT. Many women and their doctors have particular concerns about the effects of long-term HRT use on breast cancer risk.

One of the most important risk factors for developing breast cancer is a woman's lifelong exposure to naturally occurring hormones; the longer her body produces hormones, the more likely she is to develop breast cancer. Factors such as early menstruation (before age 12) and late menopause (after age 55) contribute to prolonged hormone exposure. Because of this relationship between prolonged hormone exposure and breast cancer risk, scientists have been concerned that increasing a woman's lifelong exposure to hormones with HRT would result in increased breast cancer risk.

Over the last 25 years, numerous observational studies have examined the possible relationship between HRT and breast cancer. These studies have varied widely in terms of study design; size of populations studied; and doses, timing, and types of hormones used. Results of these studies have been inconsistent. Some of the early studies that followed women who used high doses of estrogen alone showed increased breast cancer risk. Other studies have looked at the experience of women who took estrogen combined with progestin. Some have shown an increased risk, while others have not.

Two studies compared the risk of breast cancer for women who had taken estrogen-only HRT with the risk for women who had taken HRT using estrogen combined with progestin. The first study analyzed data on 46,000 women. The researchers found that the risk for breast cancer among women who had used HRT during the past 4 years was higher than the risk for women who did not use HRT. For women who had taken the combination HRT, the risk of breast cancer increased by 8 percent per year; the risk was increased by 1 percent per year for women who had taken the estrogen-only therapy. There was no increase in risk among women who had stopped using either type of HRT for 4 years or more.

The second study focused on nearly 1,900 postmenopausal women diagnosed with breast cancer and more than 1,600 controls matched for age, race, and neighborhood. The researchers found that, for combined HRT, the risk of developing breast cancer increased by 24 percent for every 5 years of use; for estrogen-only therapy, the risk

301

increased by 6 percent every 5 years. Both studies reported that the increased risk of breast cancer associated with either type of HRT was more pronounced in thin women.

In addition, data from the Postmenopausal Estrogen/Progestin Interventions (PEPI) trial indicate that about 25 percent of women who use HRT that includes a combination of progestin and estrogen have an increase in breast density on their mammograms. In the PEPI study, about 8 percent of women taking estrogen-only HRT also had increased breast density. Increased density is a concern because other studies have shown that women age 45 and older whose mammograms show at least 75 percent dense tissue are at increased risk for breast cancer. However, researchers do not know if increased breast density due to HRT carries the same risk for breast cancer as having naturally dense breasts.

Increased breast density from HRT makes it more difficult for a radiologist to read some mammograms, sometimes leading to the need for followup mammograms and breast biopsies. One study showed that stopping HRT for about 2 weeks before having a mammogram improved the readability of the mammogram. However, further research is needed to confirm the usefulness of this approach.

There is also considerable uncertainty about the relationship between a woman's risk of developing breast cancer and the length of time she receives HRT. Some women take HRT for only a few years, until the worst of their menopausal symptoms have passed, while others take it for a decade or more. Some researchers believe that there is little or no increased risk of breast cancer associated with short-term use (3 years or less) of either HRT with estrogen alone or estrogen combined with progestin, while long-term use is linked to an increased risk.

Still another area of controversy centers on whether women who have had breast cancer can take HRT, especially since treatments for breast cancer can often lead to early menopause in younger women. Use of HRT in breast cancer survivors is widely discouraged because of the concern that exposure to the estrogen in HRT would increase their risk for recurrence. Some scientists question the validity of this concern, since the prognosis of women who took HRT before developing breast cancer seems to be better than that of women who did not do so. However, this finding may be a result of increased doctor visits leading to earlier detection and may not be due to the HRT. Women with a history of breast cancer should talk with their doctor about HRT so that they can make an informed decision.

Phytoestrogens

Some women who are concerned about conventional HRT have turned to nonprescription remedies, such as foods containing phytoestrogens, to relieve their menopausal symptoms. Phytoestrogens are weak estrogen-like substances that are found in foods such as soy products, whole-grain cereals, seeds, and certain fruits and vegetables. Phytoestrogens can also be obtained in the form of soy tablets.

Researchers are studying the use of phytoestrogens as an alternative to conventional HRT, particularly in women with a history of breast cancer. However, studies conducted with breast cancer survivors have not shown a significant improvement in menopausal symptoms with increased intake of phytoestrogens. Researchers continue to study whether phytoestrogens affect a woman's risk of cancer. To make an informed decision about the use of phytoestrogens and HRT, women should talk with their doctor.

The Future of HRT

Many women decide against using HRT because they are concerned about the risk of developing cancer. Often, they prefer to take other steps (such as exercise and a well-balanced diet along with calcium supplementation) to reduce their risk of osteoporosis and heart disease.

In an effort to find definitive answers, the Women's Health Initiative (WHI) and other carefully designed studies are evaluating the effects of long-term use of HRT in postmenopausal women. Sponsored by the National Institutes of Health, the WHI is a 15-year nationwide clinical trial that is investigating heart disease, osteoporosis, and breast and colon cancers in 63,000 women ages 50 to 79. Long-term, well-designed studies such as the WHI should be able to answer many of the lingering questions about the true effects of HRT.

Weighing benefits and risks is part of all medical decisions. Some women and their doctors feel that HRT's potential beneficial effects on cardiovascular disease, osteoporosis, and general quality of life outweigh the risk of developing cancer. Others are concerned about the possible negative effects of long-term HRT use. Many women choose to reduce the risks of osteoporosis and heart disease by exercising regularly, avoiding tobacco products, eating a balanced diet, and/or taking dietary supplements or other medications.

Ultimately, physicians emphasize that each woman's decision about whether to take HRT and, if so, for how long, must be an individual one made in cooperation with her physician. This decision should be based on the woman's individual risk profile—her personal and family medical history, not only of cancer, but also of heart disease, stroke, and osteoporosis.

Resources

The following Federal Government agencies can provide information related to hormone replacement therapy:

National Heart, Lung, and Blood Institute (NHLBI)
Information Center
Post Office Box 30105
Bethesda, MD 20824-0105
Telephone: 301-592-8573
Fax: 301-592-8563
website: http://www.nhlbi.nih.gov/index.htm

The NHLBI Information Center provides printed material about heart disease and its risk factors.

National Institute on Aging (NIA)
Public Information Office
Building 31, Room 5C27
31 Center Drive, MSC 2292
Bethesda, MD 20892
Telephone: 301-496-1752 or 1-800-222-2225
TTY: 1-800-222-4225 (for deaf and hard of hearing callers)
website: http://www.nih.gov/nia

The NIA Public Information Office offers printed material about menopause, osteoporosis, heart disease, and stroke.

National Institute of Neurological Disorders and Stroke (NINDS)
Office of Communications and Public Liaison
Post Office Box 5801
Bethesda, MD 20824
website: http://www.ninds.nih.gov

The NINDS Office of Communications and Public Liaison distributes printed material about stroke and other neurological disorders.

Osteoporosis and Related Bone Diseases
National Resource Center
1232 22nd Street, NW.
Washington, DC 20037-1292
Telephone: 1-800-624-BONE (1-800-624-2663)
TTY: 202-466-4315 (for deaf and hard of hearing callers)
Fax: 202-293-2356
website: http://www.osteo.org

The Osteoporosis and Related Bone Diseases National Resource Center distributes printed material about osteoporosis prevention and treatment.

Women's Health Initiative (WHI)
Program Office
Suite 300 MS 7966
One Rockledge Centre
6705 Rockledge Drive
Bethesda, MD 20892-7966
Telephone: (301) 402-2900
Fax: (301) 480-5158
website: http://www.nhlbi.nih.gov/whi/

The WHI Program Office provides information about the WHI.

References

Andrews WC. The transitional years and beyond. *Obstetrics & Gynecology* 1995; 85(1):1-5.

Bonnier P, Romain S, Giacalone PL, et al. Clinical and biologic prognostic factors in breast cancer diagnosed during postmenopausal hormone replacement therapy. *Obstetrics & Gynecology* 1995; 85(1):11-17.

Brinton LA, Schairer C. Postmenopausal hormone-replacement therapy: time for a reappraisal? *New England Journal of Medicine* 1997; 336(25):1821-1822.

Bush TL. Feminine forever revisited: menopausal hormone therapy in the 1990s. *Journal of Women's Health* 1992; 1(1):1-4.

Bush TL, Whiteman MK. Hormone replacement therapy and risk of breast cancer. Editorial. *Journal of the American Medical Association* 1999; 281(22):2140-2141.

Davidson NE. Is hormone replacement therapy a risk? *Scientific American* 1996; 275(3):101.

Gapstur SM, Morrow M, Sellers TA. Hormone replacement therapy and risk of breast cancer with a favorable histology: results of the Iowa Women's Health Study. *Journal of the American Medical Association* 1999; 281(22):2091-2097.

Gottlieb, N. "Soybean" in a haystack? Pinpointing an anti-cancer effect. *Journal of the National Cancer Institute* 1999; 91(19):1610-1612.

Greendale GA, Reboussin BA, Sie A, et al. Effects of estrogen and estrogen-progestin on mammographic parenchymal density. Postmenopausal estrogen/progestin interventions (PEPI) investigators. *Annals of Internal Medicine* 1999; 130(4 Part 1):262-269.

Grodstein F, Stampfer MJ, Colditz GA, et al. Postmenopausal hormone therapy and mortality. *New England Journal of Medicine* 1997; 336(25):1769-1775.

Harvey JA, Pinkerton JV, Herman CR. Short-term cessation of hormone replacement therapy and improvement of mammographic specificity. *Journal of the National Cancer Institute* 1997; 89(21):1623-1625.

Hulley S, Grady D, Bush T, et al. Randomized trial of estrogen plus progestin for secondary prevention of coronary heart disease in postmenopausal women. *Journal of the American Medical Association* 1998; 280(7):605-613.

Keller C, Fullerton J, Mobley C. Supplemental and complementary alternatives to hormone replacement therapy. *Journal of the American Academy of Nurse Practitioners* 1999; 11(5):187-198.

Mayeaux EJ Jr., Johnson C. Current concepts in postmenopausal hormone replacement therapy. *The Journal of Family Practice* 1996; 43(1):69-75.

Quella SK, Loprinzi CL, Barton DL, et al. Evaluation of soy phytoestrogens for the treatment of hot flashes in breast cancer survivors: a North Central Cancer Treatment Group trial. *Journal of Clinical Oncology* 2000; 18(5):1068-1074.

Ross RK, Paganini-Hill A, Wan PC, Pike MC. Effect of hormone replacement therapy on breast cancer risk: estrogen versus estrogen plus progestin. *Journal of the National Cancer Institute* 2000; 92(4):328-332.

Schairer C, Lubin J, Troisi R, et al. Menopausal estrogen and estrogen-progestin replacement therapy and breast cancer risk. *Journal of the American Medical Association* 2000; 283(4): 485-491.

Willett W, Colditz G, Stampfer M. Postmenopausal estrogens opposed, unopposed, or none of the above. *Journal of the American Medical Association* 2000; 283(4):534-535.

Women's Health Initiative Study Group. Design of the women's health initiative clinical trial and observational study. *Controlled Clinical Trials* 1998; 19:61-109.

Writing Group for the PEPI Trial. Effects of estrogen or estrogen/progestin regimens on heart disease risk factors in postmenopausal women. The postmenopausal estrogen/progestin interventions (PEPI) trial. *Journal of the American Medical Association* 1995; 273(3):199-208.

Writing Group for the PEPI Trial. Effects of hormone therapy on bone mineral density: results from the postmenopausal estrogen/progestin interventions (PEPI) trial. *Journal of the American Medical Association* 1996; 276(17):1389-1396.

Wysowski DK, Golden L, Burke L. Use of menopausal estrogens and medroxyprogesterone in the United States, 1982-1992. *Obstetrics & Gynecology* 1995; 85(1):6-10.

Chapter 45

Questions and Answers about Diethylstilbestrol (DES)

What is DES?

DES (diethylstilbestrol) is a synthetic form of estrogen, a female hormone. It was prescribed between 1938 and 1971 to help women with certain complications of pregnancy. Use of DES declined in the 1960s after studies showed that it is not effective in preventing pregnancy complications. When given during the first 5 months of a pregnancy, DES can interfere with the development of the reproductive system in a fetus. For this reason, although DES and other estrogens may be prescribed for some medical problems, they are no longer used during pregnancy.

What health problems might DES-exposed daughters have?

In 1971, DES was linked to an uncommon cancer (called clear cell adenocarcinoma) in a small number of daughters of women who had used DES during pregnancy. This cancer of the vagina or cervix usually occurs after age 14, with most cases found at age 19 or 20 in DES-exposed daughters. The upper age limit, if any, for DES-exposed daughters to develop this type of cancer is not known, and some cases have been reported in women in their thirties and forties. The overall risk of an exposed daughter to develop this type of cancer is estimated to be approximately 1/1000 (0.1 percent). Although clear cell adenocarcinoma is extremely rare, it is important that DES-exposed daughters continue to have regular physical examinations.

Fact Sheet 3.4, Cancer Information Service, National Cancer Institute, 6/00.

Scientists found a link between DES exposure before birth and an increased risk of developing abnormal cells in the tissue of the cervix and vagina, although the significance of these findings is controversial. Physicians use a number of terms to describe these abnormal cells, including dysplasia, cervical intraepithelial neoplasia (CIN), and squamous intraepithelial lesions (SIL). These abnormal cells resemble cancer cells in appearance; however, they do not invade nearby healthy tissue as cancer cells do. These abnormal cellular changes usually occur between the ages of 25 and 35, but may appear in exposed women of other ages as well. Although this condition is not cancer, it may develop into cancer if left untreated. DES-exposed daughters should have a yearly Pap smear and pelvic exam to check for abnormal cells. DES-exposed daughters also may have structural changes in the vagina, uterus, or cervix. They also may have irregular menstruation and an increased risk of miscarriage, tubal (ectopic) pregnancy, infertility, and premature delivery.

What health problems might DES-exposed sons have?

There is some evidence that DES-exposed sons may have testicular abnormalities, such as undescended testicles or abnormally small testicles. The risk for testicular or prostate cancer is unclear; studies of the association between DES exposure *in utero* and testicular cancer have produced mixed results. In addition, investigations of abnormalities of the urogenital system among DES-exposed sons have not produced clear answers.

What health problems might DES-exposed mothers have?

Women who used DES may have a slightly increased risk of breast cancer. Current research indicates that the risk of breast cancer in DES-exposed mothers is approximately 30 percent higher than the risk for women who have not been exposed to this drug. This risk has been stable over time, and does not seem to increase as the mothers become older. Additional research is needed to clarify this issue and whether DES-exposed mothers are at higher risk for any other types of cancer.

How do you know whether you took DES during pregnancy or whether your mother took DES while pregnant with you?

It has been estimated that 5 to 10 million people were exposed to DES during pregnancy. Many of these people are not aware that they were exposed. A woman who was pregnant between 1940 and 1971

310

and had problems or a history of problems during pregnancy may have been given DES or a similar drug. If you think you or your mother used a hormone such as DES during pregnancy, you could try to contact the attending physician or the hospital where the delivery took place to ask whether there is any record that you or your mother received DES. If any pills were taken during pregnancy, obstetrical records should be checked to determine the name of the drug. Mothers and children have a right to this information.

However, finding medical records after a long period of time may be difficult. If the doctor has retired or died, another doctor may have taken over the practice as well as the records. The county medical society or health department may be able to tell you where the records are. Some pharmacies keep records for a long time. If you know where the prescription was filled, you may be able to get this information. Military medical records are kept for 25 years. In many cases, however, it may be impossible to determine whether DES was used.

What should DES-exposed daughters do?

It is important for women who believe they may have been exposed to DES before birth to be aware of the possible health effects of DES and inform their doctor of their exposure. It is important that the physician be familiar with possible problems associated with DES exposure, because some problems, such as clear cell adenocarcinoma, are likely to be found only when the doctor is looking for them. A thorough examination may include the following:

- Pelvic examination—A physical examination of the reproductive organs. An examination of the rectum also should be done.

- Palpation—As part of a pelvic examination, the doctor feels the vagina, uterus, cervix, and ovaries for any lumps. Often palpation provides the only evidence that an abnormal growth is present.

- Pap test—A routine cervical Pap test is not adequate for DES-exposed daughters. The cervical Pap test must be supplemented with a special Pap test of the vagina called a "four-quadrant" Pap test, in which cell samples are taken from all sides of the upper vagina.

- Iodine staining of the cervix and vagina—An iodine solution is used to temporarily stain the linings of the cervix and vagina to detect adenosis (a noncancerous but abnormal growth of glandular tissue) or other abnormal tissue.

311

- Colposcopy—In colposcopy, a magnifying instrument is used to view the vagina and cervix. Some doctors do not perform colposcopy routinely. However, if the Pap test result is not normal, it is very important to check for abnormal tissue.

- Biopsy—Small samples of any tissue that appear abnormal on colposcopy are removed and examined under a microscope to see whether cancer cells are present.

- Breast examinations—Thus far, DES-exposed daughters have not been shown to have a higher risk of breast cancer than unexposed daughters; however, they should follow the routine screening recommendations for their age group.

What should DES-exposed mothers do?

A woman who took DES while pregnant (or suspects she may have taken it) should inform her doctor. She should try to learn the dosage, when the medication was started, and how it was used. She also should inform her children who were exposed before birth so that this information can be included in their medical records. DES-exposed mothers should have regular breast cancer screening and yearly medical checkups that include a pelvic examination and a Pap test.

What should DES-exposed sons do?

DES-exposed sons should inform their physician of their exposure and be examined periodically. While the level of risk of developing testicular cancer is unclear among DES-exposed sons, males with undescended testicles or unusually small testicles have an increased risk of developing testicular cancer, whether or not they were exposed to DES.

Is it safe for DES-exposed daughters to use oral contraceptives or hormone replacement therapy?

Each woman should discuss this important question with her doctor. Although studies have not shown that the use of birth control pills or hormone replacement therapy are unsafe for DES-exposed daughters, some doctors believe these women should avoid these medications because they contain estrogen. Structural changes in the vagina or cervix should cause no problems with the use of other forms of contraception, such as diaphragms or spermicides.

Do DES-exposed daughters have unusual problems in pregnancy?

There is evidence that the risk of tubal (ectopic) pregnancy, miscarriage, and premature delivery is increased for a DES-exposed daughter. Although most DES-exposed daughters do not experience DES-related problems during pregnancy, the doctor should be told of the DES exposure and should monitor the pregnancy closely.

What is the focus of current research on DES exposure?

The emphasis of current research is to provide continued followup to all DES-exposed groups as they age, and to identify any cancer or other health risks that may be found in these groups. Researchers continue to study DES-exposed daughters as they move into the menopausal years. The cancer risks for exposed daughters and sons are also being studied to determine if they differ from the unexposed population. In addition, researchers are studying possible health effects on the grandchildren of mothers who were exposed to DES during pregnancy.

What kinds of education and outreach efforts are in progress?

The Centers for Disease Control and Prevention (CDC) is developing a DES National Education Campaign (DES NEC) with the assistance of the DES NEC Working Group. The campaign will focus on increasing the awareness of the general public about DES exposure and the need for careful screening and followup. It will also provide primary health care providers with up-to-date information about the health effects of DES and screening and treatment guidelines for DES-exposed groups. The campaign is currently in the research and planning stages, with plans to release the new materials in late 2001.

Where can DES-exposed people get additional information?

Resources for people who were exposed to DES include the following:

DES Action USA
Suite 510
1615 Broadway
Oakland, CA 94612
Telephone: 510-465-4011 or
1-800-DES-9288 (1-800-337-9288)

DES Action USA, continued
Fax: 510-465-4815
e-mail: desact@well.com
website: http://www.desaction.org

DES Action USA is a consumer group organized by individuals who were exposed to DES. It provides information, referrals, and support for DES-exposed people and health professionals.

DES Cancer Network
Suite 400
514 10th Street, NW.
Washington, DC 20004-1403
Telephone: 202-628-6330
1-800-DES-NET4 (1-800-337-6384)
Fax number: 202-628-6217
e-mail: DESNETWRK@aol.com
website: http:www.descancer.org

The DES Cancer Network is a national organization for DES-exposed women and their family and friends. It offers education, support, and research advocacy, with a special focus on DES cancer issues.

The Registry for Research on Hormonal Transplacental Carcinogenesis (Clear Cell Cancer Registry)
Department of Obstetrics and Gynecology
The University of Chicago
5841 South Maryland Avenue, MC 2050
Chicago, IL 60637
Telephone: 773-702-6671
Fax number: 773-702-0840
e-mail: registry@babies.bsd.uchicago.edu
website: http://cis.nci.nih.gov/asp/
disclaimernew.asp?p=obgyn.bsd.uchicago.edu/registry.html

The Registry for Research on Hormonal Transplacental Carcinogenesis (also called the Clear Cell Cancer Registry) is a worldwide registry for individuals who developed clear cell adenocarcinoma as a result of exposure to DES. Staff members also answer questions from the public.

Chapter 46

Stress and Cancer Risk

What are some of the most common causes of stress?

Stress can arise for a variety of reasons. Stress can be brought about by a traumatic accident, death, or emergency situation. Stress can also be a side effect of a serious illness or disease. There is also stress associated with daily life, the workplace, and family responsibilities.

What are some early signs of stress?

Stress can take on many different forms, and can contribute to symptoms of illness. Common symptoms include headache, sleep disorders, difficulty concentrating, short-temper, upset stomach, job dissatisfaction, low morale, depression, and anxiety.

What is post-traumatic stress disorder (PTSD)?

Post-traumatic stress disorder (PTSD) can be an extremely debilitating condition that can occur after exposure to a terrifying event or ordeal in which grave physical harm occurred or was threatened. Traumatic events that can trigger PTSD include violent personal assaults such as rape or mugging, natural or human-caused disasters, accidents, or military combat.

Department of Health and Human Services, Office on Women's Health, October 2000. This information was abstracted from the National Cancer Institute fact sheet on *Psychological Stress and Cancer* and the National Institute of Mental Health fact sheet on *Post-traumatic Stress Disorder.*

Many people with PTSD repeatedly re-experience the ordeal in the form of flashback episodes, memories, nightmares, or frightening thoughts, especially when they are exposed to events or objects that remind them of the trauma. Anniversaries of the event can also trigger symptoms. People with PTSD also experience emotional numbness and sleep disturbances, depression, anxiety, and irritability or outbursts of anger. Feelings of intense guilt are also common, particularly if others did not survive the traumatic event. Most people with PTSD try to avoid any reminders or thoughts of the ordeal. PTSD is diagnosed when these symptoms last more than 1 month.

Is there any way to relieve your stress?

There are many stress management programs that can teach you about the nature and sources of stress, the effects of stress on health, and personal skills to reduce the effects of stress. Examples of stress reducing skills include time management and physical exercise.

For more serious stress related disorders, like PTSD, research has demonstrated the effectiveness of cognitive-behavioral therapy, group therapy, and exposure therapy, in which the patient repeatedly relives the frightening experience under controlled conditions to help him or her work through the trauma. Studies have also shown that medications help ease associated symptoms of depression and anxiety and help promote sleep.

Is there a relationship between cancer and stress?

The complex relationship between physical and psychological health is not well understood. Although studies have shown that stress factors (such as death of a spouse, social isolation, and medical school examinations) alter the way the immune system (the body's defense against infection and disease, including cancer) functions, they have not provided scientific evidence of a direct cause-and-effect relationship between these immune system changes and the development of cancer. Scientists know that many types of stress activate the body's endocrine (hormone) system, which in turn can cause changes in the immune system. It has not been shown that stress-induced changes in the immune system directly cause cancer.

Several studies have indicated an increased incidence of early death, including cancer death, among people who have experienced the recent loss of a spouse or other loved one. But, most cancers have been developing for many years, and it is unlikely that cancer would be triggered by the recent death of a loved one. However, some studies of women with breast cancer have shown significantly higher rates of this disease among those women who experienced traumatic life events and losses within several years before their diagnosis.

Although the relationship between psychological stress and cancer has not been scientifically proven, stress reduction is of benefit for many other reasons.

Are hormones related to stress in women?

Scientists know that many types of stress activate the body's endocrine (hormone) system, which in turn can cause changes in the immune system, the body's defense against infection and disease (including cancer). On the positive side for women, there is some evidence that women who breast-feed their infants produce lower levels of stress response hormones, such as adrenaline, and cortisol, than do women who bottle-feed. It is also known, however, that hormone changes during pregnancy, menopause, and during the menstrual cycle can trigger symptoms of depression and stress.

For More Information

You can find out more about stress by contacting the following organizations:

American Institute of Stress
Phone: (914) 963-1200
Internet Address: http://www.stress.org

National Institute of Mental Health
Phone: (301) 443-4513
Internet Address: http://www.nimh.nih.gov

National Mental Health Services
Knowledge Exchange Network
Phone: (800) 789-2647
Internet Address: http://www.mentalhealth.org

Part Seven

Treatment Options

Chapter 47

Chemotherapy

Introduction

This text is designed to help you become an informed partner in your care, but it is only a guide. Self-help can never take the place of professional health care. Ask your doctor and nurse any questions you may have about chemotherapy. Also don't hesitate to tell them about any side effects you may have. They want and need to know.

What Is Chemotherapy?

Chemotherapy is the treatment of cancer with drugs that can destroy cancer cells. These drugs often are called "anticancer" drugs.

How Does Chemotherapy Work?

Normal cells grow and die in a controlled way. When cancer occurs, cells in the body that are not normal keep dividing and forming more cells without control. Anticancer drugs destroy cancer cells by stopping them from growing or multiplying. Healthy cells can also be harmed, especially those that divide quickly. Harm to healthy cells is what causes side effects. These cells usually repair themselves after chemotherapy.

Excerpted from "Chemotherapy and You: A Guide to Self-Help during Cancer Treatment," National Cancer Institute (NCI), NIH Pub. No. 99-1136, revised June 1999. To order a copy of the full text, or for other cancer-related information, contact NCI's Cancer Information Service at 800-4-CANCER (800-422-6237) or visit www.nci.nih.gov on the Internet.

Because some drugs work better together than alone, often two or more drugs are given at the same time. This is called combination chemotherapy.

Other types of drugs may be used to treat your cancer. These may include certain drugs that can block the effect of your body's hormones. Or doctors may use biological therapy, which is treatment with substances that boost the body's own immune system against cancer. Your body usually makes these substances in small amounts to fight cancer and other diseases. These substances can be made in the laboratory and given to patients to destroy cancer cells or change the way the body reacts to a tumor. They may also help the body repair or make new cells destroyed by chemotherapy.

What Can Chemotherapy Do?

Depending on the type of cancer and how advanced it is, chemotherapy can be used for different goals:

- *To cure the cancer.* Cancer is considered cured when the patient remains free of evidence of cancer cells.

- *To control the cancer.* This is done by keeping the cancer from spreading; slowing the cancer's growth; and killing cancer cells that may have spread to other parts of the body from the original tumor.

- *To relieve symptoms that the cancer may cause.* Relieving symptoms such as pain can help patients live more comfortably.

Is Chemotherapy Used with Other Treatments?

Sometimes chemotherapy is the only treatment a patient receives. More often, however, chemotherapy is used in addition to surgery, radiation therapy, and/or biological therapy to:

- Shrink a tumor before surgery or radiation therapy. This is called neo-adjuvant therapy.

- Help destroy any cancer cells that may remain after surgery and/or radiation therapy. This is called adjuvant chemotherapy.

- Make radiation therapy and biological therapy work better.

- Help destroy cancer if it recurs or has spread to other parts of the body from the original tumor.

Which Drugs Are Given?

Some chemotherapy drugs are used for many different types of cancer, while others might be used for just one or two types of cancer. Your doctor recommends a treatment plan based on:

- What kind of cancer you have.
- What part of the body the cancer is found.
- The effect of cancer on your normal body functions.
- Your general health.

Questions to Ask Your Doctor about Chemotherapy

- Why do I need chemotherapy?
- What are the benefits of chemotherapy?
- What are the risks of chemotherapy?
- Are there any other possible treatment methods for my type of cancer?
- What is the standard care for my type of cancer?
- Are there any clinical trials for my type of cancer?
- How many treatments will I be given?
- What drug or drugs will I be taking?
- How will the drugs be given?
- Where will I get my treatment?
- How long will each treatment last?
- What are the possible side effects of the chemotherapy? When are side effects likely to occur?
- What side effects are more likely to be related to my type of cancer?
- Are there any side effects that I should report right away?
- What can I do to relieve the side effects?
- How do I contact a health professional after hours, and when should I call?

Hints for Talking with Your Doctor

These tips might help you keep track of the information you learn during visits with your doctor:

- Bring a friend or family member to sit with you while you talk with your doctor. This person can help you understand what your doctor says during your visit and help refresh your memory afterward.

- Ask your doctor for printed information that is available on your cancer and treatment.

- You, or the person who goes with you, may want to take notes during your appointment.

- Ask your doctor to slow down when you need more time to write.

- You may want to ask if you can use a tape recorder during your visit. Take notes from the tape after the visit is finished. That way, you can review your conversation later as many times as you wish.

What Can I Expect during Chemotherapy?

Always feel free to ask your doctor, nurse, and pharmacist as many questions as you want. If you do not understand their answers, keep asking until you do. Remember, there is no such thing as a "stupid" question, especially about cancer or your treatment. To make sure you get all the answers you want, you may find it helpful to draw up a list of questions before each doctor's appointment. Some people keep a "running list" and jot down each new question as it occurs to them.

Where Will I Get Chemotherapy?

Chemotherapy can be given in many different places: at home, a doctor's office, a clinic, a hospital's outpatient department, or as an "inpatient" in a hospital. The choice of where you get chemotherapy depends on which drug or drugs you are getting, your insurance, and sometimes your own and your doctor's wishes. Most patients receive their treatment as an "outpatient" and are not hospitalized. Sometimes, a patient starting chemotherapy may need to stay at the hospital for a short time so that the medicine's effects can be watched closely and any needed changes can be made.

How Often and for How Long Will I Get Chemotherapy?

How often and how long you get chemotherapy depends on:

- The kind of cancer you have.
- The goals of the treatment.
- The drugs that are used.
- How your body responds to them.

You may get treatment every day, every week, or every month. Chemotherapy is often given in cycles that include treatment periods alternated with rest periods. Rest periods give your body a chance to build healthy new cells and regain its strength. Ask your health care provider to tell you how long and how often you may expect to get treatment.

Sticking with your treatment schedule is very important for the drugs to work right. Schedules may need to be changed for holidays and other reasons. If you miss a treatment session or skip a dose of the drug, contact your doctor.

Sometimes, your doctor may need to delay a treatment based on the results of certain blood tests. Your doctor will let you know what to do during this time and when to start your treatment again.

How Is Chemotherapy Given?

Chemotherapy can be given in several different ways: intravenously (through a vein), by mouth, through an injection (shot), or applied on the skin.

By vein (intravenous, or IV, treatment): Chemotherapy is most often given intravenously (IV), through a vein. Usually a thin needle is inserted into a vein on the hand or lower arm at the beginning of each treatment session and is removed at the end of the session. If you feel a coolness, burning, or other unusual sensation in the area of the needle stick when the IV is started, tell your doctor or nurse. Also report any pain, burning, skin redness, swelling, or discomfort that occurs during or after an IV treatment.

Chemotherapy can also be delivered by IV through catheters, ports, and pumps.

A catheter is a soft, thin, flexible tube that is placed in a large vein in the body and remains there as long as it is needed. Patients who need to have many IV treatments often have a catheter, so a needle does not have to be used each time. Drugs can be given and blood samples can be drawn through this catheter. Sometimes the catheter is attached to a port—a small round plastic or metal disc placed under the skin. The port can be used for as long as it is needed. A pump, which is used to control how fast the drug goes into a catheter or port, is sometimes used. There are two types of pumps. An external pump remains outside the body. Most are portable; they allow a person to move around while the pump is being used. An internal pump is placed inside the body during surgery, usually right under the skin. Pumps contain a small storage area for the drug and allow people to go about their normal activities. Catheters, ports, and pumps cause no pain if they are properly placed and cared for, although a person is aware they are there.

Catheters are usually placed in a large vein, most commonly to your chest, called a central venous catheter. A peripherally inserted central catheter (PICC) is inserted into a vein in the arm. Catheters can also be placed in an artery or other locations in your body, such as:

- *Intrathecal (IT) catheter.* Delivers drugs into the spinal fluid.

- *Intracavitary (IC) catheter.* Placed in the abdomen, pelvis, or chest.

By mouth (orally): The drug is given in pill, capsule, or liquid form. You swallow the drug, just as you do many other medicines.

By injection: A needle and syringe are used to give the drug in one of several ways:

- *Intramuscularly, or IM.* (Into a muscle)

- *Subcutaneously, or SQ or SC.* (Under the skin)

- *Intralesionally, or IL.* (Directly into a cancerous area in the skin)

Topically. The drug is applied on the surface of the skin.

How Will I Feel During Chemotherapy?

Most people receiving chemotherapy find that they tire easily, but many feel well enough to continue to lead active lives. Each person and treatment is different, so it is not always possible to tell exactly how you will react. Your general state of health, the type and extent of cancer you have, and the kind of drugs you are receiving can all affect how well you feel.

You may want to have someone available to drive you to and from treatment if, for example, you are taking medicine for nausea or vomiting that could make you tired. You may also feel especially tired from the chemotherapy as early as one day after a treatment and for several days. It may help to schedule your treatment when you can take off the day of and the day after your treatment. If you have young children, you may want to schedule the treatment when you have someone to help at home the day of and at least the day after your treatment. Ask your doctor when your greatest fatigue or other side effects are likely to occur.

Most people can continue working while receiving chemotherapy. However, you may need to change your work schedule for a while if your chemotherapy makes you feel very tired or have other side effects. Talk with your employer about your needs and wishes. You may be able to agree on a part-time schedule, find an area for a short nap during the day, or perhaps you can do some of your work at home.

Under Federal and state laws, some employers may be required to let you work a flexible schedule to meet your treatment needs. To find out about your on-the-job protections, check with a social worker, or your congressional or state representative. The National Cancer Institute's publication "Facing Forward: A Guide for Cancer Survivors" also has information on work-related concerns (call 800-4-CANCER to order a copy or visit www.nci.nih.gov).

Can I Take Other Medicines while I Am Getting Chemotherapy?

Some medicines may interfere or react with the effects of your chemotherapy. Give your doctor a list of all the medicines you take before you start treatment. Include:

- the name of each drug
- the dosage
- the reason you take it
- how often you take it

Remember to tell your doctor about all over-the-counter remedies, including vitamins, laxatives, medicines for allergies, indigestion, and colds, aspirin, ibuprofen, or other pain relievers, and any mineral or herbal supplements. Your doctor can tell you if you should stop taking any of these remedies before you start chemotherapy. After your treatments begin, be sure to check with your doctor before taking any new medicines or stopping the ones you are already taking.

How Will I Know If My Chemotherapy Is Working?

Your doctor and nurse will use several ways to see how well your treatments are working. You may have physical exams and tests often. Always feel free to ask your doctor about the test results and what they show about your progress.

Tests and exams can tell a lot about how chemotherapy is working; however, side effects tell very little. Sometimes people think that if they have no side effects, the drugs are not working, or, if they do have side effects, the drugs are working well. But side effects vary so much from person to person, and from drug to drug, that side effects are not a sign of whether the treatment is working or not.

Coping with Side Effects

What Causes Side Effects?

Because cancer cells may grow and divide more rapidly than normal cells, many anticancer drugs are made to kill growing cells. But certain normal, healthy cells also multiply quickly, and chemotherapy can affect these cells, too. This damage to normal cells causes side effects. The fast-growing, normal cells most likely to be affected are blood cells forming in the bone marrow and cells in the digestive tract (mouth, stomach, intestines, esophagus), reproductive system (sexual organs), and hair follicles. Some anticancer drugs may affect cells of vital organs, such as the heart, kidney, bladder, lungs, and nervous system.

You may have none of these side effects or just a few. The kinds of side effects you have and how severe they are, depend on the type and dose of chemotherapy you get and how your body reacts. Before starting chemotherapy, your doctor will discuss the side effects that you are most likely to get with the drugs you will be receiving. Before starting the treatment, you will be asked to sign a consent form. You should be given all the facts about treatment including the drugs you will be given and their side effects before you sign the consent form.

How Long Do Side Effects Last?

Normal cells usually recover when chemotherapy is over, so most side effects gradually go away after treatment ends, and the healthy cells have a chance to grow normally. The time it takes to get over side effects depends on many things, including your overall health and the kind of chemotherapy you have been taking.

Most people have no serious long-term problems from chemotherapy. However, on some occasions, chemotherapy can cause permanent changes or damage to the heart, lungs, nerves, kidneys, reproductive or other organs. And certain types of chemotherapy may have delayed effects, such as a second cancer, that show up many years later. Ask your doctor about the chances of any serious, long-term effects that can result from the treatment you are receiving (but remember to balance your concerns with the immediate threat of your cancer).

Great progress has been made in preventing and treating some of chemotherapy's common as well as rare serious side effects. Many new drugs and treatment methods destroy cancer more effectively while doing less harm to the body's healthy cells.

The side effects of chemotherapy can be unpleasant, but they must be measured against the treatment's ability to destroy cancer. Medicines can help prevent some side effects such as nausea. Sometimes people receiving chemotherapy become discouraged about the length of time their treatment is taking or the side effects they are having. If that happens to you, talk to your doctor or nurse. They may be able to suggest ways to make side effects easier to deal with or reduce them.

Below you will find suggestions for dealing with some of the more common side effects of chemotherapy.

Fatigue

Fatigue, feeling tired and lacking energy, is the most common symptom reported by cancer patients. The exact cause is not always known. It can be due to your disease, chemotherapy, radiation, surgery, low blood counts, lack of sleep, pain, stress, poor appetite, along with many other factors.

Fatigue from cancer feels different from fatigue of everyday life. Fatigue caused by chemotherapy can appear suddenly. Patients with cancer have described it as a total lack of energy and have used words such as worn out, drained, and wiped out to describe their fatigue.

And rest does not always relieve it. Not everyone feels the same kind of fatigue. You may not feel tired while someone else does or your fatigue may not last as long as someone else's does. It can last days, weeks, or months. But severe fatigue does go away gradually as the tumor responds to treatment.

How can I cope with fatigue?

- Plan your day so that you have time to rest.

- Take short naps or breaks, rather than one long rest period.

- Save your energy for the most important things.

- Try easier or shorter versions of activities you enjoy.

- Take short walks or do light exercise if possible. You may find this helps with fatigue.

- Talk to your health care provider about ways to save your energy and treat your fatigue.

- Try activities such as meditation, prayer, yoga, guided imagery, visualization, etc. You may find that these help with fatigue.

- Eat as well as you can and drink plenty of fluids. Eat small amounts at a time, if that is helpful.

- Join a support group. Sharing your feelings with others can ease the burden of fatigue. You can learn how others deal with their fatigue. Your health care provider can put you in touch with a support group in your area.

- Limit the amount of caffeine and alcohol you drink.

- Allow others to do some things for you that you usually do.

- Keep a diary of how you feel each day. This will help you plan your daily activities.

- Report any changes in energy level to your doctor or nurse.

Nausea and Vomiting

Many patients fear that they will have nausea and vomiting while receiving chemotherapy. But new drugs have made these side effects far less common and, when they do occur, much less severe. These powerful antiemetic or antinausea drugs can prevent or lessen nausea and vomiting in most patients. Different drugs work for different people, and you may need more than one drug to get relief. Do not give up. Continue to work with your doctor and nurse to find the drug or drugs that work best for you. Also, be sure to tell your doctor or nurse if you are very nauseated or have vomited for more than a day, or if your vomiting is so bad that you cannot keep liquids down.

What can I do if I have nausea and vomiting?

- Drink liquids at least an hour before or after mealtime, instead of with your meals. Drink frequently and drink small amounts.

- Eat and drink slowly.

- Eat small meals throughout the day, instead of one, two, or three large meals.

- Eat foods cold or at room temperature so you won't be bothered by strong smells.

- Chew your food well for easier digestion.

- If nausea is a problem in the morning, try eating dry foods like cereal, toast, or crackers before getting up. (Do not try this if you have mouth or throat sores or are troubled by a lack of saliva.)

- Drink cool, clear, unsweetened fruit juices, such as apple or grape juice or light-colored sodas such as ginger ale that have lost their fizz and do not have caffeine.

- Suck on mints or tart candies. (Do not use tart candies if you have mouth or throat sores.)

- Prepare and freeze meals in advance for days when you do not feel like cooking.

- Wear loose-fitting clothes.

- Breathe deeply and slowly when you feel nauseated.

- Distract yourself by chatting with friends or family members, listening to music, or watching a movie or TV show.

- Use relaxation techniques.

- Try to avoid odors that bother you, such as cooking smells, smoke, or perfume.

- Avoid sweet, fried, or fatty foods.

- Rest but do not lie flat for at least 2 hours after you finish a meal.

- Avoid eating for at least a few hours before treatment if nausea usually occurs during chemotherapy.

- Eat a light meal before treatment.

Pain

Chemotherapy drugs can cause some side effects that are painful. The drugs can damage nerves, leading to burning, numbness, tingling, or shooting pain, most often in the fingers or toes. Some drugs can also cause mouth sores, headaches, muscle pains, and stomach pains.

Not everyone with cancer or who receives chemotherapy experiences pain from the disease or its treatment. But if you do, it can be relieved. The first step to take is to talk with your doctor, nurse, and pharmacist about your pain. They need to know as many details about your pain as possible. You may want to describe your pain to your family and friends. They can help you talk to your caregivers about your pain, especially if you are too tired or in too much pain to talk to them yourself.

You need to tell your doctor, nurse, and pharmacist and family or friends:

- Where you feel pain.

- What it feels like—sharp, dull, throbbing, steady.

- How strong the pain feels.

- How long it lasts.

- What eases the pain, what makes the pain worse.

- What medicines you are taking for the pain and how much relief you get from them.

Using a pain scale is helpful in describing how much pain you are feeling. Try to assign a number from 0 to 10 to your pain level. If you have no pain, use a 0. As the numbers get higher, they stand for pain that is getting worse. A 10 means the pain is as bad as it can be. You may wish to use your own pain scale using numbers from 0 to 5 or even 0 to 100. Be sure to let others know what pain scale you are using and use the same scale each time, for example, "My pain is 7 on a scale of 0 to 10."

The goal of pain control is to prevent pain that can be prevented, and treat the pain that can't. To do this:

- If you have persistent or chronic pain, take your pain medicine on a regular schedule (by the clock).

- Do not skip doses of your scheduled pain medicine. If you wait to take pain medicine until you feel pain, it is harder to control.

- Try using relaxation exercises at the same time you take medicine for the pain. This may help to lessen tension, reduce anxiety, and manage pain.

- Some people with chronic or persistent pain that is usually controlled by medicine can have breakthrough pain. This occurs when moderate to severe pain "breaks through" or is felt for a short time. If you experience this pain, use a short-acting medicine ordered by your doctor. Don't wait for the pain to get worse. If you do, it may be harder to control.

There are many different medicines and methods available to control cancer pain. You should expect your doctor to seek all the information and resources necessary to make you as comfortable as possible. If you are in pain and your doctor has no further suggestions, ask to see a pain specialist or have your doctor consult with a pain specialist. A pain specialist may be an oncologist, anesthesiologist, neurologist, neurosurgeon, other doctor, nurse, or pharmacist.

Hair Loss

Hair loss (alopecia) is a common side effect of chemotherapy, but not all drugs cause hair loss. Your doctor can tell you if hair loss might occur with the drug or drugs you are taking. When hair loss does occur, the hair may become thinner or fall out entirely. Hair loss can occur on all parts of the body, including the head, face, arms and legs, underarms, and pubic area. The hair usually grows back after the treatments are over. Some people even start to get their hair back while they are still having treatments. Sometimes, hair may grow back a different color or texture.

Hair loss does not always happen right away. It may begin several weeks after the first treatment or after a few treatments. Many people say their head becomes sensitive before losing hair. Hair may fall out gradually or in clumps. Any hair that is still growing may become dull and dry.

How can I care for my scalp and hair during chemotherapy?

- Use a mild shampoo.

- Use a soft hair brush.

- Use low heat when drying your hair.

- Have your hair cut short. A shorter style will make your hair look thicker and fuller. It also will make hair loss easier to manage if it occurs.

- Use a sun screen, sun block, hat, or scarf to protect your scalp from the sun if you lose hair on your head.

- Avoid brush rollers to set your hair.

- Avoid dying, perming, or relaxing your hair.

Some people who lose all or most of their hair choose to wear turbans, scarves, caps, wigs, or hair pieces. Others leave their head uncovered. Still others switch back and forth, depending on whether they are in public or at home with friends and family members. There are no "right" or "wrong" choices; do whatever feels comfortable for you.

If you choose to cover your head:

- Get your wig or hairpiece before you lose a lot of hair. That way, you can match your current hair style and color. You may be able to buy a wig or hairpiece at a specialty shop just for cancer patients. Someone may even come to your home to help you. You also can buy a wig or hair piece through a catalog or by phone.

- You may also consider borrowing a wig or hairpiece, rather than buying one. Check with the nurse or social work department at your hospital about resources for free wigs in your community.

- Take your wig to your hairdresser or the shop where it was purchased for styling and cutting to frame your face.

- Some health insurance policies cover the cost of a hairpiece needed because of cancer treatment. It is also a tax-deductible expense. Be sure to check your policy and ask your doctor for a "prescription."

Losing hair from your head, face, or body can be hard to accept. Feeling angry or depressed is common and perfectly all right. At the same time, keep in mind that it is a temporary side effect. Talking about your feelings can help. If possible, share your thoughts with someone who has had a similar experience.

Anemia

Chemotherapy can reduce the bone marrow's ability to make red blood cells, which carry oxygen to all parts of your body. When there are too few red blood cells, body tissues do not get enough oxygen to do their work. This condition is called anemia. Anemia can make you feel short of breath, very weak, and tired. Call your doctor if you have any of these symptoms:

- Fatigue (feeling very weak and tired).
- Dizziness or feeling faint.
- Shortness of breath.
- Feeling as if your heart is "pounding" or beating very fast.

Your doctor will check your blood cell count often during your treatment. She or he may also prescribe a medicine that can boost the growth of your red blood cells. Discuss this with your doctor if you become anemic often. If your red count falls too low, you may need a blood transfusion or a medicine called erythropoietin to raise the number of red blood cells in your body.

Things you can do if you are anemic:

- Get plenty of rest. Sleep more at night and take naps during the day if you can.
- Limit your activities. Do only the things that are essential or most important to you.
- Ask for help when you need it. Ask family and friends to pitch in with things like child care, shopping, housework, or driving.
- Eat a well-balanced diet.
- When sitting, get up slowly. When lying down, sit first and then stand. This will help prevent dizziness.

Central Nervous System Problems

Chemotherapy can interfere with certain functions in your central nervous system (brain) causing tiredness, confusion, and depression.

These feelings will go away once the chemotherapy dose is lowered or you finish chemotherapy. Call your doctor if these symptoms occur.

Infection

Chemotherapy can make you more likely to get infections. This happens because most anticancer drugs affect the bone marrow, making it harder to make white blood cells (WBCs), the cells that fight many types of infections. Your doctor will check your blood cell count often while you are getting chemotherapy. There are medicines that help speed the recovery of white blood cells, shortening the time when the white blood count is very low. These medicines are called colony stimulating factors (CSF). Raising the white blood cell count greatly lowers the risk of serious infection.

Most infections come from bacteria normally found on your skin and in your mouth, intestines and genital tract. Sometimes, the cause of an infection may not be known. Even if you take extra care, you still may get an infection. But there are some things you can do.

How can I help prevent infections?

- Wash your hands often during the day. Be sure to wash them before you eat, after you use the bathroom, and after touching animals.

- Clean your rectal area gently but thoroughly after each bowel movement. Ask your doctor or nurse for advice if the area becomes irritated or if you have hemorrhoids. Also, check with your doctor before using enemas or suppositories.

- Stay away from people who have illnesses you can catch, such as a cold, the flu, measles, or chicken pox.

- Try to avoid crowds. For example, go shopping or to the movies when the stores or theaters are least likely to be busy.

- Stay away from children who recently have received "live virus" vaccines such as chicken pox and oral polio, since they may be contagious to people with a low blood cell count. Call your doctor or local health department if you have any questions.

- Do not cut or tear the cuticles of your nails.

- Be careful not to cut or nick yourself when using scissors, needles, or knives.

- Use an electric shaver instead of a razor to prevent breaks or cuts in your skin.

- Maintain good mouth care.

- Do not squeeze or scratch pimples.

- Take a warm (not hot) bath, shower, or sponge bath every day. Pat your skin dry using a light touch. Do not rub too hard.

- Use lotion or oil to soften and heal your skin if it becomes dry and cracked.

- Clean cuts and scrapes right away and daily until healed with warm water, soap, and an antiseptic.

- Avoid contact with animal litter boxes and waste, bird cages, and fish tanks.

- Avoid standing water, for example, bird baths, flower vases, or humidifiers.

- Wear protective gloves when gardening or cleaning up after others, especially small children.

- Do not get any immunizations, such as flu or pneumonia shots, without checking with your doctor first.

- Do not eat raw fish, seafood, meat, or eggs.

Symptoms of Infection

Call your doctor right away if you have any of these symptoms:

- Fever over 100° F or 38° C.

- Chills, especially shaking chills.

- Sweating.

- Loose bowel movements.

- Frequent urgency to urinate or a burning feeling when you urinate.

- A severe cough or sore throat.

- Unusual vaginal discharge or itching.

- Redness, swelling, or tenderness, especially around a wound, sore, ostomy, pimple, rectal area or catheter site.

- Sinus pain or pressure.

- Earaches, headaches, or stiff neck.

- Blisters on the lips or skin.

- Mouth sores.

Report any signs of infection to your doctor right away, even if it is in the middle of the night. This is especially important when your white blood cell count is low. If you have a fever, do not take aspirin, acetaminophen, or any other medicine to bring your temperature down without checking with your doctor first.

Blood Clotting Problems

Anticancer drugs can affect the bone marrow's ability to make platelets, the blood cells that help stop bleeding by making your blood clot. If your blood does not have enough platelets, you may bleed or bruise more easily than usual, even without an injury.

Call your doctor if you have any of these symptoms:

- unexpected bruising.

- small, red spots under the skin.

- reddish or pinkish urine.

- black or bloody bowel movements.

- bleeding from your gums or nose.

- vaginal bleeding that is new or lasts longer than a regular period.

- headaches or changes in vision.

- warm to hot feeling of an arm or leg.

Your doctor will check your platelet count often while you are having chemotherapy. If your platelet count falls too low, the doctor may give you a platelet transfusion to build up the count. There are also medicines called colony stimulating factors that help increase your platelets.

How to Help Prevent Problems If Your Platelet Count Is Low

- Check with your doctor or nurse before taking any vitamins, herbal remedies, including all over-the-counter medicines.

Many of these products contain aspirin, which can affect platelets.

- Before drinking any alcoholic beverages, check with your doctor.

- Use a very soft toothbrush to clean your teeth.

- When cleaning your nose blow gently into a soft tissue.

- Take extra care not to cut or nick yourself when using scissors, needles, knives, or tools.

- Be careful not to burn yourself when ironing or cooking.

- Avoid contact sports and other activities that might result in injury.

- Ask your doctor if you should avoid sexual activity.

- Use an electric shaver instead of a razor.

Mouth, Gum, and Throat Problems

Good oral care is important during cancer treatment. Some anticancer drugs can cause sores in the mouth and throat, a condition called stomatitis or mucositis. Anticancer drugs also can make these tissues dry and irritated or cause them to bleed. Patients who have not been eating well since beginning chemotherapy are more likely to get mouth sores.

In addition to being painful, mouth sores can become infected by the many germs that live in the mouth. Every step should be taken to prevent infections, because they can be hard to fight during chemotherapy and can lead to serious problems.

How can I keep my mouth, gums, and throat healthy?

- Talk to your doctor about seeing your dentist at least several weeks before you start chemotherapy. You may need to have your teeth cleaned and to take care of any problems such as cavities, gum abscesses, gum disease, or poorly fitting dentures. Ask your dentist to show you the best ways to brush and floss your teeth during chemotherapy. Chemotherapy can make you more likely to get cavities, so your dentist may suggest using a fluoride rinse or gel each day to help prevent decay.

- Brush your teeth and gums after every meal. Use a soft toothbrush and a gentle touch. Brushing too hard can damage soft mouth tissues. Ask your doctor, nurse, or dentist to suggest a special toothbrush and/or toothpaste if your gums are very sensitive. Rinse with warm salt water after meals and before bedtime.

- Rinse your toothbrush well after each use and store it in a dry place.

- Avoid mouthwashes that contain any amount of alcohol. Ask your doctor or nurse to suggest a mild or medicated mouthwash that you might use. For example, mouthwash with sodium bicarbonate (baking soda) is non-irritating.

If you develop sores in your mouth, tell your doctor or nurse. You may need medicine to treat the sores. If the sores are painful or keep you from eating, you can try these ideas:

How can I cope with mouth sores?

- Ask your doctor if there is anything you can apply directly to the sores or to prescribe a medicine you can use to ease the pain.

- Eat foods cold or at room temperature. Hot and warm foods can irritate a tender mouth and throat.

- Eat soft, soothing foods, such as ice cream, milkshakes, baby food, soft fruits (bananas and applesauce), mashed potatoes, cooked cereals, soft-boiled or scrambled eggs, yogurt, cottage cheese, macaroni and cheese, custards, puddings, and gelatin. You also can puree cooked foods in the blender to make them smoother and easier to eat.

- Avoid irritating, acidic foods and juices, such as tomato and citrus (orange, grapefruit, and lemon); spicy or salty foods; and rough or coarse foods such as raw vegetables, granola, popcorn, and toast.

How can I cope with mouth dryness?

- Ask your doctor if you should use an artificial saliva product to moisten your mouth.

- Drink plenty of liquids.

- Ask your doctor if you can suck on ice chips, popsicles, or sugarless hard candy. You can also chew sugarless gum. (Sorbitol, a sugar substitute that is in many sugar-free foods, can cause diarrhea in many people. If diarrhea is a problem for you, check the labels of sugar-free foods before you buy them and limit your use of them.)

- Moisten dry foods with butter, margarine, gravy, sauces, or broth.
- Dunk crisp, dry foods in mild liquids.
- Eat soft and pureed foods.
- Use lip balm or petroleum jelly if your lips become dry.
- Carry a water bottle with you to sip from often.

Diarrhea

When chemotherapy affects the cells lining the intestine, it can cause diarrhea (watery or loose stools). If you have diarrhea that continues for more than 24 hours, or if you have pain and cramping along with the diarrhea, call your doctor. In severe cases, the doctor may prescribe a medicine to control the diarrhea. If diarrhea persists, you may need intravenous (IV) fluids to replace the water and nutrients you have lost. Often these fluids are given as an outpatient and do not require hospitalization. Do not take any over-the-counter medicines for diarrhea without asking your doctor.

How can I help control diarrhea?

- Drink plenty of fluids. This will help replace those you have lost through diarrhea. Mild, clear liquids, such as water, clear broth, sports drinks such as Gatorade, or ginger ale, are best. If these drinks make you more thirsty or nauseous, try diluting them with water. Drink slowly and make sure drinks are at room temperature. Let carbonated drinks lose their fizz before you drink them.

- Eat small amounts of food throughout the day instead of three large meals.

- Unless your doctor has told you otherwise, eat potassium-rich foods. Diarrhea can cause you to lose this important mineral. Bananas, oranges, potatoes, and peach and apricot nectars are good sources of potassium.

- Ask your doctor if you should try a clear liquid diet to give your bowels time to rest. A clear liquid diet does not provide all the nutrients you need, so do not follow one for more than 3 to 5 days.

- Eat low-fiber foods. Low-fiber foods include white bread, white rice or noodles, creamed cereals, ripe bananas, canned or cooked fruit without skins, cottage cheese, yogurt without seeds, eggs, mashed or baked potatoes without the skin, pureed vegetables, chicken, or turkey without the skin, and fish.

- Avoid high-fiber foods, which can lead to diarrhea and cramping. High-fiber foods include whole grain breads and cereals, raw vegetables, beans, nuts, seeds, popcorn, and fresh and dried fruit.

- Avoid hot or very cold liquids, which can make diarrhea worse.

- Avoid coffee, tea with caffeine, alcohol, and sweets. Stay away from fried, greasy, or highly spiced foods, too. They are irritating and can cause diarrhea and cramping.

- Avoid milk and milk products, including ice cream, if they make your diarrhea worse.

Constipation

Some anticancer medicines, pain medicines, and other medicines can cause constipation. It can also occur if you are less active or if your diet lacks enough fluid or fiber. If you have not had a bowel movement for more than a day or two, call your doctor, who may suggest taking a laxative or stool softener. Do not take these measures without checking with your doctor, especially if your white blood cell count or platelets are low.

What can I do about constipation?

- Drink plenty of fluids to help loosen the bowels. If you do not have mouth sores, try warm and hot fluids, including water, which work especially well.

- Check with your doctor to see if you can increase the fiber in your diet (there are certain kinds of cancer and certain side effects you may have for which a high-fiber diet is not recommended). High fiber foods include bran, whole-wheat breads and cereals, raw or cooked vegetables, fresh and dried fruit, nuts, and popcorn.

- Get some exercise every day. Go for a walk or you may want to try a more structured exercise program. Talk to your doctor about the amount and type of exercise that is right for you.

Nerve and Muscle Effects

Sometimes anticancer drugs can cause problems with your body's nerves. One example of a condition affecting the nervous system is peripheral neuropathy, where you feel a tingling, burning, weakness, or numbness or pain in the hands and/or feet. Some drugs can also affect the muscles, making them weak, tired, or sore.

Sometimes, these nerve and muscle side effects, though annoying, may not be serious. In other cases, nerve and muscle symptoms may be serious and need medical attention. Be sure to report any nerve or muscle symptoms to your doctor. Most of the time, these symptoms will get better; however, it may take up to a year after your treatment ends.

Some nerve and muscle-related symptoms include:

- tingling
- burning
- weakness or numbness in the hands and/or feet
- pain when walking
- weak, sore, tired or achy muscles
- loss of balance
- clumsiness
- difficulty picking up objects and buttoning clothing
- shaking or trembling
- walking problems
- jaw pain
- hearing loss
- stomach pain
- constipation

How can I cope with nerve and muscle problems?

- If your fingers are numb, be very careful when grasping objects that are sharp, hot, or otherwise dangerous.

- If your sense of balance or muscle strength is affected, avoid falls by moving carefully, using handrails when going up or down stairs, and using bath mats in the bathtub or shower.

- Always wear shoes with rubber soles (if possible).

- Ask your doctor for pain medicine.

Effects on Skin and Nails

You may have minor skin problems while you are having chemotherapy, such as redness, rashes, itching, peeling, dryness, acne, and increased sensitivity to the sun. Certain anticancer drugs, when given intravenously, may cause the skin all along the vein to darken, especially in people who have very dark skin. Some people use makeup to cover the area, but this can take a lot of time if several veins are affected. The darkened areas will fade a few months after treatment ends.

Your nails may also become darkened, yellow, brittle, or cracked. They also may develop vertical lines or bands.

While most of these problems are not serious and you can take care of them yourself, a few need immediate attention. Certain drugs given intravenously (IV) can cause serious and permanent tissue damage if they leak out of the vein. Tell your doctor or nurse right away if you feel any burning or pain when you are getting IV drugs. These symptoms do not always mean there is a problem, but they must always be checked at once. Don't hesitate to call your doctor about even the less serious symptoms.

Some symptoms may mean you are having an allergic reaction that may need to be treated at once. Call your doctor or nurse right away if:

- you develop sudden or severe itching.

- your skin breaks out in a rash or hives.

- you have wheezing or any other trouble breathing.

How can I cope with skin and nail problems?

Acne

- Try to keep your face clean and dry.

- Ask your doctor or nurse if you can use over-the-counter medicated creams or soaps.

Itching and Dryness

- Apply corn starch as you would a dusting powder.

- To help avoid dryness, take quick showers or sponge baths. Do not take long, hot baths. Use a moisturizing soap.

- Apply cream and lotion while your skin is still moist.

- Avoid perfume, cologne, or aftershave lotion that contains alcohol.

- Use a colloid oatmeal bath or diphenhydramine for generalized pruritis.

Nail Problems

- You can buy nail-strengthening products in a drug store. Be aware that these products may bother your skin and nails.

- Protect your nails by wearing gloves when washing dishes, gardening, or doing other work around the house.

- Be sure to let your doctor know if you have redness, pain, or changes around the cuticles.

Sunlight Sensitivity

- Avoid direct sunlight as much as possible, especially between 10 a.m. and 4 p.m. when the sun's rays are the strongest.

- Use a sun screen lotion with a skin protection factor (SPF) of 15 or higher to protect against sun damage. A product such as zinc oxide, sold over the counter, can block the sun's rays completely.

- Use a lip balm with a sun protection factor.

- Wear long-sleeve cotton shirts, pants, and hats with a wide brim (particularly if you are having hair loss), to block the sun.

- Even people with dark skin need to protect themselves from the sun during chemotherapy.

Radiation Recall

Some people who have had radiation therapy develop "radiation recall" during their chemotherapy. During or shortly after certain anticancer drugs are given, the skin over an area that had received radiation turns red—a shade anywhere from light to very bright. The skin may blister and peel. This reaction may last hours or even days. Report radiation recall reactions to your doctor or nurse. You can soothe the itching and burning by:

- Placing a cool, wet compress over the affected area.

- Wearing soft, non-irritating fabrics. Women who have radiation for breast cancer following lumpectomy often find cotton bras the most comfortable.

Kidney and Bladder Effects

Some anticancer drugs can irritate the bladder or cause temporary or permanent damage to the bladder or kidneys. If you are taking one or more of these drugs, your doctor may ask you to collect a 24-hour urine sample. A blood sample may also be obtained before you begin chemotherapy to check your kidney function. Some anticancer drugs cause the urine to change color (orange, red, green, or yellow) or take on a strong or medicine-like odor for 24-72 hours. Check with your doctor to see if the drugs you are taking may have any of these effects.

Always drink plenty of fluids to ensure good urine flow and help prevent problems. This is very important if you are taking drugs that affect the kidney and bladder. Water, juice, soft drinks, broth, ice cream, soup, popsicles, and gelatin are all considered fluids.

Tell your doctor if you have any of these symptoms:

- Pain or burning when you urinate (pass your water).

- Frequent urination.

- Not being able to urinate.

- A feeling that you must urinate right away ("urgency").

- Reddish or bloody urine.

- Fever.

- Chills, especially shaking chills.

Flu-Like Symptoms

Some people feel as though they have the flu for a few hours to a few days after chemotherapy. This may be especially true if you are receiving chemotherapy in combination with biological therapy. Flu-like symptoms—muscle and joint aches, headache, tiredness, nausea, slight fever (usually less than 100° F), chills, and poor appetite—may last from 1 to 3 days. An infection or the cancer itself can also cause these symptoms. Check with your doctor if you have flu-like symptoms.

Fluid Retention

Your body may retain fluid when you are having chemotherapy. This may be due to hormonal changes from your therapy, to the drugs themselves, or to your cancer. Check with your doctor or nurse if you notice swelling or puffiness in your face, hands, feet, or abdomen. You may need to avoid table salt and foods that have a lot of salt. If the problem is severe, your doctor may prescribe a diuretic, medicine to help your body get rid of excess fluids.

Effects on Sexual Organs

Chemotherapy may—but does not always—affect sexual organs and functioning. The side effects that might occur depend on the drugs used and the person's age and general health.

Effects on the ovaries. Anticancer drugs can affect the ovaries and reduce the amount of hormones they produce. Some women find that their menstrual periods become irregular or stop completely while having chemotherapy. Related side effects may be temporary or permanent.

- *Infertility.* Damage to the ovaries may result in infertility, the inability to become pregnant. The infertility can be either temporary or permanent. Whether infertility occurs, and how long it lasts, depends on many factors, including the type of drug, the dosage given, and the woman's age.

- *Menopause.* A woman's age and the drugs and dosages used will determine whether she experiences menopause while on chemotherapy. Chemotherapy may also cause menopause-like symptoms such as hot flashes and dry vaginal tissues. These tissue changes can make intercourse uncomfortable and can make a woman more prone to bladder and/or vaginal infections. Any infection should be treated right away. Menopause may be temporary or permanent.

Help for Hot Flashes

- Dress in layers.

- Avoid caffeine and alcohol.

- Exercise.

- Try meditation or other relaxation methods.

Relieving Vaginal Symptoms and Preventing Infection

- Use a water or mineral oil-based vaginal lubricant at the time of intercourse.

- There are products that can be used to stop vaginal dryness. Ask your pharmacist about vaginal gels that can be applied to the vagina.

- Avoid using petroleum jelly, which is difficult for the body to get rid of and increases the risk of infection.

- Wear cotton underwear and pantyhose with a ventilated cotton lining.

- Avoid wearing tight slacks or shorts.

- Ask your doctor about prescribing a vaginal cream or suppository to reduce the chances of infection.

- Ask your doctor about using a vaginal dilator if painful intercourse continues.

Pregnancy. Although pregnancy may be possible during chemotherapy, it still is not advisable because some anticancer drugs may cause birth defects. Doctors advise women of childbearing age, from the teens through the end of menopause, to use some method of birth control throughout their treatment, such as condoms, spermicidal agents, diaphragms, or birth control pills. Birth control pills may not be appropriate for some women, such as those with breast cancer. Ask your doctor about these contraceptive options.

If a woman is pregnant when her cancer is discovered, it may be possible to delay chemotherapy until after the baby is born. For a woman who needs treatment sooner, the possible effects of chemotherapy on the fetus need to be evaluated.

Feelings about Sexuality

Sexual feelings and attitudes vary among people during chemotherapy. Some people find that they feel closer than ever to their partners and have an increased desire for sexual activity. Others experience little or no change in their sexual desire and energy level. Still others find that their sexual interest declines because of the physical and emotional stresses of having cancer and getting chemotherapy. These stresses may include:

- worries about changes in appearance.

- anxiety about health, family, or finances.

- side effects of treatment, including fatigue, and hormonal changes.

A partner's concerns or fears also can affect the sexual relationship. Some may worry that physical intimacy will harm the person who has cancer. Others may fear that they might "catch" the cancer or be affected by the drugs. Both you and your partner should feel free to discuss sexual concerns with your doctor, nurse, social worker, or other counselor who can give you the information and the reassurance you need.

You and your partner also should try to share your feelings with each other. If talking to each other about sex, cancer, or both, is hard, you may want to speak to a counselor who can help you talk more openly. People who can help include psychiatrists, psychologists, social workers, marriage counselors, sex therapists, and members of the clergy.

If you were comfortable with and enjoyed sexual relations before starting chemotherapy, chances are you will still find pleasure in physical intimacy during your treatment. You may discover, however, that intimacy changes during treatment. Hugging, touching, holding, and cuddling may become more important, while sexual intercourse may become less important. Remember that what was true before you started chemotherapy remains true now: There is no one "right" way to express your sexuality. You and your partner should decide together what gives both of you pleasure.

Eating Well during Chemotherapy

It is very important to eat well while you are getting chemotherapy. Eating well during chemotherapy means choosing a balanced diet that contains all the nutrients the body needs. Eating well also means having a diet high enough in calories to keep your weight up and high enough in protein to rebuild tissues that cancer treatment may harm. People who eat well can cope with side effects and fight infection better. Also, their bodies can rebuild healthy tissues faster.

What If I Don't Feel Like Eating?

On some days you may feel you just cannot eat. You can lose your appetite if you feel depressed or tired. Or, side effects such as nausea or mouth and throat problems may make it difficult or painful to eat. In some cases, if you cannot eat for a long period of time, your doctor may recommend that you be given nutrition intravenously until you are able to eat again.

When a poor appetite is the problem, try these suggestions:

- Eat frequent, small meals or snacks whenever you want, perhaps four to six times a day. You do not have to eat three regular meals each day.

- Keep snacks within easy reach, so you can have something whenever you feel like it.

- Even if you do not want to eat solid foods, try to drink beverages during the day. Juice, soup, and other fluids like these can give you important calories and nutrients.

- Vary your diet by trying new foods and recipes.

- When possible, take a walk before meals; this may make you feel hungrier.

- Try changing your mealtime routine. For example, eat in a different location.

- Eat with friends or family members. When eating alone, listen to the radio or watch TV.

- Ask your doctor or nurse about nutrition supplements.

- Speak with your dietician about your specific nutrition needs.

The National Cancer Institute's booklet, "Eating Hints for Cancer Patients: Before, During and After Treatment" provides more tips about how to make eating easier and more enjoyable. It also gives many ideas about how to eat well and get extra protein and calories during cancer treatment. For a free copy of this booklet, ask your nurse or call the Cancer Information Service at 1-800-4-CANCER (1-800-422-6237).

Can I Drink Alcoholic Beverages?

Small amounts of alcohol can help you relax and increase your appetite. On the other hand, alcohol may interfere with how some drugs work and/or worsen their side effects. For this reason, some people must drink less alcohol or avoid alcohol completely during chemotherapy. Ask your doctor if and how much beer, wine, or other alcoholic beverages you can drink during treatment.

Can I Take Extra Vitamins and Minerals?

You can usually get all the vitamins and minerals you need by eating a healthy diet. Talk to your doctor, nurse, registered dietician, or a pharmacist before taking any vitamin or mineral supplements. Too much of some vitamins and minerals can be just as dangerous as too little. Find out what is recommended for you.

Paying for Chemotherapy

The cost of chemotherapy varies with the kinds and doses of drugs used, how long and how often they are given, and whether you get them at home, in a clinic or office, or in the hospital. Most health insurance policies cover at least part of the cost of many kinds of chemotherapy. There are also organizations who will help with the cost of chemotherapy and with transportation costs. Ask your nurse or social worker about these organizations. Finding the answers to the questions below will help avoid problems in receiving payment later on.

What Questions Should I Be Able to Answer about My Insurance?

- What are the benefits of my insurance plan?

- What cancer treatments/care does it cover?

- Do I have a primary care provider? Can I use only certain "preferred providers" under my plan?

- Am I entitled to a yearly checkup or does my plan only cover office visits when I am sick?

- What are the benefits if I go outside of my health plan to obtain care?

- What are the rules of my insurance plan?

- Do I need a referral from a primary care provider?

- Do I need a written referral form?

- Do I need to get approval from my health plan (pre-certification) before seeing a specialist, obtaining treatment, tests, and medical equipment or physical therapy services or going to the emergency room or a hospital?

- Does my lab work, including blood work, or pap smear need to go to a special lab?

- Do I have to pay a certain amount (co-pay) at the time of my visit?

- Do I have an amount that I must pay for medical expenses (annual deductible) before the insurance pays for services?

- Do I have a lifetime or annual limit on how much is covered for medical expenses?

- Is there a special pharmacy where I need to get my medications?

- Are all tests and procedures covered both as an in-patient and out-patient?

Getting Maximum Coverage of Clinical Trials Costs

Many clinical trials (treatment studies) offer some part of care free of charge. But some insurers will not cover certain costs when a new treatment is under study. Your doctor can work with you to try to help you. If you are taking part in or considering a clinical trial:

- Ask your doctor about other patients in the trial. Have their insurers paid for their care? Have there been any consistent problems?

- Talk to your doctor about the paperwork he or she submits to your insurer. Often the way the doctor describes a treatment can help or hurt your chances of insurance coverage.

- Find out what is in your policy. Check to see if there is a specific exclusion for "experimental treatment."

Getting the Most From Your Insurance

- Get a copy of your insurance policies before treatment and find out exactly what your coverage includes.

- Keep careful records of all your covered expenses and claims.

- File claims for all covered costs.

- Get help in filing a claim if you need it. If friends or family cannot help you, ask a social worker for help. Private companies and some community organizations offer insurance-filing aid.

- If your claim is turned down, file again and inquire about the reasons. Ask your doctor to explain to the company why the services meet the requirements for coverage under your policy. If you are turned down again, find out if the company has an appeals process.

Many insurance companies handle new treatments on a case-by-case basis, rather than having a blanket policy. You can always ask about their coverage of specific therapies. However, some patients say that their questions may have hurt their chances for coverage by raising a red flag. A call from your nurse or social worker to your insurance company about specific coverage may be helpful.

In some states, Medicaid (which makes health care services available for people with financial need) may help pay for certain treatments. Contact the office that handles social services in your city or county to find out whether you are eligible for Medicaid and whether your chemotherapy is a covered expense.

For more information on paying for chemotherapy, call the Cancer Information Service at 1-800-4-CANCER (1-800-422-6237) and ask for the booklet "Facing Forward: A Guide for Cancer Survivors."

Chapter 48

Radiation Therapy

Introduction

Radiation therapy may vary somewhat among different doctors, hospitals, and treatment centers. Therefore, your treatment or the advice of your doctor (the radiation oncologist) may be different from what you read here. Be sure to ask questions and discuss your concerns with your doctor, nurse, or radiation therapist. Ask whether they have any additional written information that might help you.

Radiation in Cancer Treatment

How Does Radiation Therapy Work?

Radiation in high doses kills cells or keeps them from growing and dividing. Because cancer cells grow and divide more rapidly than most of the normal cells around them, radiation therapy can successfully treat many kinds of cancer. Normal cells are also affected by radiation but, unlike cancer cells, most of them recover from the effects of radiation.

To protect normal cells, doctors carefully limit the doses of radiation and spread the treatment out over time. They also shield as much

Excerpted from "Radiation Therapy and You," National Cancer Institute (NCI), last updated September 22, 1999. To order a copy of the full text, or for other cancer-related information, contact NCI's Cancer Information Service at 800-4-CANCER (800-422-6237) or visit www.nci.nih.gov on the Internet.

normal tissue as possible while they aim the radiation at the site of the cancer.

What Are the Goals and Benefits of Radiation Therapy?

The goal of radiation therapy is to kill the cancer cells with as little risk as possible to normal cells. Radiation therapy can be used to treat many kinds of cancer in almost any part of the body. In fact, more than half of all people with cancer are treated with some form of radiation. For many cancer patients, radiation is the only kind of treatment they need. Thousands of people who have had radiation therapy alone or in combination with other types of cancer treatment are free of cancer.

Radiation treatment, like surgery, is a local treatment—it affects the cancer cells only in a specific area of the body. Sometimes doctors add radiation therapy to treatments that reach all parts of the body (systemic treatment) such as chemotherapy, or biological therapy to improve treatment results. You may hear your doctor use the term, adjuvant therapy, for a treatment that is added to, and given after, the primary therapy.

Radiation therapy is often used with surgery to treat cancer. Doctors may use radiation before surgery to shrink a tumor. This makes it easier to remove the cancerous tissue and may allow the surgeon to perform less radical surgery.

Radiation therapy may be used after surgery to stop the growth of cancer cells that may remain. Your doctor may choose to use radiation therapy and surgery at the same time. This procedure, known as intraoperative radiation.

In some cases, instead of surgery, doctors use radiation along with anticancer drugs (chemotherapy) to destroy the cancer. Radiation may be given before, during, or after chemotherapy. Doctors carefully tailor this combination treatment to each patient's needs depending on the type of cancer, its location, and its size. The purpose of radiation treatment before or during chemotherapy is to make the tumor smaller and thus improve the effectiveness of the anticancer drugs. Doctors sometimes recommend that a patient complete chemotherapy and then have radiation treatment to kill any cancer cells that might remain.

When curing the cancer is not possible, radiation therapy can be used to shrink tumors and reduce pressure, pain, and other symptoms of cancer. This is called palliative care or palliation. Many cancer patients find that they have a better quality of life when radiation is used for this purpose.

Who Gives Radiation Treatments?

A doctor who specializes in using radiation to treat cancer—a radiation oncologist—will prescribe the type and amount of treatment that is right for you. The radiation oncologist works closely with the other doctors and health care professionals involved in your care. This highly trained health care team may include:

- The radiation physicist, who makes sure that the equipment is working properly and that the machines deliver the right dose of radiation. The physicist also works closely with your doctor to plan your treatment.

- The dosimetrist, who works under the direction of your doctor and the radiation physicist and helps carry out your treatment plan by calculating the amount of radiation to be delivered to the cancer and normal tissues that are nearby.

- The radiation therapist, who positions you for your treatments and runs the equipment that delivers the radiation.

- The radiation nurse, who will coordinate your care, help you learn about treatment, and tell you how to manage side effects. The nurse can also answer questions you or family members may have about your treatment.

Your health care team also may include a physician assistant, radiologist, dietitian, physical therapist, social worker, or other health care professional.

Is Radiation Treatment Expensive?

Treatment of cancer with radiation can be costly. It requires very complex equipment and the services of many health care professionals. The exact cost of your radiation therapy will depend on the type and number of treatments you need.

Most health insurance policies, including Part B of Medicare, cover charges for radiation therapy. It's a good idea to talk with your doctor's office staff or the hospital business office about your policy and how expected costs will be paid.

In some states, the Medicaid program may help you pay for treatments. You can find out from the office that handles social services in your city or county whether you are eligible for Medicaid and whether your radiation therapy is a covered expense.

If you need financial aid, contact the hospital social service office or the National Cancer Institute's (NCI) Cancer Information Service at 1-800-4-CANCER. They may be able to direct you to sources of help.

External Radiation Therapy: What to Expect

How Does the Doctor Plan My Treatment?

The high energy rays used for radiation therapy can come from a variety of sources. Your doctor may choose to use x-rays, an electron beam, or cobalt-60 gamma rays. Some cancer treatment centers have special equipment that produces beams of protons or neutrons for radiation therapy. The type of radiation your doctor decides to use depends on what kind of cancer you have and how far into your body the radiation should go. High-energy radiation is used to treat many types of cancer. Low-energy x-rays are used to treat some kinds of skin diseases.

After a physical exam and a review of your medical history, the doctor plans your treatment. In a process called simulation, you will be asked to lie very still on an examining table while the radiation therapist uses a special x-ray machine to define your treatment port or field. This is the exact place on your body where the radiation will be aimed. Depending on the location of your cancer, you may have more than one treatment port.

Simulation may also involve CT scans or other imaging studies to plan how to direct the radiation. Depending on the type of treatment you will be receiving, body molds or other devices that keep you from moving during treatment (immobilization devices) may be made at this time. They will be used each time you have treatment to be sure that you are positioned correctly. Simulation may take from a half hour to about 2 hours.

The radiation therapist often will mark the treatment port on your skin with tattoos or tiny dots of colored, permanent ink. It's important that the radiation be targeted at the same area each time. If the dots appear to be fading, tell your radiation therapist who will darken them so that they can be seen easily.

Once simulation has been done, your doctor will meet with the radiation physicist and the dosimetrist. Based on the results of your medical history, lab tests, x-rays, other treatments you may have had, and the location and kind of cancer you have, they will decide how much radiation is needed, what kind of machine to use to deliver it, and how many treatments you should have.

How Long Does the Treatment Take?

For most types of cancer, radiation therapy usually is given 5 days a week for 6 or 7 weeks. (When radiation is used for palliative care, the course of treatment is shorter, usually 2 to 3 weeks.) The total dose of radiation and the number of treatments you need will depend on the size, location, and kind of cancer you have, your general health, and other medical treatments you may be receiving.

Using many small doses of daily radiation rather than a few large doses helps protect normal body tissues in the treatment area. Weekend rest breaks allow normal cells to recover.

It's very important that you have all of your scheduled treatments to get the most benefit from your therapy. Missing or delaying treatments can lessen the effectiveness of your radiation treatment.

What Happens during the Treatment Visits?

Before each treatment, you may need to change into a hospital gown or robe. It's best to wear clothing that is easy to take off and put on again.

In the treatment room, the radiation therapist will use the marks on your skin to locate the treatment area and to position you correctly. You may sit in a special chair or lie down on a treatment table. For each external radiation therapy session, you will be in the treatment room about 15 to 30 minutes, but you will be getting radiation for only about 1 to 5 minutes of that time. Receiving external radiation treatments is painless, just like having an x-ray taken. You will not hear, see, or smell the radiation.

The radiation therapist may put special shields (or blocks) between the machine and certain parts of your body to help protect normal tissues and organs. There might also be plastic or plaster forms that help you stay in exactly the right place. You need to remain very still during the treatment so that the radiation reaches only the area where it's needed and the same area is treated each time. You don't have to hold your breath—just breathe normally.

The radiation therapist will leave the treatment room before your treatment begins. The radiation machine is controlled from a nearby area. You will be watched on a television screen or through a window in the control room. Although you may feel alone, keep in mind that the therapist can see and hear you and even talk with you using an intercom in the treatment room. If you should feel ill or very uncomfortable during the treatment, tell your therapist at once. The machine can be stopped at any time.

The machines used for radiation treatments are very large, and they make noises as they move around your body to aim at the treatment area from different angles. Their size and motion may be frightening at first. Remember that the machines are being moved and controlled by your radiation therapist. They are checked constantly to be sure they're working right. If you have concerns about anything that happens in the treatment room, discuss these concerns with the radiation therapist.

What Is Hyperfractionated Radiation Therapy?

Radiation is usually given once daily in a dose that is based on the type and location of the tumor. In hyperfractionated radiation therapy, the daily dose is divided into smaller doses that are given more than once a day. The treatments usually are separated by 4 to 6 hours. Doctors are studying hyperfractionated therapy to learn if it is equal to, or perhaps more effective than, once-a-day therapy and whether there are fewer long-term side effects. Early results of treatment studies of some kinds of tumors are encouraging, and hyperfractionated therapy is becoming a more common way to give radiation treatments for some types of cancer.

What Is Intraoperative Radiation?

Intraoperative radiation combines surgery and radiation therapy. The surgeon first removes as much of the tumor as possible. Before the surgery is completed, a large dose of radiation is given directly to the tumor bed (the area from which the tumor has been removed) and nearby areas where cancer cells might have spread. Sometimes intraoperative radiation is used in addition to external radiation therapy. This gives the cancer cells a larger amount of radiation than would be possible using external radiation alone.

What Are the Side Effects of Treatment?

External radiation therapy does not cause your body to become radioactive. There is no need to avoid being with other people because you are undergoing treatment. Even hugging, kissing, or having sexual relations with others poses no risk of radiation exposure.

Most side effects of radiation therapy are related to the area that is being treated. Many patients have no side effects at all. Your doctor and nurse will tell you about the possible side effects you might expect and how you should deal with them. You should contact your doctor or nurse if you have any unusual symptoms during your treatment, such as coughing, sweating, fever, or pain.

The side effects of radiation therapy, although unpleasant, are usually not serious and can be controlled with medication or diet. They usually go away within a few weeks after treatment ends, although some side effects can last longer.

What Can I Do to Take Care of Myself During Therapy?

- Before starting treatment, be sure your doctor knows about any medicines you are taking and if you have any allergies. Do not start taking any medicine (whether prescription or over-the-counter) during your radiation therapy without first telling your doctor or nurse.

- Fatigue is common during radiation therapy. Your body will use a lot of extra energy over the course of your treatment, and you may feel very tired. Be sure to get plenty of rest and sleep as often as you feel the need. It's common for fatigue to last for 4 to 6 weeks after your treatment has been completed.

- Good nutrition is very important. Try to eat a balanced diet that will prevent weight loss.

- Check with your doctor before taking vitamin supplements or herbal preparations during treatment.

- Avoid wearing tight clothes such as girdles or close-fitting collars over the treatment area.

- Be extra kind to your skin in the treatment area.

- Ask your doctor or nurse if you may use soaps, lotions, deodorants, sun blocks, medicines, perfumes, cosmetics, talcum powder, or other substances in the treated area.

- Wear loose, soft cotton clothing over the treated area.

- Do not wear starched or stiff clothing over the treated area.

- Do not scratch, rub, or scrub treated skin.

- Do not use adhesive tape on treated skin. If bandaging is necessary, use paper tape and apply it outside of the treatment area.

Your nurse can help you place dressings so that you can avoid irritating the treated area.

- Do not apply heat or cold (heating pad, ice pack, etc.) to the treated area. Use only lukewarm water for bathing the area.

- Use an electric shaver if you must shave the treated area but only after checking with your doctor or nurse. Do not use a preshave lotion or hair removal products on the treated area.

- Protect the treatment area from the sun. Do not apply sunscreens just before a radiation treatment. If possible, cover treated skin (with light clothing) before going outside. Ask your doctor if you should use a sunscreen or a sunblocking product. If so, select one with a protection factor of at least 15 and reapply it often. Ask your doctor or nurse how long after your treatments are completed you should continue to protect the treated skin from sunlight.

- If you have questions, ask your doctor or nurse. They are the only ones who can properly advise you about your treatment, its side effects, home care, and any other medical concerns you may have.

Internal Radiation Therapy: What to Expect

When Is Internal Radiation Therapy Used?

Your doctor may decide that a high dose of radiation given to a small area of your body is the best way to treat your cancer. Internal radiation therapy allows the doctor to give a higher total dose of radiation in a shorter time than is possible with external treatment.

Internal radiation therapy places the radiation source as close as possible to the cancer cells. Instead of using a large radiation machine, the radioactive material, sealed in a thin wire, catheter, or tube (implant), is placed directly into the affected tissue. This method of treatment concentrates the radiation on the cancer cells and lessens radiation damage to some of the normal tissue near the cancer. Some of the radioactive substances used for internal radiation treatment include cesium, iridium, iodine, phosphorus, and palladium.

Internal radiation therapy may be used for cancers of the head and neck, breast, uterus, thyroid, cervix, and prostate. Your doctor may suggest using both internal and external radiation therapy.

In this chapter, 'internal radiation treatment' refers to implant radiation. Health professionals prefer to use the term "brachytherapy" for implant radiation therapy. You may hear your doctor or nurse use the terms, interstitial radiation or intracavitary radiation; each is a form of internal radiation therapy. Sometimes radioactive implants are called "capsules" or "seeds."

How Is the Implant Placed in the Body?

The type of implant and the method of placing it depend on the size and location of the cancer. Implants may be put right into the tumor (interstitial radiation), in special applicators inside a body cavity (intracavitary radiation) or passage (intraluminal radiation), on the surface of a tumor, or in the area from which the tumor has been removed. Implants may be removed after a short time or left in place permanently. If they are to be left in place, the radioactive substance used will lose radiation quickly and become non-radioactive in a short time.

When interstitial radiation is given, the radiation source is placed in the tumor in catheters, seeds, or capsules. When intracavitary radiation is used, a container or applicator of radioactive material is placed in a body cavity such as the uterus. In surface brachytherapy the radioactive source is sealed in a small holder and placed in or against the tumor. In intraluminal brachytherapy the radioactive source is placed in a body lumen or tube, such as the bronchus or esophagus.

Internal radiation also may be given by injecting a solution of radioactive substance into the bloodstream or a body cavity. This form of radiation therapy may be called unsealed internal radiation therapy.

For most types of implants, you will need to be in the hospital. You will be given general or local anesthesia so that you will not feel any pain when the doctor places the holder for the radioactive material in your body. In many hospitals, the radioactive material is placed in its holder or applicator after you return to your room so that other patients, staff, and visitors are not exposed to radiation.

How Are Other People Protected from Radiation while the Implant Is in Place?

Sometimes the radiation source in your implant sends its high energy rays outside your body. To protect others while you are having implant therapy, the hospital will have you stay in a private room. Although the nurses and other people caring for you will not be able to spend a long time in your room, they will give you all of the care you need. You should call for a nurse when you need one, but keep in

363

mind that the nurse will work quickly and speak to you from the doorway more often than from your bedside. In most cases, your urine and stool will contain no radioactivity unless you are having unsealed internal radiation therapy.

There also will be limits on visitors while your implant is in place. Children younger than 18 or pregnant women should not visit patients who are having internal radiation therapy. Be sure to tell your visitors to ask the hospital staff for any special instructions before they come into your room. Visitors should sit at least 6 feet from your bed and the radiation oncology staff will determine how long your visitors may stay. The time can vary from 30 minutes to several hours per day. In some hospitals a rolling lead shield is placed beside the bed and kept between the patient and visitors or staff members.

What Are the Side Effects of Internal Radiation Therapy?

The side effects of implant therapy depend on the area being treated. You are not likely to have severe pain or feel ill during implant therapy. However, if an applicator is holding your implant in place, it may be somewhat uncomfortable. If you need it, the doctor will order medicine to help you relax or to relieve pain. If general anesthesia was used while your implant was put in place, you may feel drowsy, weak, or nauseated but these effects do not last long. If necessary, medications can be ordered to relieve nausea.

How Long Does the Implant Stay in Place?

Your doctor will decide the amount of time that an implant is to be left in place. It depends on the dose (amount) of radioactivity needed for effective treatment. Your treatment schedule will depend on the type of cancer, where it is located, your general health, and other cancer treatments you have had. Depending on where the implant is placed, you may have to keep it from shifting by staying in bed and lying fairly still.

Temporary implants may be either low dose-rate (LDR) or high dose-rate (HDR). Low dose-rate implants are left in place for several days; high dose-rate implants are removed after a few minutes.

For some cancer sites, the implant is left in place permanently. If your implant is permanent, you may need to stay in your hospital room away from other people for a few days while the radiation is most active. The implant becomes less radioactive each day; by the time you are ready to go home, the radiation in your body will be much weaker. Your doctor will advise you if there are any special precautions you need to use at home.

What Happens after the Implant Is Removed?

Usually, an anesthetic is not needed when the doctor removes a temporary implant. Most can be taken out right in the patient's hospital room. Once the implant is removed, there is no radioactivity in your body. The hospital staff and your visitors will no longer have to limit the time they stay with you.

Your doctor will tell you if you need to limit your activities after you leave the hospital. Most patients are allowed to do as much as they feel like doing. You may need some extra sleep or rest breaks during your days at home, but you should feel stronger quickly.

The area that has been treated with an implant may be sore or sensitive for some time. If any particular activity such as sports or sexual intercourse cause irritation in the treatment area, your doctor may suggest that you limit these activities for a while.

Remote Brachytherapy

In remote brachytherapy, a computer sends the radioactive source through a tube to a catheter that has been placed near the tumor by the patient's doctor. The procedure is directed by the brachytherapy team who watch the patient on closed-circuit television and communicate with the patient using an intercom. The radioactivity remains at the tumor for only a few minutes. In some cases, several remote treatments may be required and the catheter may stay in place between treatments.

Remote brachytherapy may be used for low dose-rate (LDR) treatments in an inpatient setting. High dose-rate (HDR) remote brachytherapy allows a person to have internal radiation therapy in an outpatient setting. High dose-rate treatments take only a few minutes. Because no radioactive material is left in the body, the patient can return home after the treatment. Remote brachytherapy has been used to treat cancers of the cervix, breast, lung, pancreas, prostate, and esophagus.

Managing Side Effects

Are Side Effects the Same for Everyone?

The side effects of radiation treatment vary from patient to patient. You may have no side effects or only a few mild ones through your course of treatment. Some people do experience serious side effects, however. The side effects that you have depend mostly on the radiation dose and the part of your body that is treated. Your general health also can affect how your body reacts to radiation therapy and whether you have side effects. Before beginning your treatment, your doctor and nurse will discuss the side effects you might experience, how long they might last, and how serious they might be.

Side effects may be acute or chronic. Acute side effects are sometimes referred to as "early side effects." They occur soon after the treatment begins and usually are gone within a few weeks of finishing therapy. Chronic side effects, sometimes called "late side effects," may take months or years to develop and usually are permanent.

The most common early side effects of radiation therapy are fatigue and skin changes. They can result from radiation to any treatment site. Other side effects are related to treatment of specific areas. For example, temporary or permanent hair loss may be a side effect of radiation treatment to the head. Appetite can be altered if treatment affects the mouth, stomach, or intestine.

Fortunately, most side effects will go away in time. In the meantime, there are ways to reduce discomfort. If you have a side effect that is especially severe, the doctor may prescribe a break in your treatments or change your treatment in some way.

Be sure to tell your doctor, nurse, or radiation therapist about any side effects that you notice. They can help you treat the problems and tell you how to lessen the chances that the side effects will come back. The information in this chapter can serve as a guide to handling some side effects, but it cannot take the place of talking with the members of your health care team.

Will Side Effects Limit My Activity?

Not necessarily. It will depend on which side effects you have and how severe they are. Many patients are able to work, prepare meals, and enjoy their usual leisure activities while they are having radiation therapy. Others find that they need more rest than usual and therefore cannot do as much. Try to continue doing the things you enjoy as long as you don't become too tired.

Your doctor may suggest that you limit activities that might irritate the area being treated. In most cases, you can have sexual relations if you wish. You may find that your desire for physical intimacy is lower because radiation therapy may cause you to feel more tired than usual. For most patients, these feelings are temporary.

What Causes Fatigue?

Fatigue, feeling tired and lacking energy, is the most common symptom reported by cancer patients. The exact cause is not always known. It may be due to the disease itself or to treatment. It may also result from lowered blood counts, lack of sleep, pain, and poor appetite.

Most people begin to feel tired after a few weeks of radiation therapy. During radiation therapy, the body uses a lot of energy for healing. You also may be tired because of stress related to your illness, daily trips for treatment, and the effects of radiation on normal cells. Feelings of weakness or weariness will go away gradually after your treatment has been completed.

You can help yourself during radiation therapy by not trying to do too much. If you do feel tired, limit your activities and use your leisure time in a restful way. Save your energy for doing the things that you feel are most important. Do not feel that you have to do everything you normally do. Try to get more sleep at night, and plan your day so that you have time to rest if you need it. Several short naps or breaks may be more helpful than a long rest period.

Sometimes, light exercise such as walking may combat fatigue. Talk with your doctor or nurse about how much exercise you may do while you are having therapy. Talking with other cancer patients in a support group may also help you learn how to deal with fatigue.

If you have a full-time job, you may want to try to continue to work your normal schedule. However, some patients prefer to take time off while they're receiving radiation therapy; others work a reduced number of hours. Speak frankly with your employer about your needs and wishes during this time. A part-time schedule may be possible or perhaps you can do some work at home. Ask your doctor's office or the radiation therapy department to help by trying to schedule treatments with your workday in mind.

Whether you're going to work or not, it's a good idea to ask family members or friends to help with daily chores, shopping, child care, housework, or driving. Neighbors may be able to help by picking up groceries for you when they do their own shopping. You also could ask someone to drive you to and from your treatment visits to help conserve your energy.

How Are Skin Problems Treated?

You may notice that your skin in the treatment area is red or irritated. It may look as if it is sunburned, or tanned. After a few weeks your skin may be very dry from the therapy. Ask your doctor or nurse for advice on how to relieve itching or discomfort.

With some kinds of radiation therapy, treated skin may develop a "moist reaction," especially in areas where there are skin folds. When this happens, the skin is wet and it may become very sore. It's important to notify your doctor or nurse if your skin develops a moist reaction. They can give you suggestions on how to care for these areas and prevent them from becoming infected.

During radiation therapy you will need to be very gentle with the skin in the treatment area. The following suggestions may be helpful:

- Avoid irritating treated skin.

- When you wash, use only lukewarm water and mild soap; pat dry.

- Do not wear tight clothing over the area.

- Do not rub, scrub, or scratch the skin in the treatment area.

- Avoid putting anything that is hot or cold, such as heating pads or ice packs, on your treated skin.

- Ask your doctor or nurse to recommend skin care products that will not cause skin irritation. Do not use any powders, creams, perfumes, deodorants, body oils, ointments, lotions, or home remedies in the treatment area while you're being treated and for several weeks afterward unless approved by your doctor or nurse.

- Do not apply any skin lotions within 2 hours of a treatment.

- Avoid exposing the radiated area to the sun during treatment. If you expect to be in the sun for more than a few minutes you will need to be very careful. Wear protective clothing (such as a hat with a broad brim and a shirt with long sleeves) and use a sunscreen. Ask your doctor or nurse about using sunblocking lotions. After your treatment is over, ask your doctor or nurse how long you should continue to take extra precautions in the sun.

The majority of skin reactions to radiation therapy go away a few weeks after treatment is completed. In some cases, though, the treated skin will remain slightly darker than it was before and it may continue to be more sensitive to sun exposure.

What Can Be Done about Hair Loss?

Radiation therapy can cause hair loss, also known as alopecia, but only in the area being treated. For example, if you are receiving treatment to your hip, you will not lose the hair from your head. Radiation of your head may cause you to lose some or all of the hair on your scalp. Many patients find that their hair grows back again after the treatments are finished. The amount of hair that grows back will depend on how much and what kind of radiation you receive. You may notice that your hair has a slightly different texture or color when it grows back. Other types of cancer treatment, such as chemotherapy, also can affect how your hair grows back.

Although your scalp may be tender after the hair is lost, it's a good idea to cover your head with a hat, turban, or scarf. You should wear a protective cap or scarf when you're in the sun or outdoors in cold weather. If you prefer a wig or toupee, be sure the lining does not irritate your scalp. The cost of a hairpiece that you need because of cancer treatment is a tax-deductible expense and may be covered in part by your health insurance. If you plan to buy a wig, it's a good idea to select it early in your treatment if you want to match the color and style to your own hair.

How are Side Effects on the Blood Managed?

Radiation therapy can cause low levels of white blood cells and platelets. These blood cells normally help your body fight infection and prevent bleeding. If large areas of active bone marrow are treated, your red blood cell count may be low as well. If your blood tests show these side effects, your doctor may wait until your blood counts increase to continue treatments. Your doctor will check your blood counts regularly and change your treatment schedule if it is necessary.

Will Eating Be a Problem?

Sometimes radiation treatment causes loss of appetite and interferes with eating, digesting, and absorbing food. Try to eat enough to help damaged tissues rebuild themselves. It is not unusual to lose 1 or 2 pounds a week during radiation therapy. You will be weighed weekly to monitor your weight.

It is very important to eat a balanced diet. You may find it helpful to eat small meals often and to try to eat a variety of different foods. Your doctor or nurse can tell you whether you should eat a special diet, and a dietitian will have some ideas that will help you maintain your weight.

Coping with short-term diet problems may be easier than you expect. There are a number of diet guides and recipe booklets for patients who need help with eating problems. A National Cancer Institute booklet, "Eating Hints for Cancer Patients" explains how to get more calories and protein without eating more food. It also has many tips that should help you enjoy eating. The recipes it contains can be used for the whole family and are marked for people with special concerns, such as low-salt diets. (To obtain this booklet, call the National Cancer Institute's Cancer Information Service at 800-4-CANCER.)

Will Radiation Therapy Affect Me Emotionally?

Nearly all patients being treated for cancer report feeling emotionally upset at different times during their therapy. It's not unusual to feel anxious, depressed, afraid, angry, frustrated, alone, or helpless. Radiation therapy may affect your emotions indirectly through fatigue or changes in hormone balance, but the treatment itself is not a direct cause of mental distress.

You may find that it's helpful to talk about your feelings with a close friend, family member, chaplain, nurse, social worker, or psychologist with whom you feel at ease. You may want to ask your doctor or nurse about meditation or relaxation exercises that might help you unwind and feel calmer.

Nationwide support programs can help cancer patients to meet others who share common problems and concerns. Some medical centers have formed peer support groups so that patients can meet to discuss their feelings and inspire each other.

There are several helpful books, tapes, and videos on dealing with the emotional effects of having cancer. You may find that the National Cancer Institute publication, "Taking Time," is a good resource for this kind of information. You can obtain this booklet from the Cancer Information Service (1-800-4-CANCER). They can also direct you to reading matter and other resources in your area for emotional support.

Are There Side Effects with Radiation Therapy for Breast Cancer?

The most common side effects with radiation therapy for breast cancer are fatigue and skin changes. However there may be other side effects as well. If you notice that your shoulder feels stiff, ask your doctor or nurse about exercises to keep your arm moving freely. Other side effects include breast or nipple soreness, swelling from fluid buildup in the treated area, and skin reddening or tanning. Except for tanning which may take up to 6 months to fade, these side effects will most likely disappear in 4 to 6 weeks.

If you are being treated for breast cancer and you are having radiation therapy after a lumpectomy or mastectomy, it's a good idea to go without your bra whenever possible or, if this makes you more uncomfortable, wear a soft cotton bra without underwires. This will help reduce skin irritation in the treatment area.

Radiation therapy after a lumpectomy may cause additional changes in the treated breast after therapy is complete. These long-term side effects may continue for a year or longer after treatment. The skin redness will fade, leaving your skin slightly darker, just as when a sunburn fades to a sun tan. The pores in the skin of your breast may be enlarged and more noticeable. Some women report increased sensitivity of the skin on the breast; others have decreased feeling. The skin and the fatty tissue of the breast may feel thicker and firmer than it was before your radiation treatment. Sometimes the size of your breast changes—it may become larger because of fluid buildup or smaller because of the development of scar tissue. Many women have little or no change in size.

Your radiation therapy plan may include temporary implants of radioactive material in the area around your lumpectomy. A week or two after external treatment is completed, these implants are inserted during a short hospitalization. The implants may cause breast tenderness or a feeling of tightness. After they are removed, you are likely to notice some of the same effects that occur with external treatment. If so, let your doctor or nurse know about any problems that persist.

Most changes resulting from radiation therapy for breast cancer are seen within 10 to 12 months after completing therapy. Occasionally small red areas called telangiectasias appear. These are areas of dilated blood vessels and the color may fade with time. If you see new changes in breast size, shape, appearance, or texture after this time, report them to your doctor at once.

What Side Effects Occur with Radiation Therapy to the Stomach and Abdomen?

If you are having radiation treatment to the stomach or some portion of the abdomen, you may have an upset stomach, nausea, or diarrhea. Your doctor can prescribe medicines to relieve these problems. Do not take any medications for these symptoms unless you first check with your doctor or nurse.

Managing Nausea. It's not unusual to feel queasy for a few hours right after radiation treatment to the stomach or abdomen. Some patients find that they have less nausea if they have their treatment with an empty stomach. Others report that eating a light meal 1 to 2 hours before treatment lessens queasiness. You may find that nausea is less of a problem if you wait 1 to 2 hours after your treatment before you eat. If this problem persists, ask your doctor to prescribe a medicine (an antiemetic) to prevent nausea. If antiemetics are prescribed, take them within the hour before treatment or when your doctor or nurse suggests, even if you sometimes feel that they are not needed.

If your stomach feels upset just before every treatment, the queasiness or nausea may be caused by anxiety and concerns about cancer treatment. Try having a bland snack such as toast or crackers and apple juice before your appointment. It may also help to try to unwind before your treatment. Reading a book, writing a letter, or working a crossword puzzle may help you relax.

Here are some other tips to help an unsettled stomach:

- Stick to any special diet that your doctor, nurse, or dietitian gives you.

- Eat small meals.

- Eat often and try to eat and drink slowly.

- Avoid foods that are fried or are high in fat.

- Drink cool liquids between meals.

- Eat foods that have only a mild aroma and can be served cool or at room temperature.

For severe nausea and vomiting, try a clear liquid diet (broth and clear juices) or bland foods that are easy to digest, such as dry toast and gelatin.

What to Do about Diarrhea. Diarrhea may begin in the third or fourth week of radiation therapy to the abdomen or pelvis. You may be able to prevent diarrhea by eating a low fiber diet when you start therapy: avoid foods such as raw fruits and vegetables, beans, cabbage, and whole grain breads and cereals. Your doctor or nurse may suggest other changes to your diet, prescribe antidiarrhea medicine, or give you special instructions to help with the problem. Tell the doctor or nurse if these changes fail to control your diarrhea. The following changes in your diet may help:

- Try a clear liquid diet (water, weak tea, apple juice, clear broth, plain gelatin) as soon as diarrhea starts or when you feel that it's going to start.

- Ask your doctor or nurse to advise you about liquids that won't make your diarrhea worse. Weak tea and clear broth are frequent suggestions.

- Avoid foods that are high in fiber or can cause cramps or a gassy feeling such as raw fruits and vegetables, coffee and other beverages that contain caffeine, beans, cabbage, whole grain breads and cereals, sweets, and spicy foods.

- Eat frequent small meals.

- If milk and milk products irritate your digestive system, avoid them or use lactose-free dairy products.

- Continue a diet that is low in fat and fiber and lactose-free for 2 weeks after you have finished your radiation therapy. Gradually re-introduce other foods. You may want to start with small amounts of low-fiber foods such as rice, bananas, applesauce, mashed potatoes, low-fat cottage cheese, and dry toast.

- Be sure your diet includes foods that are high in potassium (bananas, potatoes, apricots), an important mineral that you may lose through diarrhea.

Diet planning is very important for patients who are having radiation treatment of the stomach and abdomen. Try to pack the highest possible food value into every meal and snack so that you will be eating enough calories and vital nutrients. Remember that nausea, vomiting, and diarrhea are likely to disappear once your treatment is over.

What Side Effects Occur with Radiation Therapy to the Pelvis?

If you are having radiation therapy to any part of the pelvis (the area between your hips), you might have some of the digestive problems already described. You also may have bladder irritation which can cause discomfort or frequent urination. Drinking a lot of fluid can help relieve some of this discomfort. Avoid caffeine and carbonated beverages. Your doctor also can prescribe some medicine to help relieve these problems.

The effects of radiation therapy on sexual and reproductive functions depend on which organs are in the radiation treatment area. Some of the more common side effects do not last long after treatment is finished. Others may be long-term or permanent. Before your treatment begins, ask your doctor about possible side effects and how long they might last.

Depending on the radiation dose, women having radiation therapy in the pelvic area may stop menstruating and have other symptoms of menopause such as vaginal itching, burning, and dryness. You should report these symptoms to your doctor or nurse, who can suggest treatment.

Effects on Fertility. Scientists are still studying how radiation treatment affects fertility. If you are a woman in your childbearing years, it's important to discuss birth control and fertility issues with your doctor. You should not become pregnant during radiation therapy because radiation treatment during pregnancy may injure the fetus, especially in the first three months. If you are pregnant before your therapy begins, be sure to tell your doctor so that the fetus can be protected from radiation, if possible.

Sexual Relations. With most types of radiation therapy, women are not likely to notice any change in their ability to enjoy sex, however, they may notice a decrease in their level of desire. This is more likely to be due to the stress of having cancer than to the effects of radiation therapy. Once the treatment ends, sexual desire is likely to return to previous levels.

During radiation treatment to the pelvis, some women are advised not to have intercourse. Others may find that intercourse is uncomfortable or painful. Within a few weeks after treatment ends, these symptoms usually disappear. If shrinking of vaginal tissues occurs as a side effect of radiation therapy, your doctor or nurse can explain how to use a dilator, a device that gently stretches the tissues of the vagina.

If you have questions or concerns about sexual activity during and after cancer treatment, discuss them with your nurse or doctor. Ask them to recommend booklets that may be helpful.

Chapter 49

Lasers in Cancer Treatment

Laser therapy involves the use of high-intensity light to destroy cancer cells. This technique is often used to relieve symptoms of cancer such as bleeding or obstruction, especially when the cancer cannot be cured by other treatments. It may also be used to treat cancer by shrinking or destroying tumors.

What Is Laser Light?

The term "laser" stands for light amplification by stimulated emission of radiation. Ordinary light, such as that from a light bulb, has many wavelengths and spreads in all directions. Laser light, on the other hand, has a specific wavelength and is focused in a narrow beam. This type of high-intensity light contains a lot of energy. Lasers are very powerful and may be used to cut through steel or to shape diamonds. Lasers also can be used for very precise surgical work, such as repairing a damaged retina in the eye or cutting through tissue (in place of a scalpel).

Types of Lasers

Although there are several different kinds of lasers, only three kinds have gained wide use in medicine:

- **Carbon dioxide (CO2) laser:** This type of laser can remove thin layers from the skin's surface without penetrating the

Fact Sheet 7.8, Cancer Info. Service, National Cancer Institute, July 1999.

deeper layers. This technique is particularly useful in treating tumors that have not spread deep into the skin and certain precancerous conditions. As an alternative to traditional scalpel surgery, the CO2 laser is also able to cut the skin. The laser is used in this way to remove skin cancers.

- **Neodymium:yttrium-aluminum-garnet (Nd:YAG) laser:** Light from this laser can penetrate deeper into tissue than light from the other types of lasers, and it can cause blood to clot quickly. It can be carried through optical fibers to less accessible parts of the body. This type of laser is sometimes used to treat throat cancers.

- **Argon laser:** This laser can pass through only superficial layers of tissue and is therefore useful in dermatology and in eye surgery. It also is used with light-sensitive dyes to treat tumors in a procedure known as photodynamic therapy (PDT).

Advantages and Disadvantages of Laser Use in Medicine

Lasers have several advantages over standard surgical tools:

- Lasers are more precise than scalpels. Tissue near an incision is protected, since there is little contact with surrounding skin or other tissue.

- The heat produced by lasers sterilizes the surgery site, thus reducing the risk of infection.

- Less operating time may be needed because the precision of the laser allows for a smaller incision.

- Healing time is often shortened; since laser heat seals blood vessels, there is less bleeding, swelling, or scarring.

- Laser surgery may be less complicated. For example, with fiber optics, laser light can be directed to parts of the body without making a large incision.

- More procedures may be done on an outpatient basis.

There are also disadvantages with laser surgery:

- Relatively few surgeons are trained in laser use.

- Laser equipment is expensive and bulky compared with the usual surgical tools, such as scalpels.

- Strict safety precautions must be observed in the operating room. (For example, the surgical team and the patient must use eye protection.)

Treating Cancer with Lasers

Lasers can be used in two ways to treat cancer: by shrinking or destroying a tumor with heat, or by activating a chemical—known as a photosensitizing agent—that destroys cancer cells. In PDT, a photosensitizing agent is retained in cancer cells and can be stimulated by light to cause a reaction that kills cancer cells.

CO_2 and Nd:YAG lasers are used to shrink or destroy tumors. They may be used with endoscopes, tubes that allow physicians to see into certain areas of the body, such as the bladder. The light from some lasers can be transmitted through a flexible endoscope fitted with fiber optics. This allows physicians to see and work in parts of the body that could not otherwise be reached except by surgery and therefore allows very precise aiming of the laser beam. Lasers also may be used with low-power microscopes, giving the doctor a clear view of the site being treated. Used with other instruments, laser systems can produce a cutting area as small as 200 microns in diameter—less than the width of a very fine thread.

Lasers are used to treat many types of cancer. Laser surgery is a standard treatment for certain stages of glottis (vocal cord), cervical, skin, lung, vaginal, vulvar, and penile cancers.

In addition to its use to destroy the cancer, laser surgery is also used to help relieve symptoms caused by cancer (palliative care). For example, lasers may be used to shrink or destroy a tumor that is blocking a patient's trachea (windpipe), making it easier to breathe. It is also sometimes used for palliation in colorectal and anal cancer.

Laser-Induced Interstitial Thermotherapy

Laser-induced interstitial thermotherapy (LITT) is one of the most recent developments in laser therapy. LITT uses the same idea as a cancer treatment called hyperthermia; that heat may help shrink tumors by damaging cells or depriving them of substances they need to live. In this treatment, lasers are directed to interstitial areas (areas between organs) in the body. The laser light then raises the temperature of the tumor, which damages or destroys cancer cells.

Photodynamic Therapy

Photodynamic therapy (PDT) is based on the discovery that certain chemicals can kill one-celled organisms in the presence of light. Recent interest in photosensitizing agents stems from research showing that some of these substances have a tendency to collect in cancer cells.

The photosensitizing agent injected into the body is absorbed by all cells. The agent remains in or around tumor cells for a longer time than it does in normal tissue. When treated cancer cells are exposed to red light from a laser, the light is absorbed by the photosensitizing agent. This light absorption causes a chemical reaction that destroys the tumor cells. Light exposure must be carefully timed to coincide with the period when most of the agent has left healthy cells but still remains in cancer cells. There are several promising features of PDT: (1) Cancer cells can be selectively destroyed while most normal cells are spared, (2) the damaging effect of the photosensitizing agent occurs only when the substance is exposed to light, and (3) the side effects are relatively mild.

A disadvantage of PDT is that argon laser light cannot pass through more than 3 centimeters of tissue (a little more than one and an eighth inch). PDT is mainly used to treat tumors on or just under the skin, or on the lining of internal organs. It can be used in the treatment of skin cancers just under the skin; or it can be directed through a bronchoscope into the lungs, through an endoscope into the esophagus and gastrointestinal tract, or through a cystoscope into the bladder. The National Cancer Institute and other institutions are supporting clinical trials (research studies) to evaluate the use of photodynamic therapy for other cancers. Researchers are also looking at different laser types and new photosensitizers that may increase the effectiveness of PDT against cancers that are located further below the skin or inside an organ.

The Outlook for Lasers in Cancer Treatment

Doctors are trying to find new and better ways to use lasers in cancer surgery. As more cancer surgeons become trained in laser use and the technology improves, lasers may make increasing contributions to cancer treatment. Doctors are currently studying the effects of lasers in treating breast, esophageal, skin, colon, lung, brain, vulva, vaginal, cervical, and head and neck cancers.

Chapter 50

Cryosurgery in Cancer Treatment

What is cryosurgery?

Cryosurgery (also called cryotherapy) is the use of extreme cold to destroy cancer cells. Traditionally, it has been used to treat external tumors, such as those on the skin, but recently some physicians have begun using it as a treatment for tumors that occur inside the body. Cryosurgery for internal tumors is increasing as a result of developments in technology over the past several years.

For external tumors, liquid nitrogen (-196 degrees Celsius, -320.8 degrees Fahrenheit) is applied directly to the cancer cells with a cotton swab or spraying device. For internal tumors, liquid nitrogen is circulated through an instrument called a cryoprobe, which is placed in contact with the tumor. To guide the cryoprobe and to monitor the freezing of the cells, the physician uses ultrasound (computerized moving pictures of the body generated by high-frequency sound waves). By using ultrasound, physicians hope to spare nearby healthy tissue.

Cryosurgery often involves a cycle of treatments in which the tumor is frozen, allowed to thaw, and then refrozen.

What types of cancer can be treated with cryosurgery?

Cryosurgery is being evaluated in the treatment of a number of cancers, including prostate cancer and cancer that affects the liver

Fact Sheet 7.34, Cancer Info. Service, National Cancer Institute, 1/97.

(both primary liver cancer and cancer that has spread to the liver from another site). Researchers also are studying its effectiveness as a treatment for some tumors of the bone, for brain and spinal tumors, and for tumors in the windpipe that may develop with non-small cell lung cancer. In addition, some researchers are using cryosurgery in combination with other cancer treatments such as radiation, surgery, and hormone therapy. While initial results of cryosurgical treatment are encouraging, researchers have not yet drawn any solid conclusions regarding its long-term effectiveness.

For certain types of cancer and precancerous conditions, however, cryosurgery has proven to be an effective therapy. It has tradition-ally been used to treat retinoblastoma (a childhood cancer that affects the retina of the eye) and early-stage skin cancers (both basal cell and squamous cell carcinomas). Precancerous skin growths known as ac-tinic keratosis and the precancerous condition cervical intraepithelial neoplasia (abnormal cell changes in the cervix that can develop into cervical cancer) also can be treated with cryosurgery.

Does cryosurgery have any complications or side effects?

Cryosurgery does have side effects, although they may be less se-vere than those associated with surgery or radiation therapy. Cryosurgery in the liver may cause damage to the bile ducts and/or major blood vessels, which can lead to hemorrhage (heavy bleeding) or infection. Cryosurgery for prostate cancer may affect the urinary system. It also may cause incontinence (lack of control over urine flow) and impotence (loss of sexual function), although these side effects are often temporary. Cryosurgery for cervical intraepithelial neopla-sia has not been shown to affect fertility, but this possibility is under study. More studies must be conducted to determine the long-term effects of cryosurgery.

What are the advantages of cryosurgery?

Cryosurgery offers some advantages over other methods of cancer treatment. It is less invasive than surgery, involving only a small in-cision or insertion of the cryoprobe through the skin. Consequently, pain, bleeding, and other complications of surgery are minimized. Cryosurgery is less expensive than other treatments and requires shorter recovery time and a shorter hospital stay.

Because physicians can focus cryosurgical treatment on a limited area, they can avoid the destruction of nearby healthy tissue. The treatment can be safely repeated and may be used along with standard treatments such as surgery, chemotherapy, and radiation. Furthermore, cryosurgery may offer an option for treating cancers that are considered inoperable or that do not respond to standard treatments.

What are the disadvantages of cryosurgery?

The major disadvantage of cryosurgery is the uncertainty surrounding its long-term effectiveness. While cryosurgery may be effective in treating tumors made visible to the physician through imaging tests (tests that produce pictures of areas inside the body), it can miss microscopic cancer spread. Furthermore, because the effectiveness of the technique is still being assessed, insurance coverage issues may arise.

What does the future hold for cryosurgery?

Additional studies are needed to determine the effectiveness of cryosurgery in controlling cancer and improving survival. Data from these studies will allow physicians to compare cryosurgery with standard treatment options such as surgery, chemotherapy, and radiation. Moreover, physicians continue to examine the possibility of using cryosurgery in combination with other treatments.

Where is cryosurgery currently available?

Cryosurgery is widely available in gynecologists' offices for the treatment of cervical neoplasias. A limited number of hospitals and cancer centers throughout the country currently have skilled physicians and the necessary technology to perform cryosurgery for other precancerous and cancerous conditions. Individuals can consult with their doctors or contact hospitals and cancer centers in their area to find out where cryosurgery is being used.

Chapter 51

Taxanes in Cancer Treatment

The taxanes are a group of drugs that includes paclitaxel (Taxol®) and docetaxel (Taxotere®), which are used in the treatment of cancer. Taxanes have a unique way of preventing the growth of cancer cells: they affect cell structures called microtubules, which play an important role in cell functions. In normal cell growth, microtubules are formed when a cell starts dividing. Once the cell stops dividing, the microtubules are broken down or destroyed. Taxanes stop the microtubules from breaking down; cancer cells become so clogged with microtubules that they cannot grow and divide.

Paclitaxel

In 1984, NCI began clinical trials (research studies with people) that looked at paclitaxel's safety and how well it worked to treat certain cancers. In 1989, NCI-supported researchers at The Johns Hopkins Oncology Center reported that tumors shrank or disappeared in 30 percent of patients who received paclitaxel for the treatment of advanced ovarian cancer. Although the responses to paclitaxel were not permanent (they lasted an average of 5 months, some up to 9 months), it was clear that advanced ovarian cancer patients could benefit from this treatment. In December 1992, the U.S. Food and Drug Administration (FDA) approved the use of paclitaxel for ovarian cancer that was resistant to treatment (refractory). Paclitaxel was later approved as initial treatment for ovarian cancer in combination

Fact Sheet 7.15, Cancer Info. Service, National Cancer Institute, 1/01.

with cisplatin. Women with epithelial ovarian cancer are now generally treated with surgery followed by a taxane and a platinum (another type of anticancer drug).

The FDA has also approved paclitaxel for the treatment of breast cancer that recurred within 6 months after adjuvant chemotherapy (chemotherapy that is given after the primary treatment to enhance the effectiveness of the primary treatment), or that spread (metastasized) to nearby lymph nodes or other parts of the body. Paclitaxel is also used for other cancers, including AIDS-related Kaposi's sarcoma and lung cancer.

Side Effects of Paclitaxel

Like most cancer drugs, paclitaxel has side effects that can be serious. It is important for patients to talk with their doctor about possible side effects. For example, paclitaxel can cause hypersensitivity (allergic) reactions such as flushing of the face, skin rash, or shortness of breath. Patients often receive medication to prevent hypersensitivity reactions before they take paclitaxel. Paclitaxel can also cause temporary damage to the bone marrow. The bone marrow is the soft, sponge-like tissue in the center of large bones that produces blood cells, which fight infection, carry oxygen, and help prevent bleeding by causing blood clots to form. Bone marrow damage can cause a person to be more susceptible to infection, anemia (a condition in which the number of red blood cells is below normal), and bruise or bleed easily. Other side effects may include joint or muscle pain in the arms or legs; diarrhea; nausea and vomiting; numbness, burning, or tingling in the hands or feet; and loss of hair. Nevertheless, for many patients with cancer, the benefits outweigh the risks associated with this drug.

Paclitaxel Supplies: Old Problems and New Approaches

Paclitaxel is a compound that was originally isolated from the bark of the Pacific yew tree (Taxus brevifolia). Early research using paclitaxel was limited due to difficulties in obtaining the drug. The amount of paclitaxel in yew bark is small, and extracting it is a complicated and expensive process. In addition, bark collection is restricted because the Pacific yew is a limited resource located in forests that are home to the endangered spotted owl.

As demand for paclitaxel grew, NCI, in collaboration with other Government agencies and the pharmaceutical company Bristol-Myers

Squibb, worked to increase the availability and find other sources of paclitaxel besides the bark of the Pacific yew tree. This work led to the production of a semi-synthetic form of paclitaxel derived from the needles and twigs of the Himalayan yew tree (Taxus bacatta), which is a renewable resource. The FDA approved the semi-synthetic form of paclitaxel in the spring of 1995. This form of paclitaxel has now replaced the drug derived from the bark of the Pacific yew tree.

Docetaxel

Docetaxel, a compound that is similar to paclitaxel, is also used to treat cancer. Docetaxel, like the semi-synthetic paclitaxel, comes from the needles of the yew tree. The FDA has approved docetaxel to treat advanced breast, lung, and ovarian cancer.

Side Effects of Docetaxel

The side effects of docetaxel are similar to those related to paclitaxel. Additionally, docetaxel can cause fluid retention, which is the accumulation of fluid in the body. This can result in shortness of breath, swelling of hands or feet, or unexplained weight gain. Before receiving docetaxel, patients are often given medication to prevent fluid retention.

Current Clinical Trials with Taxanes

Researchers continue to look for new and better ways to use taxanes to treat cancer. They are studying paclitaxel in combination with other anticancer drugs to treat many different types of cancer, including lymphoma and cancers of the head and neck, breast, esophagus, stomach, bladder, prostate, endometrium (uterus), and cervix. In addition, researchers are studying ways to overcome some cancers' resistance to paclitaxel. Clinical trials are also in progress to test the effectiveness of docetaxel, alone or in combination with other anticancer drugs, for several types of cancer, including cancers of the head and neck, prostate, breast, lung, and endometrium (uterus).

Chapter 52

Questions and Answers about Tamoxifen

What is tamoxifen?

Tamoxifen (Nolvadex®) is a medication in pill form that interferes with the activity of estrogen (a hormone). Tamoxifen has been used for more than 20 years to treat patients with advanced breast cancer. It is used as adjuvant, or additional, therapy following primary treatment for early stage breast cancer. In women at high risk of developing breast cancer, tamoxifen reduces the chance of developing the disease. Tamoxifen continues to be studied for the prevention of breast cancer. It is also being studied in the treatment of several other types of cancer. It is important to note that tamoxifen is also used to treat men with breast cancer.

How does tamoxifen work on breast cancer?

Estrogen promotes the growth of breast cancer cells. Tamoxifen works against the effects of estrogen on these cells. It is often called an "anti-estrogen." As a treatment for breast cancer, the drug slows or stops the growth of cancer cells that are present in the body. As adjuvant therapy, tamoxifen helps prevent the original breast cancer from returning and also helps prevent the development of new cancers in the other breast.

National Cancer Institute, December 2000

Are there other beneficial effects of tamoxifen?

While tamoxifen acts against the effects of estrogen in breast tissue, it acts like estrogen in other tissue. This means that women who take tamoxifen may derive many of the beneficial effects of menopausal estrogen replacement therapy, such as lower blood cholesterol and slower bone loss (osteoporosis).

Can tamoxifen prevent breast cancer?

Research has shown that when tamoxifen is used as adjuvant therapy for early stage breast cancer, it not only prevents the recurrence of the original cancer but also prevents the development of new cancers in the other breast. Based on these findings, the National Cancer Institute (NCI) funded a large research study to determine the usefulness of tamoxifen in preventing breast cancer in women who have an increased risk of developing the disease. This study, known as the Breast Cancer Prevention Trial (BCPT), was conducted by the National Surgical Adjuvant Breast and Bowel Project (NSABP), a component of the NCI's Clinical Trials Cooperative Group Program. This study found a 49 percent reduction in diagnoses of invasive breast cancer among women who took tamoxifen. Women who took tamoxifen also had 50 percent fewer diagnoses of noninvasive breast tumors, such as ductal or lobular carcinoma *in situ*. However, there are risks associated with tamoxifen. Some are even life threatening. The decision to take tamoxifen is an individual one: The woman and her doctor must carefully consider the benefits and risks of therapy.

Women with an increased risk of developing breast cancer have the option to consider taking tamoxifen to reduce their chance of developing this disease. They may also consider participating in the Study of Tamoxifen and Raloxifene (see below).

At this time, there is no evidence that tamoxifen is beneficial for women who do not have an increased risk of developing breast cancer.

What is the Study of Tamoxifen and Raloxifene (STAR), and how can a woman learn more about it?

The Study of Tamoxifen and Raloxifene (STAR) is a clinical trial (a research study conducted with people) designed to see whether the osteoporosis drug raloxifene (Evista®) is more or less effective than tamoxifen in reducing the chance of developing breast cancer in women who are at an increased risk of developing the disease.

Raloxifene may have breast cancer risk reduction properties similar to those found in tamoxifen. This study will also examine whether raloxifene has benefits over tamoxifen, such as fewer side effects.

The STAR trial, which began in June 1999, is being conducted by the NSABP. It will involve about 22,000 postmenopausal women who are at least 35 years old and are at increased risk for developing breast cancer.

Women can learn more about the STAR trial in several ways. They can call NCI's Cancer Information Service at 1-800-4-CANCER (1-800-422-6237). The number for deaf and hard of hearing callers with TTY equipment is 1-800-332-8615. Information is also available on NSABP's Web site at http://www.nsabp.pitt.edu/ or NCI's cancerTrials™ website at http://cancertrials.nci.nih.gov/ on the Internet.

What are some of the more common side effects of taking tamoxifen?

In general, the side effects of tamoxifen are similar to some of the symptoms of menopause. The most common side effects are hot flashes and vaginal discharge. Some women experience irregular menstrual periods, headaches, fatigue, nausea and/or vomiting, vaginal dryness or itching, irritation of the skin around the vagina, and skin rash. As is the case with menopause, not all women who take tamoxifen have these symptoms. Men who take tamoxifen may experience headaches, nausea and/or vomiting, skin rash, impotence, or a decrease in sexual interest.

Does tamoxifen cause uterine cancer?

The BCPT found that women taking tamoxifen had more than twice the chance of developing uterine cancer compared with women who took a placebo (an inactive substance that looks the same as, and is administered in the same way as, tamoxifen). The risk of uterine cancer in women taking tamoxifen was in the same range as (or less than) the risk in postmenopausal women taking single-agent estrogen replacement therapy. Additional studies are under way to define more clearly the role of other risk factors for uterine cancer, such as prior hormone use, in women receiving tamoxifen.

Most of the uterine cancers that have occurred during studies of women taking tamoxifen have been found in the early stages, and treatment was usually effective. However, tamoxifen was life threatening for some breast cancer patients who developed uterine cancer while taking tamoxifen.

Abnormal vaginal bleeding and lower abdominal (pelvic) pain are two symptoms of uterine cancer. Women who are taking tamoxifen should talk with their doctor about having regular pelvic examinations, and should also be checked promptly if they have any abnormal vaginal bleeding between scheduled exams.

Does tamoxifen cause blood clots or stroke?

Data from large treatment studies suggest that there is a small increase in the number of blood clots in women taking tamoxifen, particularly in women who are receiving anticancer drugs (chemotherapy) along with tamoxifen. The total number of women who have experienced this side effect is small. The risk of having a blood clot due to tamoxifen is similar to the risk of a blood clot when taking estrogen replacement therapy.

Women in the BCPT who took tamoxifen also had an increased chance of developing blood clots and an increased chance of stroke.

Does tamoxifen cause eye problems?

As women age, they are more likely to develop cataracts (a clouding of the lens inside the eye). Women taking tamoxifen appear to be at increased risk for developing cataracts. Other eye problems, such as corneal scarring or retinal changes, have been reported in a few patients.

Does tamoxifen cause other types of cancer?

Although tamoxifen can cause liver cancer in particular strains of rats, it is not known to cause liver cancer in humans. It is clear, however, that tamoxifen can sometimes cause other liver toxicities in patients, which can be severe or life threatening. Doctors may order blood tests from time to time to check liver function.

One study suggested a possible increase in cancers of the digestive tract among women receiving tamoxifen for breast cancer. Other trials, including the BCPT, have not shown an association between tamoxifen and these cancers.

Studies such as the BCPT show no increase in cancers other than uterine cancer. This potential risk is being evaluated.

Should women taking tamoxifen avoid pregnancy?

Yes. Tamoxifen may make premenopausal women more fertile, but doctors advise women on tamoxifen to avoid pregnancy because animal studies have suggested that the use of tamoxifen in pregnancy can cause fetal harm. Women who have questions about fertility, birth control, or pregnancy should discuss their concerns with their doctor.

Does tamoxifen cause a woman to begin menopause?

Tamoxifen does not cause a woman to begin menopause, although it can cause some symptoms that are similar to those that may occur during menopause. In most premenopausal women taking tamoxifen, the ovaries continue to act normally and produce estrogen in the same or slightly increased amounts.

Do the benefits of tamoxifen in treating breast cancer outweigh its risks?

The benefits of tamoxifen as a treatment for breast cancer are firmly established and far outweigh the potential risks. Patients who are concerned about the risks and benefits of tamoxifen or any other medications are encouraged to discuss these concerns with their doctor.

How long should a patient take tamoxifen for the treatment of breast cancer?

Patients with advanced breast cancer may take tamoxifen for varying lengths of time, depending on their response to this treatment and other factors. When used as adjuvant therapy for early stage breast cancer, tamoxifen is generally prescribed for 5 years. However, the ideal length of treatment with tamoxifen is not known.

Two studies have confirmed the benefit of taking adjuvant tamoxifen daily for 5 years. These studies compared 5 years of treatment with tamoxifen with 10 years of treatment. When taken for 5 years, the drug prevents the recurrence of the original breast cancer and also prevents the development of a second primary cancer in the other breast. Taking tamoxifen for longer than 5 years is not more effective than 5 years of therapy.

Chapter 53

Considering Complementary and Alternative Therapies

What is complementary and alternative medicine?

Complementary and alternative medicine (CAM)—also referred to as integrative medicine—includes a broad range of healing philosophies, approaches, and therapies. A therapy is generally called complementary when it is used in addition to conventional treatments; it is often called alternative when it is used instead of conventional treatment. (Conventional treatments are those that are widely accepted and practiced by the mainstream medical community.) Depending on how they are used, some therapies can be considered either complementary or alternative.

Complementary and alternative therapies are used in an effort to prevent illness, reduce stress, prevent or reduce side effects and symptoms, or control or cure disease. Some commonly used methods of complementary or alternative therapy include mind/body control interventions such as visualization or relaxation; manual healing, including acupressure and massage; homeopathy; vitamins or herbal products; and acupuncture.

Are complementary and alternative therapies widely used?

Research indicates that the use of complementary and alternative therapies is increasing. A large-scale study published in the November 11, 1998, issue of the *Journal of the American Medical Association* found that CAM use among the general public increased from 34 percent in 1990 to 42 percent in 1997.

Fact Sheet 9.14, Cancer Info. Service, National Cancer Institute, 12/00.

Several surveys of CAM use by cancer patients have been conducted with small numbers of patients. One study published in the February 2000 issue of the journal *Cancer* reported that 37 percent of 46 patients with prostate cancer used one or more CAM therapies as part of their cancer treatment. These therapies included herbal remedies, old-time remedies, vitamins, and special diets. A larger study of CAM use in patients with different types of cancer was published in the July 2000 issue of the *Journal of Clinical Oncology*. That study found that 83 percent of 453 cancer patients had used at least one CAM therapy as part of their cancer treatment. The study included CAM therapies such as special diets, psychotherapy, spiritual practices, and vitamin supplements. When psychotherapy and spiritual practices were excluded, 69 percent of patients had used at least one CAM therapy in their cancer treatment.

How are complementary and alternative approaches evaluated?

It is important that the same scientific evaluation which is used to assess conventional approaches be used to evaluate complementary and alternative therapies. A number of medical centers are evaluating complementary and alternative therapies by developing clinical trials (research studies with people) to test them.

Conventional approaches to cancer treatment have generally been studied for safety and effectiveness through a rigorous scientific process, including clinical trials with large numbers of patients. Often, less is known about the safety and effectiveness of complementary and alternative methods. Some of these complementary and alternative therapies have not undergone rigorous evaluation. Others, once considered unorthodox, are finding a place in cancer treatment—not as cures, but as complementary therapies that may help patients feel better and recover faster. One example is acupuncture. According to a panel of experts at a National Institutes of Health (NIH) Consensus Conference in November 1997, acupuncture has been found to be effective in the management of chemotherapy-associated nausea and vomiting and in controlling pain associated with surgery. Some approaches, such as laetrile, have been studied and found ineffective or potentially harmful.

What is the Best Case Series Program?

The Best Case Series Program, which was started by the National Cancer Institute (NCI) in 1991, is another way that early data about complementary and alternative approaches are evaluated. The Best Case Series Program is overseen by the NCI's Office of Cancer Complementary and Alternative Medicine (OCCAM). Through the Best Case Series Program, health care professionals who offer CAM services submit their patients' medical records and related materials to OCCAM. The OCCAM conducts a critical review of the materials and presents the approaches that have the most therapeutic potential to the Cancer Advisory Panel for Complementary and Alternative Medicine (CAPCAM) for further review.

CAPCAM was jointly created in 1999 by the NCI and the NIH National Center for Complementary and Alternative Medicine (NCCAM). CAPCAM's membership is drawn from a broad range of experts from the conventional and CAM cancer research and practice communities. CAPCAM evaluates CAM cancer approaches that are submitted through the Best Case Series Program, and makes recommendations to NCCAM on whether and how these approaches should be followed up.

Is NCI sponsoring clinical trials in complementary and alternative medicine?

The NCI is currently sponsoring several clinical trials (research studies with patients) that study complementary and alternative treatments for cancer. Current trials include enzyme therapy with nutritional support for the treatment of inoperable pancreatic cancer, shark cartilage therapy for the treatment of non-small cell lung cancer, and studies of the effects of diet on prostate and breast cancers. Some of these trials compare alternative therapies with conventional treatments, while others study the effects of complementary approaches used in addition to conventional treatments. Patients who are interested in taking part in these or any clinical trials should talk with their doctor.

More information about clinical trials sponsored by the NCI can be obtained from NCCAM, OCCAM, and the NCI's Cancer Information Service (CIS) (see below).

What should patients do when considering complementary and alternative therapies?

Cancer patients considering complementary and alternative therapies should discuss this decision with their doctor or nurse, as they would any therapeutic approach, because some complementary and alternative therapies may interfere with their standard treatment or may be harmful when used with conventional treatment.

When considering complementary and alternative therapies, what questions should patients ask their health care provider?

- What benefits can be expected from this therapy?
- What are the risks associated with this therapy?
- Do the known benefits outweigh the risks?
- What side effects can be expected?
- Will the therapy interfere with conventional treatment?
- Is this therapy part of a clinical trial? If so, who is sponsoring the trial?
- Will the therapy be covered by health insurance?

How can patients and their health care providers learn more about complementary and alternative therapies?

Patients and their doctor or nurse can learn about complementary and alternative therapies from the following Government agencies:

NCCAM Clearinghouse
Post Office Box 8218
Silver Spring, MD 20907–8218
Telephone: 1-888-644-6226
TTY/TDY (for deaf and hard of hearing callers): 1-888-644-6226
Web site: http://nccam.nih.gov

The NIH National Center for Complementary and Alternative Medicine (NCCAM) facilitates research and evaluation of complementary and alternative practices, and provides information about a variety of approaches to health professionals and the public.

Office of Cancer Complementary and Alternative Medicine (OCCAM)
Web site: http://occam.nci.nih.gov

The NCI Office of Cancer Complementary and Alternative Medicine (OCCAM) coordinates the activities of the NCI in the area of complementary and alternative medicine (CAM). OCCAM supports CAM cancer research and provides information about cancer-related CAM to health providers and the general public.

Food and Drug Administration
5600 Fishers Lane
Rockville, MD 20857
Telephone: 1-888-463-6332
Web site: http://www.fda.gov

The Food and Drug Administration (FDA) regulates drugs and medical devices to ensure that they are safe and effective.

Federal Trade Commission
Consumer Response Center
CRC-240
Washington, DC 20580
Telephone: 1-877-FTC-HELP (1-877-382-4357)
TTY (for deaf and hard of hearing callers): 202-326-2502
Web site: http://www.ftc.gov

The Federal Trade Commission (FTC) enforces consumer protection laws. Publications available from the FTC include:

- "Who Cares: Sources of Information About Health Care Products and Services"

- "Fraudulent Health Claims: Don't Be Fooled"

References

Bennet M, Lengacher C. Use of Complementary Therapies in a Rural Cancer Population. *Oncology Nursing Forum* 1999;26(8):1287–1294.

Cassileth B, Chapman C. Alternative and Complementary Cancer Therapies. *Cancer* 1996; 77(6):1026–1033.

Eisenberg DM, Davis RB, Ettner SL, et al. Trends in Alternative Medicine Use in the United States, 1990–1997. *Journal of the American Medical Association* 2000;280(18):1569–1675.

Jacobs J. Unproven Alternative Methods of Cancer Treatment. In: DeVita, Hellman, Rosenberg, editors. *Cancer: Principles and Practice of Oncology*. 5th edition. Philadelphia: Lippincott-Raven Publishers; 1997. 2993–3001.

Kao GD, Devine P. Use of Complementary Health Practices by Prostate Carcinoma Patients Undergoing Radiation Therapy. *Cancer* 2000;88(3):615–619.

Nelson W. Alternative Cancer Treatments. *Highlights in Oncology Practice* 1998;15(4):85–93.

Richardson MA, Sanders T, Palmer JL, Greisinger A, Singletary SE. Complementary/Alternative Medicine Use in a Comprehensive Cancer Center and the Implications for Oncology. *Journal of Clinical Oncology* 2000;18(13):2505–2514.

Sparber A, Bauer L, Curt G, et al. Use of Complementary Medicine by Adult Patients Participating in Cancer Clinical Trials. *Oncology Nursing Forum* 2000;27(4):623–630.

Part Eight

Recent Research and Clinical Trials

Chapter 54

The Women's Health Initiative

What Is the Women's Health Initiative?

The Women's Health Initiative (WHI) is a long-term national health study that focuses on strategies for preventing heart disease, breast and colorectal cancer, and osteoporosis in postmenopausal women. These chronic diseases are the major causes of death, disability, and frailty in older women of all races and socioeconomic backgrounds.

This multi-million dollar, 15-year project, sponsored by the National Institutes of Health (NIH), National Heart, Lung, and Blood Institute (NHLBI), involves over 161,000 women aged 50-79, and is one of the most definitive, far reaching clinical trials of women's health ever undertaken in the U.S. The WHI Clinical Trial and Observational Study will attempt to address many of the inequities in women's health research and provide practical information to women and their physicians about hormone replacement therapy, dietary patterns and calcium/vitamin D supplements, and their effects on the prevention of heart disease, cancer and osteoporosis.

A Community Prevention Study (CPS), a 5-year cooperative venture with CDC, is a study of strategies to enhance adoption of healthful behaviors through a multi-disciplinary approach. The purpose of the CPS is to develop community-based public health interventions

This chapter includes text from "Backgrounder," and "Why WHI?" undated documents produced by the National Heart, Lung, and Blood Institute (NHLBI).

401

models which will achieve healthful behaviors in women aged 40 and over.

How Is WHI Being Conducted?

The WHI study has three components: a randomized clinical trial, an observational study, and a community prevention study.

The randomized controlled clinical trial (CT) has enrolled over 68,000 postmenopausal women between the ages of 50-79. The clinical trial has three study components. If eligible, women could choose to enroll in one, two, or all three of the components. The components are:

- **Hormone Replacement Therapy (HRT):** This component will examine the effect of HRT on the prevention of heart disease and osteoporosis, and any associated risk for breast cancer. Women participating in this component take hormone pills or a placebo (inactive pill).

- **Dietary Modification:** The Dietary Modification component will evaluate the effect of a low-fat, high fruit, vegetable and grain diet on the prevention of breast and colorectal cancer and heart disease. Study participants follow either their usual eating pattern or a low-fat eating program.

- **Calcium/Vitamin D:** This component starts up to 2 years after a woman joins one or both of the other studies. It will evaluate the effect of calcium and vitamin D supplementation on the prevention of osteoporosis-related fractures and colorectal cancer. Women in this component take calcium and vitamin D pills or a placebo.

The observational study (OS) will examine the relationship between lifestyle, health and risk factors and specific disease outcomes. This component will track the medical history and health habits of approximately 100,000 women.

Recruitment for the observational study was completed in 1998 and participants will be followed for 8 to 12 years.

The community prevention study (CPS) is a unique collaborative venture between the Centers for Disease Control and Prevention (CDC), and the National Institutes of Health. Eight University-based Prevention Centers underwritten by CDC will conduct and evaluate health programs that encourage women of all races and socioeconomic backgrounds to adopt healthful behaviors such as improved diet, nutritional supplementation, smoking cessation, exercise, and early detection of treatable health problems. The goal of the community prevention study is to develop carefully evaluated, model programs that can be implemented in a wide range of communities throughout the U.S.

Where Is WHI CT/OS Taking Place?

The WHI clinical trial and observational study is being conducted at 40 clinical centers nationwide. The Fred Hutchinson Cancer Research Center in Seattle, WA serves as the WHI Clinical Coordinating Center for data collection, management, and analysis. Recruitment began in September 1993 and continued through July 1998 for those women who chose to "be part of the answer." The OS enrolled through December 1998.

Study participants get the personal satisfaction of knowing that they are contributing to their own health and the health of women for generations to come.

Why WHI?

The WHI is focusing on the major causes of death, disability and frailty in postmenopausal women. The overall goal of WHI is to reduce coronary heart disease, breast, and colorectal cancer, and osteoporotic-fractures among postmenopausal women via prevention strategies and risk factor identification.

Scientific knowledge about prevention and treatment of diseases common in or unique to women is insufficient. Successful prevention strategies will have major public health implications.

WHI and Cancer-Related Concerns

Breast Cancer

- Second leading cause of cancer deaths in U.S. women.
- Over 46,000 women die of breast cancer annually.
- Approximately 183,000 new cases of breast cancer each year.
- Inconclusive data on dietary fat intake and breast cancer.
- Inconsistent data on hormones and breast cancer risk.

Colon Cancer

- Third leading cause of cancer deaths in U.S. women.

- Over 28,000 women die of colorectal cancer each year.

- Approximately 51,000 women per year are diagnosed with colon cancer; 16,500 new cases of rectal cancer in women each year.

- Studies suggest increased calcium and Vitamin D intake may decrease risk of colorectal cancer.

Chapter 55

Taking Part in Clinical Trials

Understanding Clinical Trials

Clinical trials, also called cancer treatment or research studies, test new treatments in people with cancer. The goal of this research is to find better ways to treat cancer and help cancer patients. Clinical trials test many types of treatment such as new drugs, new approaches to surgery or radiation therapy, new combinations of treatments, or new methods such as gene therapy.

A clinical trial is one of the final stages of a long and careful cancer research process. The search for new treatments begins in the laboratory, where scientists first develop and test new ideas. If an approach seems promising, the next step may be testing a treatment in animals to see how it affects cancer in a living being and whether it has harmful effects. Of course, treatments that work well in the lab or in animals do not always work well in people. Studies are done with cancer patients to find out whether promising treatments are safe and effective.

What Happens in a Clinical Trial?

In a clinical trial, patients receive treatment and doctors carry out research on how the treatment affects the patients. While clinical trials

Excerpted from "Taking Part in Clinical Trials: What Cancer Patients Should Know," National Cancer Institute (NCI), NIH Pub. No. 97-4250, revised May 1998. To order a complete copy of this publication, call 1-800-4CANCER (422-6237).

have risks for the people who take part, each study also takes steps to protect patients.

When you take part in a clinical trial, you receive your treatment in a cancer center, hospital, clinic, and/or doctor's office. Doctors, nurses, social workers, and other health professionals may be part of your treatment team. They will follow your progress closely. You may have more tests and doctor visits than you would if you were not taking part in a study. You will follow a treatment plan your doctor prescribes, and you may also have other responsibilities such as keeping a log or filling out forms about your health. Some studies continue to check on patients even after their treatment is over.

In clinical trials, both research concerns and patient well-being are important. To help protect patients and produce sound results, research with people is carried out according to strict scientific and ethical principles. These include:

1. Each clinical trial has an action plan (protocol) that explains how it will work. The study's investigator, usually a doctor, prepares an action plan for the study. Known as a protocol, this plan explains what will be done in the study and why. It outlines how many people will take part in the study, what medical tests they will receive and how often, and the treatment plan. The same protocol is used by each doctor that takes part. For patient safety, each protocol must be approved by the organization that sponsors the study (such as the National Cancer Institute) and the Institutional Review Board (IRB) at each hospital or other study site. This board, which includes consumers, clergy, and health professionals, reviews the protocol to try to be sure that the research will not expose patients to extreme or unethical risks.

2. Each study enrolls people who are alike in key ways. Each study's protocol describes the characteristics that all patients in the study must have. Called eligibility criteria, these guidelines differ from study to study, depending on the research purpose. They may include age, gender, the type and stage of cancer, and whether cancer patients who have had prior cancer treatment or who have other health problems can take part. Using eligibility criteria is an important principle of medical research that helps produce reliable results. During a study, they help protect patient safety, so that people who are likely to be harmed by study drugs or other treatments are

406

not exposed to the risk. After results are in, they also help doctors know which patient groups will benefit if the new treatment being studied is proven to work. For instance, a new treatment may work for one type of cancer but not for another, or it may be more effective for men than women.

3. Cancer clinical trials include research at three different phases. Each phase answers different questions about the new treatment.

   Phase I trials are the first step in testing a new treatment in humans. In these studies, researchers look for the best way to give a new treatment (e.g., by mouth, IV drip, or injection? how many times a day?). They also try to find out if and how the treatment can be given safely (e.g., best dose?); and they watch for any harmful side effects. Because less is known about the possible risks and benefits in Phase I, these studies usually include only a limited number of patients who would not be helped by other known treatments.

   Phase II trials focus on learning whether the new treatment has an anticancer effect (e.g., Does it shrink a tumor? improve blood test results?). As in Phase I, only a small number of people take part because of the risks and unknowns involved.

   Phase III trials compare the results of people taking the new treatment with results of people taking standard treatment (e.g., Which group has better survival rates? fewer side effects?). In most cases, studies move into Phase III testing only after a treatment shows promise in Phases I and II. Phase III trials may include hundreds of people around the country.

4. In Phase III trials, people are assigned at random to receive either the new treatment or standard treatment. Researchers assign patients by chance either to a group taking the new treatment (called the treatment group) or to a group taking standard treatment (called the control group). This method, called randomization, helps avoid bias: having the study's results affected by human choices or other factors not related to the treatments being tested.

   In some studies, researchers do not tell the patient whether he or she is in the treatment or control group (called a single blind study). This approach is another way to avoid bias, because when people know what drug they are taking, it might change the way they react. For instance, patients who knew they were taking the new treatment might expect it to work better and report hopeful signs because they want to believe they are getting well. This could bias the study by making results look better than they really were.

Why Do Phase III Clinical Trials Compare Treatment Groups?

Comparing similar groups of people taking different treatments for the same type of cancer is another way to make sure that study results are real and caused by the treatment rather than by chance or other factors. Comparing treatments with each other often shows clearly which one is more effective or has fewer side effects.

Another reason Phase III trials compare the new treatment with standard treatment is so that no one in a study is left without any treatment when standard treatment is available—which would be unethical. When no standard treatment exists for a cancer, some studies compare a new treatment with a placebo (a look-alike pill that contains no active drug). However, you will be told if this is a possibility before you decide whether to take part in a study.

Should I Take Part in a Clinical Trial?

This is a question only you, those close to you, and your health professionals can answer together. Learning you have cancer and deciding what to do about it is often overwhelming. This section has information you can use in thinking about your choices and making your decision. While a clinical trial is a good choice for some people, this treatment option has possible benefits and drawbacks. Here are some factors to consider. You may want to discuss them with your doctor and the people close to you.

Possible Benefits

- Clinical trials offer high-quality cancer care. If you are in a study and do not receive the new treatment being tested, you will receive the best standard treatment. This may be as good as, or better than, the new approach.

- If a new treatment approach is proven to work and you are taking it, you may be among the first to benefit.

- By looking at the pros and cons of clinical trials and your other treatment choices, you are taking an active role in a decision that affects your life.

- You have the chance to help others and improve cancer treatment.

Possible Drawbacks

- New treatments under study are not always better than, or even as good as, standard care. They may have side effects that doctors do not expect or that are worse than those of standard treatment.

- Even if a new treatment has benefits, it may not work for you. Even standard treatments, proven effective for many people, do not help everyone.

- If you receive standard treatment instead of the new treatment being tested, it may not be as effective as the new approach.

- Health insurance and managed care providers do not always cover all patient care costs in a study. What they cover varies by plan and by study. To find out in advance what costs are likely to be paid in your case, talk to a doctor, nurse or social worker from the study.

Your Rights, Your Protections

Before and during a cancer treatment study, you have a number of rights. Knowing these can help protect you from harm.

- Taking part in a treatment study is up to you. It may be only one of your treatment choices. Talk with your doctor. Together, you can make the best choice for you.

- If you do enter a study, doctors and nurses will follow your response to treatment carefully throughout the research.

- If researchers learn that a treatment harms you, you will be taken off the study right away. You may then receive other treatment from your own doctor.

- You have the right to leave a study at any time.

One of your key rights is the right to informed consent. Informed consent means that you must be given all the facts about a study before you decide whether to take part. This includes details about the treatments and tests you may receive and the possible benefits and risks they may have. The doctor or nurse will give you an informed consent form that goes over key facts. If you agree to take part in the study, you will be asked to sign this informed consent form.

The informed consent process continues throughout the study. For instance, you will be told of any new findings regarding your clinical trial, such as new risks. You may be asked to sign a new consent form if you want to stay in the study.

Signing a consent form does not mean you must stay in the study. In fact, you can leave at any time. If you choose to leave the study, you will have the chance to discuss other treatments and care with your own doctor or a doctor from the study.

Questions You Should Ask

Finding answers and making choices may be hard for people with cancer and those who care about them. It is important to discuss your treatment choices with your doctor, a cancer specialist (an oncologist) to whom your doctor may refer you, and the staff of any clinical trial you consider entering. Here are some questions you may want to ask about:

The Study

- What is the purpose of the study? In what phase is this study?

- Why do researchers believe the new treatment being tested may be effective? Has it been tested before?

- Who sponsors the study, and who has reviewed and approved it?

- How are the study data and patient safety being checked?

- When and where will study results and information go?

Possible Risks and Benefits

- What are the possible short- and long-term risks, side effects, and benefits to me?

- Are there standard treatments for my type of cancer?

- How do the possible risks, side effects, and benefits in the study compare with standard treatment?

Your Care

- What kinds of treatments, medical tests, or procedures will I have during the study? Will they be painful? How do they compare with what I would receive outside the study?

- How often and for how long will I receive the treatment, and how long will I need to remain in the study? Will there be follow-up after the study?

- Where will my treatment take place? Will I have to be in the hospital? If so, how often and for how long?

- How will I know if the treatment is working?

- Will I be able to see my own doctor? Who will be in charge of my care?

Personal Issues

- How could the study affect my daily life?

- Can you put me in touch with other people who are in this study?

- What support is there for me and my family in the community?

Cost Issues

- Will I have to pay for any treatment, tests, or other charges?

- What is my health insurance likely to cover?

- Who can help answer any questions from my insurance company or managed care plan?

Terms Related to Clinical Trials

Bias: Human choices or any other factors beside the treatments being tested that affect a study's results. Clinical trials use many methods to avoid bias, because biased results may not be correct.

Clinical trials: Research studies that involve people. Each study tries to answer scientific questions and to find better ways to prevent or treat cancer.

Control group: In a clinical trial, the group of people that receives standard treatment for their cancer.

Informed consent: The process in which a person learns key facts about a clinical trial or research study and then agrees voluntarily to take part or decides against it. This process includes signing a form that describes the benefits and risks that may occur if the person decides to take part.

Institutional Review Board (IRB): Groups of scientists, doctors, clergy, and consumers at each health care facility at which a clinical trial takes place. Designed to protect patients who take part in studies, IRBs review and must approve the protocols for all clinical trials funded by the Federal Govern-ment. They check to see that the study is well-designed, does not involve undue risks, and includes safeguards for patients.

Investigator: A researcher in a treatment study.

Oncologist: A doctor who specializes in treating cancer.

Placebo: A tablet, capsule, or injection that looks like the drug or other substance being tested but contains no drug.

Protocol: An action plan for a clinical trial. The plan states what will be done in the study and why. It outlines how many people will take part in the study, what types of patients may take part, what tests they will receive and how often, and the treatment plan.

Randomization: A method used to prevent bias in research. People are assigned by chance to either the treatment or control group.

Remission: When the signs and symptoms of cancer go away, the disease is said to be "in remission." A remission can be temporary or permanent.

Side effects: Problems that occur when treatment affects healthy cells. Common side effects of standard cancer treatments are fatigue, nausea, vomiting, decreased blood cell counts, hair loss, and mouth sores. New treatments being tested may have these or other unknown side effects.

Single blind study: A method used to prevent bias in treatment studies. In a single blind study, the patient is not told whether he/she is taking the standard treatment or the new treatment being tested. Only the doctors know.

Stage: The extent of a cancer and whether the disease has spread from the original site to other parts of the body. Numbers with or without letters are used to define cancer stages (e.g., Stage IIb).

Standard treatment: The best treatment currently known for a cancer, based on results of past research.

Treatment group: The group that receives the new treatment being tested during a study.

Chapter 56

Atypical Squamous Cells of Undetermined Significance (ASCUS)/ Low-Grade Squamous Intraepithelial Lesions (LSIL) Triage Study

Questions and Answers about the ALTS Findings

What Is ALTS?

ALTS is a clinical trial designed to find the best way to manage the mild abnormalities that often show up on Pap tests. The study began enrolling patients in November 1996 and completed enrollment in December 1998. Analysis of the data is under way.

ALTS, which stands for the ASCUS/LSIL Triage Study, was organized and funded by the National Cancer Institute (NCI), the U.S. government's principal agency for cancer research. It was conducted at four major medical centers: the University of Alabama at Birmingham; the University of Oklahoma in Oklahoma City; Magee-Womens Hospital of the University of Pittsburgh Medical Center in Pittsburgh, Pennsylvania; and the University of Washington in Seattle.

What are ASCUS and LSIL?

ASCUS and LSIL are acronyms for two mild abnormalities detected by Pap tests. ASCUS stands for atypical squamous cells of undetermined significance and LSIL for low-grade squamous intraepithelial lesion.

A diagnosis of ASCUS means that the nature of the abnormality is uncertain or equivocal. A diagnosis of LSIL means that there is a more definite, but still mild, abnormality.

National Cancer Institute, February 2001.

415

Why did NCI initiate ALTS?

NCI initiated this trial to help resolve the controversy over what physicians and women should do about ASCUS and LSIL Pap test results. Most of these mild abnormalities will go away without treatment, but some may lead to a precancerous condition or cancer.

Many physicians in the United States now opt for aggressive management of ASCUS and LSIL, referring women to a colposcopic exam with biopsies of suspicious abnormalities. This approach carries a small risk of medical complications and is expensive. Other doctors opt for a more conservative, wait-and-see approach, recommending frequent, repeat Pap tests to see if the abnormalities go away without treatment.

The ALTS study looked at three different ways to manage ASCUS and LSIL: immediate colposcopy, conservative management, and HPV triage.

How was the study designed?

Women who enrolled in the study were divided into those with ASCUS and those with LSIL diagnoses. Patients in each category were then assigned randomly to one of three groups or study arms.

Immediate Colposcopy: Women in this arm were referred to colposcopy (examination with a magnifying instrument) to identify abnormal tissue for biopsy and, if necessary, treatment. This is the aggressive management option used commonly in the United States. Women in this arm, as in the others, also had a repeat Pap test every six months.

Conservative Management: Women in this arm were closely followed with repeat Pap tests (or, to use the more scientific term, cervical cytology) every six months. Patients had a colposcopy and a biopsy only if the repeat Pap test results suggested they had more severe abnormalities. This conservative approach is now common in Canada and in some European countries.

HPV Triage: Women in this arm were managed based on results of the Pap test plus a test for the human papillomavirus (HPV), which is the cause of most cervical cancers. If their Pap test showed more severe abnormalities or if their cervical cells contained DNA from certain HPV types associated with cancer, they had colposcopy. The

HPV Triage arm tested the hypothesis that HPV testing is effective at determining which women with ASCUS need colposcopy.

What specifically do the researchers expect to learn from ALTS?

Researchers are comparing the three different groups to learn 1) how effective each management option is in early detection of the serious abnormalities that can progress to cancer; 2) how acceptable each option is to patients; and 3) how cost effective each option is. These are the trial's three main objectives, or "endpoints."

In addition, the investigators are analyzing the ALTS data to learn more about mild cervical abnormalities and their relationship to cancer. For instance, they hope to gain information about immune system factors that may help determine whether a mild abnormality goes away without treatment or progresses to a more severe abnormality.

What are the principal findings of ALTS?

Analysis of the ALTS data is ongoing. To date, the results show:

For women with an ASCUS diagnosis, the HPV test identified virtually all women with underlying abnormalities that need immediate attention.

To conduct this analysis, the researchers looked at results from women who received a colposcopy when they enrolled in the trial. They compared the HPV test results, the colposcopy results, and the results of the repeat Pap test at enrollment (the initial Pap test was done before the patient entered the trial). The data showed that:

- About 5 percent to 10 percent of women with ASCUS turned out, on colposcopy, to have precancer or (rarely) cancer.

- Of the women who had precancer or cancer on colposcopy, 96.3 percent also had a positive HPV test. Thus the test had a 96-percent sensitivity in triaging women with precancer or cancer to colposcopy. [Sensitivity: The percent of people with disease who have a positive test.]

- About 55 percent of women with ASCUS were HPV positive and thus would have been referred to colposcopy if the HPV test had been used for triage in all cases.

- About 10 percent to 20 percent of women with a positive HPV test had precancer or, rarely, cancer. In scientific terms, the test's positive predictive value was 10 percent to 20 percent. [Positive predictive value: For positive test results, the percent of cases in which disease is present.]

- About 99.5 percent of the women with a negative HPV test did not have precancer or cancer. The test's negative predictive value was 99.5 percent. [Negative predictive value: For negative test results, the percent of cases in which disease is absent. A high negative predictive value provides strong reassurance that disease is absent.]

- About 57 percent of women with ASCUS had the same or a more serious result on a repeat Pap test using a thin-layer slide preparation method, done when they enrolled in the study. If these ASCUS-or-worse Pap test results had been used as a basis for assigning women to colposcopy (a current method for managing ASCUS), about 85 percent of those with precancerous abnormalities would have been triaged to colposcopy. Thus, the sensitivity of the repeat, thin-layer Pap test, using ASCUS or a more serious abnormality as the basis for referral to colposcopy, was 85 percent.

Conclusion: HPV testing is highly sensitive in detecting the underlying abnormalities that need immediate attention.

Reference: D. Solomon, M. Schiffman, R. Tarone for the ALTS Group, Comparison of Three Management Strategies for Patients With Atypical Squamous Cells of Undetermined Significance: Baseline Results From a Randomized Trial, *Journal of the National Cancer Institute*, Vol. 93, No. 4, Feb. 21, 2001.

For women with an LSIL diagnosis, the HPV test is positive in a large majority of cases.

This analysis focused on the 642 women in ALTS with an initial LSIL diagnosis. The investigators looked at the HPV test results in this group and also at data that had been collected through questionnaires and interviews. They found that:

- The HPV test was positive for 82.9 percent of these patients. The high frequency of HPV, as measured by the HPV test, was confirmed by another sensitive test, known as polymerase chain reaction or PCR, in a subset of this group.

- Women 30 years of age and older were less likely to be HPV positive.

- Women with three or more lifetime sex partners were more likely to be HPV positive than those with one or two partners.

Conclusion: The high prevalence of HPV infection in women with LSIL limits the usefulness of HPV testing in deciding how to manage these abnormalities.

Reference: The ASCUS/LSIL Study (ALTS) Group, Human Papillomavirus Testing for Triage of Women With Cytologic Evidence of Low-Grade Squamous Intraepithelial Lesions: Baseline Data From a Randomized Trial, *Journal of the National Cancer Institute*, Vol. 92, No. 5, March 1, 2000.

Chapter 57

Angiogenesis Inhibitors as a Possible Cancer Treatment

Angiogenesis means the formation of new blood vessels. Angiogenesis is a process controlled by certain chemicals produced in the body. These chemicals stimulate cells to repair damaged blood vessels or form new ones. Other chemicals, called angiogenesis inhibitors, signal the process to stop.

Angiogenesis plays an important role in the growth and spread of cancer. New blood vessels "feed" the cancer cells with oxygen and nutrients, allowing these cells to grow, invade nearby tissue, spread to other parts of the body, and form new colonies of cancer cells.

Because cancer cannot grow or spread without the formation of new blood vessels, scientists are trying to find ways to stop angiogenesis. They are studying natural and synthetic angiogenesis inhibitors, also called anti-angiogenesis agents, in the hope that these chemicals will prevent the growth of cancer by blocking the formation of new blood vessels. In animal studies, angiogenesis inhibitors have successfully stopped the formation of new blood vessels, causing the cancer to shrink and die.

Whether angiogenesis inhibitors will be effective against cancer in humans is not yet known. Various angiogenesis inhibitors are currently being evaluated in clinical trials (research studies in humans). These studies include patients with cancers of the breast, prostate, brain, pancreas, lung, stomach, ovary, and cervix; some leukemias and lymphomas; and AIDS-related Kaposi's sarcoma. If the results of

Fact Sheet 7.42, Cancer Info. Service, National Cancer Institute, July 1998.

clinical trials show that angiogenesis inhibitors are both safe and effective in treating cancer in humans, these agents may be approved by the Food and Drug Administration (FDA) and made available for widespread use. The process of producing and testing angiogenesis inhibitors is likely to take several years.

Detailed information about ongoing clinical trials evaluating angiogenesis inhibitors and other promising new treatments is available from the Cancer Information Service (CIS). The CIS, a national information and education network, is a free public service of the National Cancer Institute (NCI), the Nation's primary agency for cancer research. The CIS meets the information needs of patients, the public, and health professionals. The toll-free phone number is 1-800-4-CANCER (1-800-422-6237). For callers with TTY equipment, the number is 1-800-332-8615. The NCI's clinical trials website also provides a listing of NCI-sponsored clinical trials at http://cancertrials.nci.nih.gov/ on the Internet.

Chapter 58

Researching Biological Therapies

Biological therapy (sometimes called immunotherapy, biotherapy, or biological response modifier therapy) is a relatively new addition to the family of cancer treatments that also includes surgery, chemotherapy, and radiation therapy. Biological therapies use the body's immune system, either directly or indirectly, to fight cancer or to lessen the side effects that may be caused by some cancer treatments.

The immune system is a complex network of cells and organs that work together to defend the body against attacks by "foreign," or "nonself," invaders. This network is one of the body's main defenses against disease. It works against disease, including cancer, in a variety of ways. For example, the immune system may recognize the difference between healthy cells and cancer cells in the body and work to eliminate those that become cancerous.

Cancer may develop when the immune system breaks down or is not functioning adequately. Biological therapies are designed to repair, stimulate, or enhance the immune system's responses.

Immune system cells include the following:

- Lymphocytes are a type of white blood cell found in the blood and many other parts of the body. Types of lymphocytes include B cells, T cells, and Natural Killer cells.

    B cells (B lymphocytes) mature into plasma cells that secrete antibodies (immunoglobulins), the proteins that recognize and

Fact Sheet 7.2, Cancer Info. Service, National Cancer Institute, 1/01.

attach to foreign substances known as antigens. Each type of B cell makes one specific antibody, which recognizes one specific antigen.

T cells (T lymphocytes) directly attack infected, foreign, or cancerous cells. T cells also regulate the immune response by signaling other immune system defenders. T cells work primarily by producing proteins called lymphokines.

Natural Killer cells (NK cells) produce powerful chemical substances that bind to and kill any foreign invader. They attack without first having to recognize a specific antigen.

- Monocytes are white blood cells that can swallow and digest microscopic organisms and particles in a process known as phagocytosis. Monocytes can also travel into tissue and become macrophages, or "big eaters."

Cells in the immune system secrete two types of proteins: antibodies and cytokines. Antibodies respond to antigens by latching onto, or binding with, the antigens. Specific antibodies match specific antigens, fitting together much the way a key fits a lock. Cytokines are substances produced by some immune system cells to communicate with other cells. Types of cytokines include lymphokines, interferons, interleukins, and colony-stimulating factors. Cytotoxic cytokines are released by a type of T-cell called a cytotoxic T-cell. These cytokines attack cancer cells directly.

Nonspecific Immunomodulating Agents

Nonspecific immunomodulating agents are substances that stimulate or indirectly augment the immune system. Often, these agents target key immune system cells and cause secondary responses such as increased production of cytokines and immunoglobulins. Two nonspecific immunomodulating agents used in cancer treatment are bacillus Calmette-Guerin (BCG) and levamisole.

BCG, which has been widely used as a tuberculosis vaccine, is used in the treatment of superficial bladder cancer following surgery. BCG may work by stimulating an inflammatory, and possibly an immune, response. A solution of BCG is instilled in the bladder and stays there for about 2 hours before the patient is allowed to empty the bladder by urinating. This treatment is usually performed once a week for 6 weeks.

Levamisole is used along with fluorouracil (5-FU) chemotherapy in the treatment of stage III (Dukes' C) colon cancer following surgery. Levamisole may act to restore depressed immune function.

Biological Response Modifiers

Some antibodies, cytokines, and other immune system substances can be produced in the laboratory for use in cancer treatment. These substances are often called biological response modifiers (BRMs). They alter the interaction between the body's immune defenses and cancer cells to boost, direct, or restore the body's ability to fight the disease. BRMs include interferons, interleukins, colony-stimulating factors, monoclonal antibodies, and vaccines.

Researchers continue to discover new BRMs, learn more about how they function, and develop ways to use them in cancer therapy. Biological therapies may be used to:

- Stop, control, or suppress processes that permit cancer growth;

- Make cancer cells more recognizable, and therefore more susceptible, to destruction by the immune system;

- Boost the killing power of immune system cells, such as T cells, NK cells, and macrophages;

- Alter cancer cells' growth patterns to promote behavior like that of healthy cells;

- Block or reverse the process that changes a normal cell or a precancerous cell into a cancerous cell;

- Enhance the body's ability to repair or replace normal cells damaged or destroyed by other forms of cancer treatment, such as chemotherapy or radiation; and

- Prevent cancer cells from spreading to other parts of the body.

Some BRMs are a standard part of treatment for certain types of cancer, while others are being studied in clinical trials (research studies with people). BRMs are being used alone or in combination with each other. They are also being used with other treatments, such as radiation therapy and chemotherapy.

Interferons (IFN)

Interferons are types of cytokines that occur naturally in the body. They were the first cytokines produced in the laboratory for use as BRMs. There are three major types of interferons—interferon alpha, interferon beta, and interferon gamma; interferon alpha is the type most widely used in cancer treatment.

Researchers have found that interferons can improve the way a cancer patient's immune system acts against cancer cells. In addition, interferons may act directly on cancer cells by slowing their growth or promoting their development into cells with more normal behavior. Researchers believe that some interferons may also stimulate NK cells, T cells, and macrophages, boosting the immune system's anti-cancer function.

The U.S. Food and Drug Administration (FDA) has approved the use of interferon alpha for the treatment of certain types of cancer, including hairy cell leukemia, melanoma, chronic myeloid leukemia, and AIDS-related Kaposi's sarcoma. Studies have shown that interferon alpha may also be effective in treating other cancers such as metastatic kidney cancer and non-Hodgkin's lymphoma. Researchers are exploring combinations of interferon alpha and other BRMs or chemotherapy in clinical trials to treat a number of cancers.

Interleukins (IL)

Like interferons, interleukins are cytokines that occur naturally in the body and can be made in the laboratory. Many interleukins have been identified; interleukin-2 (IL-2 or aldesleukin) has been the most widely studied in cancer treatment. IL-2 stimulates the growth and activity of many immune cells, such as lymphocytes, that can destroy cancer cells. The FDA has approved IL-2 for the treatment of metastatic kidney cancer and metastatic melanoma.

Researchers continue to study the benefits of interleukins to treat a number of other cancers, including colorectal, ovarian, lung, brain, breast, prostate, some leukemias, and some lymphomas.

Colony-Stimulating Factors (CSFs)

Colony-stimulating factors (CSFs) (sometimes called hematopoietic growth factors) usually do not directly affect tumor cells; rather, they encourage bone marrow stem cells to divide and develop into white blood cells, platelets, and red blood cells. Bone marrow is critical to the body's immune system because it is the source of all blood cells.

The CSFs' stimulation of the immune system may benefit patients undergoing cancer treatment. Because anticancer drugs can damage the body's ability to make white blood cells, red blood cells, and platelets, patients receiving anticancer drugs have an increased risk of developing infections, becoming anemic, and bleeding more easily. By using CSFs to stimulate blood cell production, doctors can increase the doses of anticancer drugs without increasing the risk of infection or the need for transfusion with blood products. As a result, researchers have found CSFs particularly useful when combined with high-dose chemotherapy.

Some examples of CSFs and their use in cancer therapy are as follows:

- G-CSF (filgrastim) and GM-CSF (sargramostim) can increase the number of white blood cells, thereby reducing the risk of infection in patients receiving chemotherapy. G-CSF and GM-CSF can also stimulate the production of stem cells in preparation for stem cell or bone marrow transplants;

- Erythropoietin can increase the number of red blood cells and reduce the need for red blood cell transfusions in patients receiving chemotherapy; and

- Oprelvekin can reduce the need for platelet transfusions in patients receiving chemotherapy.

Researchers are studying CSFs in clinical trials to treat some types of leukemia, metastatic colorectal cancer, melanoma, lung cancer, and other types of cancer.

Monoclonal Antibodies (MOABs)

Researchers are evaluating the effectiveness of certain antibodies made in the laboratory called monoclonal antibodies (MOABs or MoABs). These antibodies are produced by a single type of cell and are specific for a particular antigen. Researchers are examining ways to create MOABs specific to the antigens found on the surface of the cancer cell being treated.

MOABs are made by injecting human cancer cells into mice so that their immune systems will make antibodies against these cancer cells. The mouse cells producing the antibodies are then removed and fused with laboratory-grown cells to create "hybrid" cells called hybridomas. Hybridomas can indefinitely produce large quantities of these pure antibodies, or MOABs.

MOABs may be used in cancer treatment in a number of ways:

- MOABs that react with specific types of cancer may enhance a patient's immune response to the cancer.

- MOABs can be programmed to act against cell growth factors, thus interfering with the growth of cancer cells.

- MOABs may be linked to anticancer drugs, radioisotopes (radioactive substances), other BRMs, or other toxins. When the antibodies latch onto cancer cells, they deliver these poisons directly to the tumor, helping to destroy it.

- MOABs may help destroy cancer cells in bone marrow that has been removed from a patient in preparation for a bone marrow transplant.

MOABs carrying radioisotopes may also prove useful in diagnosing certain cancers, such as colorectal, ovarian, and prostate.

Rituxan® (rituximab) and Herceptin® (trastuzumab) are examples of monoclonal antibodies that have been approved by the FDA. Rituxan is used for the treatment of B-cell non-Hodgkin's lymphoma that has returned after a period of improvement or has not responded to chemotherapy. Herceptin is used to treat metastatic breast cancer in patients with tumors that produce excess amounts of a protein called HER-2. (Approximately 25 percent of breast cancer tumors produce excess amounts of HER-2.) Researchers are testing MOABs in clinical trials to treat lymphomas, leukemias, colorectal cancer, lung cancer, brain tumors, prostate cancer, and other types of cancer.

Cancer Vaccines

Cancer vaccines are another form of biological therapy currently under study. Vaccines for infectious diseases, such as measles, mumps, and tetanus, are effective because they expose the body's immune cells to weakened forms of antigens that are present on the surface of the infectious agent. This exposure causes the immune cells to produce more plasma cells, which make antibodies. T-cells that recognize the infectious agent also multiply. These activated T-cells later remember the exposure. The next time the agent enters the body, cells in the immune system are already prepared to respond and stop the infection.

For cancer treatment, researchers are developing vaccines that may encourage the patient's immune system to recognize cancer cells. These vaccines may help the body reject tumors and prevent cancer from recurring. In contrast to vaccines against infectious diseases, cancer vaccines are designed to be injected after the disease is diagnosed, rather than before it develops. Cancer vaccines given when the tumor is small may be able to eradicate the cancer. Early cancer vaccine clinical trials (research studies with people) involved mainly patients with melanoma. Currently, cancer vaccines are also being studied in the treatment of many other types of cancer, including lymphomas and cancers of the kidney, breast, ovary, prostate, colon, and rectum. Researchers are also investigating ways that cancer vaccines can be used in combination with other BRMs.

Side Effects

Like other forms of cancer treatment, biological therapies can cause a number of side effects, which can vary widely from patient to patient. Rashes or swelling may develop at the site where the BRMs are injected. Several BRMs, including interferons and interleukins, may cause flu-like symptoms including fever, chills, nausea, vomiting, and appetite loss. Fatigue is another common side effect of BRMs. Blood pressure may also be affected. The side effects of IL-2 can often be severe, depending on the dosage given. Patients need to be closely monitored during treatment. Side effects of CSFs may include bone pain, fatigue, fever, and appetite loss. The side effects of MOABs vary, and serious allergic reactions may occur. Cancer vaccines can cause muscle aches and fever.

Clinical Trials

Information about ongoing clinical trials involving these and other biological therapies is available from the Cancer Information Service or from the National Cancer Institute's cancerTrials™ website.

National Cancer Institutes' Cancer Information Service
Telephone: 1-800-4-CANCER (1-800-422-6237)
TTY: (for deaf and hard of hearing callers): 1-800-332-8615
Website: http://cancertrials.nci.nih.gov

Chapter 59

The Study of Estrogen Replacement Therapy

What is the Estrogen Replacement Therapy Study?

The Estrogen Replacement Therapy (ERT) Study is a clinical trial (research study) designed to resolve the debate over whether women who have had early stage cancer of the uterus, or endometrial cancer, can safely take ERT. It is one of many research studies sponsored by the National Cancer Institute (NCI) and carried out in medical centers around the country.

What is a clinical trial?

A clinical trial is a study with people that is designed to answer a question related to the diagnosis, treatment, prevention, or course of a disease. Such studies are designed to show how a particular approach—for instance, a promising treatment for a particular kind of cancer or a possible way to improve quality of life for cancer survivors—affects those who receive it. The study design is specified in a document called a protocol. Clinical trials are sometimes simply called protocols.

What is endometrial cancer?

Endometrial cancer is a form of cancer that originates in the endometrium (inner lining) of the uterus. Because most cancers of the

Fact Sheet 6.27, Cancer Info. Service, National Cancer Institute, April 2000.

uterus develop in this inner lining, the terms "cancer of the uterus" and "endometrial cancer" are often used interchangeably. Most women with endometrial cancer are treated with surgery to remove the uterus (hysterectomy) and bilateral salpingo-oophorectomy (removal of the ovaries and fallopian tubes).

What is ERT?

ERT is treatment often prescribed to reduce the discomforts of menopause, such as hot flashes, and to reduce the risk of osteoporosis (fragile bones) and heart disease in women after menopause.

Why is ERT after endometrial cancer controversial?

It has been commonly assumed that ERT is not safe for women with a history of endometrial cancer. Many physicians fear that ERT will increase a woman's chances of having the cancer reappear. (Even though the uterus has been removed, the cancer can recur in nearby tissues or spread to other parts of the body.)

There are several reasons for this assumption. One is that estrogen makes endometrial cancer cells grow in the laboratory. In addition, there is a good deal of evidence that estrogen, taken without progestins (another female hormone), can contribute to the first development of endometrial cancer.

However, two studies of patients with a history of endometrial cancer have suggested that ERT does not increase the risk of recurrence in selected patients. These findings have led to the current debate.

What is the evidence linking ERT with the first development of endometrial cancer?

Several large studies have found that women who take estrogen without progestins have a higher risk of developing endometrial cancer than women who do not use ERT. The risk for estrogen users is estimated to be 5 to 10 times higher than that for nonusers.

What is the evidence that ERT does not cause a recurrence of endometrial cancer?

Two studies have looked at data from groups of endometrial cancer survivors who used ERT. In one study, scientists analyzed data for 221 patients with stage I endometrial cancer, 47 of whom received estrogen for about 26 months after the tumor was removed. This study found that the cancer recurred in 15 percent of the women who did not receive estrogen and in 2 percent of those who did take estrogen.

In the other study, scientists analyzed data from 144 women who had stage I endometrial cancer, including 45 who were at low risk of recurrence and who had taken ERT for about 64 months. None of the estrogen users in this study had the cancer recur.

How will the new study be carried out?

More than 2,000 women who have had recent surgery for early stage uterine cancer (stage I or II) will take part in the study. Participants will be divided randomly (as in a flip of a coin) into two groups. One group will receive pills containing estrogen and the other will receive identical-appearing pills that do not contain estrogen (a placebo) for 3 years. The study is double-blinded—that is, neither physicians nor patients will know which women are taking the placebo and which are taking estrogen. Women in both groups will have check-ups every 6 months for 3 years and then annually for 2 more years.

Who is eligible for this study?

Women with endometrial cancer who were treated with a total hysterectomy and bilateral salpingo-oophorectomy and found to be at surgical stage IA, IB, IC, IIA, or IIB may be eligible for this study. These women must have at least one indication for ERT, including hot flashes, vaginal atrophy (dryness), increased risk of cardiovascular disease, or increased risk of osteoporosis. Women must have recovered from the effects of the recent surgery and be entered in the study within 12 weeks of surgery.

Women not eligible for this study include those with known or suspected breast cancer; those with a history of breast cancer, acute liver disease, or thromboembolic disease (blood clots); or those receiving other forms of hormonal therapy.

How can patients enroll in this study?

As in all NCI-sponsored clinical studies, patients are referred by a physician. Any health care provider can enroll patients in this study by contacting physicians who are members of NCI's Community Clinical Oncology Program (CCOP) or Cancer Therapy Evaluation Program (CTEP). For more information, health care providers may contact their nearest participating Gynecologic Oncology Group (GOG) or

CCOP institution or call the GOG administrative office at 1-800-225-3053.

Patients may learn more about this study by calling the NCI's Cancer Information Service at 1-800-4-CANCER.

How can people learn more about endometrial cancer?

The NCI's PDQ database has information for patients and physicians on diagnosing and treating endometrial cancer. In addition, a booklet for patients, called *What You Need To Know About*™ *Cancer of the Uterus*, is available from the NCI. Call 1-800-4-CANCER to ask for both the PDQ information and the booklet. PDQ is also accessible through the NCI Web site http://cancer.gov/

Single, free copies of the pamphlets *Cancer of the Uterus* (APO97) or *Hormone Replacement Therapy* (APO66) are available from the American College of Obstetricians and Gynecologists (ACOG). For each pamphlet, send a stamped, self-addressed, business-size envelope along with the name of the pamphlet to ACOG, Resource Center, 409 12th Street, SW., Post Office Box 96920, Washington, DC 20090–6920. The ACOG Resource Center may also be reached by telephone at 202-863-2518, and requests may be faxed to 202-484-1595.

Chapter 60

Tamoxifen and the Breast Cancer Prevention Trial

Questions and Answers about Tamoxifen

What is tamoxifen?

Tamoxifen is a medication in pill form that interferes with the activity of estrogen (a female hormone). Tamoxifen has been used for more than 20 years to treat patients with advanced breast cancer. It has also been used as adjuvant, or additional, therapy following surgery or radiation therapy for early stage breast cancer. Tamoxifen has recently been found to reduce the incidence of breast cancer in women at high risk of developing this disease. Tamoxifen continues to be studied for the prevention of breast cancer. It is also being studied in the treatment of several other types of cancer.

How does tamoxifen work on breast cancer?

Estrogen promotes the growth of breast cancer cells. Tamoxifen works against the effects of estrogen on these cells. It is often called an "anti-estrogen." As a treatment for breast cancer, the drug slows or stops the growth of cancer cells that are already present in the body. As adjuvant therapy, tamoxifen has been shown to help prevent the

This chapter includes text from "Questions and Answers about Tamoxifen," Cancer Facts, National Cancer Institute (NCI), June 1999; and "Tamoxifen Approved for DCIS: More Trials On the Way," Cancer Trials, National Cancer Institute, August 2000.

original breast cancer from returning and also prevent the development of new cancers in the opposite breast.

Are there other beneficial effects of tamoxifen?

While tamoxifen acts against the effects of estrogen in breast tissue, it acts like estrogen in other body systems. This means that women who take tamoxifen may derive many of the beneficial effects of menopausal estrogen replacement therapy, such as a lowering of blood cholesterol and a slowing of bone loss (osteoporosis).

Can tamoxifen prevent breast cancer?

Research has shown that when tamoxifen is used as adjuvant therapy for early stage breast cancer, it not only prevents the recurrence of the original cancer but also prevents the development of new cancers in the opposite breast.

Based on these findings, the National Cancer Institute (NCI) funded a large research study, the Breast Cancer Prevention Trial (BCPT) conducted by the National Surgical Adjuvant Breast and Bowel Project (NSABP), to determine the usefulness of tamoxifen in preventing breast cancer in women who have an increased risk of developing the disease.

Results from this study showed a 49 percent reduction in diagnoses of invasive breast cancer among women who took tamoxifen. Women who took tamoxifen also had 50 percent fewer diagnoses of non-invasive breast tumors, such as ductal or lobular carcinoma in situ. However, there are some risks associated with tamoxifen, some even life threatening.

The decision to take tamoxifen is an individual one in which the woman and her doctor must carefully consider the benefits and risks of therapy.

Women with an increased risk of developing breast cancer have the option to consider taking tamoxifen to reduce their chance of developing this disease. They may also consider participating in the Study of Tamoxifen and Raloxifene that will compare tamoxifen with the osteoporosis prevention drug raloxifene, which could have similar breast cancer risk reduction properties, but might be associated with fewer adverse effects.

At this time, there is no evidence that tamoxifen is beneficial for women who do not have an increased risk of breast cancer.

What is the Study of Tamoxifen and Raloxifene (STAR), and how can a woman learn more about it?

The National Surgical Adjuvant Breast and Bowel Project (NSABP), a component of NCI's Clinical Trials Cooperative Group Program, has launched a new breast cancer study. The new trial, known as STAR, began recruiting participants in June 1999. It will involve about 22,000 postmenopausal women who are at least 35 years old and are at increased risk for developing breast cancer. The study is designed to determine whether raloxifene, a drug similar to tamoxifen, is also effective in reducing the chance of developing breast cancer in women who have not had the disease, and whether the drug has benefits over tamoxifen, such as fewer side effects.

Women can learn more about the STAR trial in several ways. They can call NCI's Cancer Information Service at 1-800-4-CANCER (1-800-422-6237). The number for deaf and hard of hearing callers with TTY equipment is 1-800-332-8615. Information is also available on NSABP'S Web site at http://www.nsabp.pitt.edu or NCI's clinical trials Web site at http://cancertrials.nci.nih.gov on the Internet.

Does tamoxifen cause blood clots?

Data from large treatment studies suggest that there is a small increase in the number of blood clots in women taking tamoxifen, particularly in women who are receiving anticancer drugs (chemotherapy) along with tamoxifen. The total number of women who have experienced this side effect is small. Women in the BCPT who took tamoxifen also had an increased chance of developing blood clots. The risk of having a blood clot due to tamoxifen is similar to the risk of blood clots for women on single-agent estrogen replacement therapy.

Does tamoxifen cause uterine cancer?

The BCPT found that women taking tamoxifen had more than twice the chance of developing uterine cancer compared with women on placebo (an inactive substance that looks the same as, and is administered in the same way as, tamoxifen). The risk of uterine cancer in women taking tamoxifen was in the same range as (or less than) the risk in postmenopausal women taking single-agent estrogen replacement therapy. Additional studies are under way to define more clearly the role of other risk factors for uterine cancer, such as prior hormone use, in women receiving tamoxifen.

Like many cancers, uterine cancer is potentially life threatening. Most of the uterine cancers that have occurred during studies of women taking tamoxifen have been found in the early stages, and treatment was usually effective. However, breast cancer patients who developed uterine cancer while taking tamoxifen have died from the disease. Abnormal vaginal bleeding and lower abdominal (pelvic) pain are two symptoms of the disease. Women on tamoxifen should see their doctor if they experience these symptoms.

Does tamoxifen cause eye problems?

As women age, they are more likely to develop cataracts (a clouding of the lens inside the eye). Women taking tamoxifen appear to be at increased risk for developing cataracts. Other eye problems, such as corneal scarring or retinal changes, have been reported in a few patients.

Does tamoxifen cause other types of cancer?

There have been a few reports of liver cancer and reports of other liver toxicities that have occurred in women taking tamoxifen. Although tamoxifen can cause liver cancer in particular strains of rats, it is not known to cause liver cancer in humans. Tamoxifen did not cause liver cancer in the BCPT. It is clear that tamoxifen can sometimes cause other liver toxicities in women, which rarely can be severe or life threatening. Doctors may order blood tests from time to time to check liver function.

Although one study suggested a possible increase in cancers of the digestive tract among women receiving tamoxifen for breast cancer, other trials, including the BCPT, have not shown an association between tamoxifen and these cancers.

Studies such as the BCPT show no increase in cancers other than uterine cancer. This potential risk is being evaluated.

Should women taking tamoxifen avoid pregnancy?

Yes. Tamoxifen may make premenopausal women more fertile, but doctors advise women on tamoxifen to avoid pregnancy because animal studies have suggested that the use of tamoxifen in pregnancy can cause fetal harm. Women who have questions about fertility, birth control, or pregnancy should discuss their concerns with their doctor.

What are some of the more common side effects of taking tamoxifen?

In general, the side effects of tamoxifen are similar to some of the symptoms of menopause. The most common side effects are hot flashes and vaginal discharge. Some women experience irregular menstrual periods, dizziness, headaches, fatigue, loss of appetite, nausea and/or vomiting, vaginal dryness or bleeding, and irritation of the skin around the vagina. As is the case with menopause, not all women who take tamoxifen have these symptoms.

Does tamoxifen cause a woman to begin menopause?

Tamoxifen does not cause a woman to begin menopause, although it can cause some symptoms that are similar to those that may occur during menopause. In most premenopausal women taking tamoxifen, the ovaries continue to act normally and produce female hormones (estrogens) in the same or slightly increased amounts.

Do the benefits of tamoxifen in treating breast cancer outweigh its risks?

The benefits of tamoxifen as a treatment for breast cancer are firmly established and far outweigh the potential risks. Women concerned about the risks and benefits of medications they are taking are encouraged to discuss these concerns with their doctor.

How long should a woman take tamoxifen for the treatment of breast cancer?

Women with advanced breast cancer may take tamoxifen for varying lengths of time depending on their response to prior treatment and other factors. When used as adjuvant therapy for early stage breast cancer, tamoxifen is generally prescribed for 5 years. However, the ideal length of treatment with tamoxifen is not known.

Two studies have confirmed the benefit of taking tamoxifen daily for 5 years. These studies compared 5 years of treatment with tamoxifen with 10 years of treatment. When taken for 5 years, the drug prevents the recurrence of the original breast cancer and also prevents the development of a second primary cancer in the opposite breast. Taking tamoxifen for longer than 5 years is not more effective than 5 years of therapy.

Tamoxifen Approved for DCIS; More Trials On the Way

The drug tamoxifen reached another milestone in June 2000 with its approval by the Food and Drug Administration for ductal carconoma in situ, or DCIS. Women who have had DCIS—a small, non-invasive group of abnormal cells—are at high risk of developing invasive breast cancer. Tamoxifen reduces that risk substantially, according to the clinical trial that led to FDA approval.

In this 1,804-patient trial, women first received lumpectomy and radiation therapy, a standard treatment for DCIS, and then were randomly divided into two groups to receive either tamoxifen or a placebo. After five years, the tamoxifen group had 43% percent fewer cases of invasive breast cancer.

The study is the latest, but by no means last, in a series of findings from clinical trials exploring the uses of tamoxifen. First studied as a treatment for advanced breast cancer, the drug later moved into studies to treat early breast cancer, and then into primary prevention trials.

But even with FDA approval in these three settings, the tamoxifen story is not yet over. Researchers continue to ask questions about the drug. For instance, when used for prevention of breast cancer, will it reduce overall death rates from that disease? The landmark Breast Cancer Prevention Trial in the United States showed that tamoxifen reduced incidence (number of new cases) of breast cancer in postmenopausal women at increased risk who had been taking the drug for about four years. The study was not designed to show whether the tamoxifen would reduce breast cancer death rates, however.

Some information on mortality may come from the International Breast Cancer Intervention Study, which is comparing tamoxifen to a placebo in 7,000 women at increased risk of the disease. The primary aim of this trial is to compare the incidence of breast cancer in the two groups, but it will also assess mortality, other cancers, cardiovascular disease, and fractures according to Jack Cuzick, Ph.D., of the Imperial Cancer Research Fund, London.

Cuzick spoke at a workshop at the National Institutes of Health, Bethesda, Maryland, in April, 2000, when enrollment had passed the 6000 mark. He projected all 7000 participants needed would be enrolled by the end of the year.

New Combinations

For some investigators, tamoxifen's success in both prevention and treatment studies has set the stage for its use in combination with other agents that may also span these two uses. "It helps to think of breast cancer as a continuum," said JoAnne Zujewski, M.D., who leads several breast cancer clinical trials at the National Cancer Institute in Bethesda. "I'm interested in compounds that may be useful from prevention to in situ disease to invasive cancer."

Such compounds include a class of drugs known as retinoids—4HPR or Fenretidine is one of most-studied—and another group known as farnesyl transferase inhibitors. In a pilot prevention trial, Zujewski and colleagues have shown that Fenretidine combined with tamoxifen is safe and, they concluded, warrants further study as a preventive agent.

Treatment studies have also combined tamoxifen and Fenretidine. In metastatic disease, these include a phase I/II study by Melody Cobleigh, M.D., and colleagues at the University of Chicago and a phase II trial by Zujewski and colleagues at NCI. In early breast cancer, studies of the combination are under way in Chicago and in Italy, at the National Institute for Cancer Research, where A. Decenzi, M.D. has been working with the two drugs.

Another retinoid, 9-cis-retinoic acid, has also been studied in combination with tamoxifen to treat metastic breast cancer. Zujewski said that a phase I trial showed the combination is safe and holds some promise and that phase II trials of tamoxifen in combination with 9-cis or similar retinoids are under consideration.

Comparisons

In other studies, tamoxifen now serves as the benchmark against which newer therapies are measured. Perhaps the most widely watched of the current tamoxifen trials is the one comparing it to raloxifene for the primary prevention of breast cancer in women at increased risk. The Study of Tamoxifen and Raloxifene (STAR), launched in July 1999, has enrolled about 6,000 of the 22,000 women needed for the study.

Raloxifene is also an estrogen-like drug—both it and tamoxifen are called selective estrogen receptor modulators or SERMS—and was originally developed to prevent osteoporosis. Other novel SERMs are in development, including one known as LY353381, which is now being tested against tamoxifen in a small phase I study.

Treatment studies have compared tamoxifen to Arimidex, an aromatase inhibitor, and a randomized trial of the two drugs has been under way for several years. This trial has completed enrolling patients and preliminary results could be available next year, according to a spokesperson for AstraZeneca Pharmaceuticals, maker of both drugs and sponsor of the trial.

Another DCIS Trial

Also under way is more tamoxifen research in DCIS. Approved by the FDA for use with radiotherapy, the drug will now be tested without radiotherapy in a large trial conducted by the Radiation Therapy Oncology Group and the Cancer and Leukemia Group B, both NCI-sponsored Cooperative Clinical Trials Groups. Patients in this trial will be randomized, after lumpectomy, to receive either tamoxifen with radiation therapy—the combination that was just approved by the FDA—or tamoxifen alone.

This trial is one of the first to be open to members of all NCI-sponsored Groups through the new Cancer Trial Support Unit (CTSU). One aim of the CTSU is to speed and facilitate the completion of trials, so enrollment in this trial may proceed rapidly.

Chapter 61

The Study of Tamoxifen and Raloxifene (STAR)

Questions and Answers about the Study of Tamoxifen and Raloxifene (STAR)

What is the Study of Tamoxifen and Raloxifene (STAR)?

The Study of Tamoxifen and Raloxifene (STAR) is a clinical trial (a research study conducted with people) designed to see how the drug raloxifene (Evista®) compares with the drug tamoxifen (Nolvadex®) in reducing the incidence of breast cancer in women who are at an increased risk of developing the disease. Researchers with the National Surgical Adjuvant Breast and Bowel Project (NSABP) are conducting the study at more than 400 centers across the United States, Puerto Rico, and Canada. The study is primarily funded by the National Cancer Institute (NCI), the U.S. Government's main agency for cancer research.

What is tamoxifen?

Tamoxifen is a drug, taken by mouth as a pill. It has been used for more than 20 years to treat patients with breast cancer. Tamoxifen works against breast cancer, in part, by interfering with the activity

This chapter includes text from "Questions and Answers About the Study of Tamoxifen and Raloxifene (STAR)," Cancer Facts, National Cancer Institute, June 1999; and "STAR Enrolls 6,139 Women in First Year," Press Release, National Cancer Institute, July 27, 2000.

of estrogen, a female hormone that promotes the growth of breast cancer cells. In October 1998, the U.S. Food and Drug Administration (FDA) approved tamoxifen to reduce the incidence of breast cancer in women at high risk of the disease based on the results of the Breast Cancer Prevention Trial (BCPT). The BCPT is a study of more than 13,000 pre- and postmenopausal high-risk women ages 35 and older who took either tamoxifen or a placebo (an inactive pill that looked like tamoxifen) for up to 5 years. NSABP conducted the BCPT, which also showed that tamoxifen works like estrogen to preserve bone strength, decreasing fractures of the hip, wrist, and spine in the women who took the drug.

What is raloxifene?

Raloxifene is a drug, taken by mouth as a pill. In December 1997, it was approved by the FDA for the prevention of osteoporosis in postmenopausal women. Raloxifene is being studied because large studies testing its effectiveness against osteoporosis have shown that women taking the drug developed fewer breast cancers than women taking a placebo.

Who is eligible to participate in STAR?

Women at increased risk for developing breast cancer, who have gone through menopause and are at least 35 years old, can participate in STAR. All women must have an increased risk of breast cancer equivalent to or greater than that of an average 60- to 64-year-old woman. At that age, about 17 of every 1,000 women are expected to develop breast cancer within 5 years.

Why can't premenopausal women participate in STAR?

STAR is limited to postmenopausal women because the drug raloxifene has yet to be adequately tested for long-term safety in premenopausal women. NCI recently launched a separate study to evaluate the safety of raloxifene in premenopausal woman.

What factors are used to determine increased risk of breast cancer for the participants?

Increased risk of breast cancer is determined in one of two ways. The risk for most women is determined by a computer calculation based on the following factors:

- Current age;

- Number of first-degree relatives (mother, daughters, or sisters) diagnosed with breast cancer;

- Whether a woman had any children and her age at her first delivery;

- The number of breast biopsies a woman has had, especially if the tissue showed a condition known as atypical hyperplasia; and

- The woman's age at her first menstrual period.

Women diagnosed as having lobular carcinoma in situ (LCIS), a condition that is not cancer but indicates an increased chance of developing invasive breast cancer, are eligible based on that diagnosis alone, as long as any treatment for the condition was limited to local excision. Mastectomy, radiation, or systemic therapy would disqualify a woman with LCIS from the study.

How will a potential participant's risk of breast cancer be determined?

Each potential participant will complete a one-page questionnaire (risk assessment form), which will be forwarded to NSABP by the local STAR clinical staff. The NSABP will use computer software to generate an individualized risk profile based on the information provided and will return the profile to the local STAR site so that it can be given to the potential participant. The profile will estimate the woman's chance of developing breast cancer over the next 5 years and will also present the potential risks and benefits of the study drugs. The woman can then use this information to help her decide whether or not she is interested in participating in STAR.

What other factors affect eligibility for the study?

Certain existing health conditions affect eligibility for the study. Health professionals at the STAR site will discuss these with each potential participant. For example, women with a history of cancer (except basal or squamous cell skin cancer), blood clots, stroke, or certain types of heartbeat irregularities cannot participate. Women whose high blood pressure or diabetes is not controlled also cannot participate.

Also, women taking hormone replacement therapy (estrogen or an estrogen/progesterone combination) cannot take part in the trial unless they stop taking this medication. Those who stop taking these hormones are eligible for the study 3 months after they discontinue the drugs. Women who have taken tamoxifen or raloxifene for no more than 3 months are eligible for the study, but they must also stop the medication for 3 months before joining STAR.

What are the common side effects of tamoxifen and raloxifene?

Like most medications, including over-the-counter medications, prescription drugs, or drugs in clinical trials, tamoxifen and raloxifene cause adverse effects in some women. The effects experienced most often by women taking either drug are hot flashes and vaginal symptoms, including discharge, dryness, or itching. It is possible that some women may experience leg cramps, constipation, pain with intercourse, sinus irritation or infection, or problems controlling the bladder upon exertion. Treatments that may minimize or eliminate most of these side effects will be available to the participants.

Does tamoxifen have any serious side effects?

The best information available about the serious side effects of tamoxifen comes from 30 years of clinical trials, including the BCPT. In the BCPT, women taking tamoxifen had more than twice the chance of developing endometrial cancer (cancer of the lining of the uterus or womb) compared with women who took the placebo (36 of the 6,600 women taking tamoxifen versus 15 of the 6,600 women taking placebo). The risk was higher in women over the age of 50. The increased risk is in the same range as the risk for postmenopausal women taking single-agent estrogen replacement therapy. Like all cancers, endometrial cancer is potentially life-threatening. Women who have had a hysterectomy (surgery to remove the uterus) are not at risk for endometrial cancer.

Women taking tamoxifen in the BCPT had three times the chance of developing a pulmonary embolism (blood clot in the lung) as women who took the placebo (18 women taking tamoxifen versus 6 on placebo). Three women taking tamoxifen died from these embolisms. Women in the tamoxifen group were also more likely to have a deep vein thrombosis (a blood clot in a major vein) than women on placebo (35 women on tamoxifen versus 22 on placebo). Women taking tamoxifen also appeared to have an increased chance of stroke (38 women on tamoxifen versus 24 on placebo).

Does raloxifene have any serious side effects?

Information about raloxifene is limited compared with the data available on tamoxifen because of the shorter time it has been studied (about 5 years) and the smaller number of women who have been studied. Studies of raloxifene have generally involved women who received the drug to determine its effect on osteoporosis, and the duration of both therapy and followup have been short. Women taking raloxifene in clinical trials have about three times the chance of developing a deep vein thrombosis or pulmonary embolism as women on a placebo. In osteoporosis studies of raloxifene, the drug did not increase the risk of endometrial cancer. An important part of STAR will be to assess the long-term safety of raloxifene versus tamoxifen in women at increased risk of breast cancer.

Who will get which drug?

Participants in STAR will be randomized (assigned by chance) to receive either tamoxifen or raloxifene. In a process known as "double blinding", neither the participant nor her physician will know which pill she is receiving. Setting up a study in this way allows the researchers to directly compare the true benefits and side effects of each drug without the influence of other factors. All women in the study will take two pills a day for 5 years: half will take active tamoxifen and a raloxifene placebo (an inactive pill that looks like raloxifene); the other half will take active raloxifene and a tamoxifen placebo (an inactive pill that looks like tamoxifen). All women will receive one of the active drugs; no one in STAR will receive only the placebo. The dosages are 20 mg of tamoxifen and 60 mg raloxifene.

Why does everyone have to take two pills?

Tamoxifen and raloxifene have different shapes. The trial would not be double blinded if participants or physicians could tell which drug they were receiving because of its shape. The maker of tamoxifen, Zeneca Pharmaceuticals in Wilmington, Delaware, and the maker of raloxifene, Eli Lilly and Company in Indianapolis, Indiana, are providing the active pills and the look-alike placebos without charge.

447

Are participants required to have any medical exams? Who will pay for these exams?

Participants are required to have blood tests, a mammogram, a breast exam, and a gynecologic exam before they are accepted into the study. These tests will be repeated at intervals during the trial. Physicians' fees and the costs of medical tests will be charged to the participant in the same fashion as if she were not part of the trial; however, the costs for these tests generally are covered by insurance. Every effort is made to contain the costs specifically associated with participation in this trial, and financial assistance is available for some women.

How is the safety of participants ensured? Is the trial monitored?

The safety of participants is of primary importance to STAR investigators. There are strict requirements about who can join the trial as well as frequent monitoring of participants' health status. An independent Data Safety and Monitoring Committee (DSMC) will provide oversight of the trial. The DSMC includes medical and cancer specialists, biostatisticians, and bioethicists who have no other connection to NSABP. The DSMC will meet semiannually and review unblinded data from all participants. Two other committees will also provide oversight. The Participant Advisory Board (PAB) is made up of 16 women from the BCPT. As women join STAR, board membership will change to include STAR participants. The PAB meets semiannually with professionals from NSABP and NCI and provides feedback on many study-related functions such as informed consent, participant recruitment, and communications issues. The STAR Steering Committee is made up of NSABP investigators, breast cancer advocates, experts from other medical disciplines, as well as NCI and NSABP personnel. The committee, which also meets semiannually, is charged with providing overall administrative oversight of the trial.

In addition, NSABP provides the FDA, NCI, Zeneca Pharmaceuticals, and Eli Lilly and Company with annual reports on STAR that summarize the overall data collected to date (only the DSMC receives unblinded data).

What is the National Surgical Adjuvant Breast and Bowel Project?

The NSABP is a cooperative group with a 40-year history of designing and conducting clinical trials, the results of which have changed the way breast cancer is treated and, now, prevented. Results of clinical trials conducted by NSABP researchers have been the dominant force in altering the standard surgical treatment of breast cancer from radical mastectomy to lumpectomy plus radiation. This group was also the first to demonstrate that adjuvant therapy could alter the natural history of breast cancer, thus increasing survival rates.

STAR Enrolls 6,139 Women in First Year

The first year of the Study of Tamoxifen and Raloxifene (STAR) saw 6,139 postmenopausal women at increased risk of breast cancer enroll in this landmark prevention study—and more than 47,000 women went through an individualized, no-obligation risk assessment to determine their risk of breast cancer and weigh the pros and cons of joining the trial. Enrollment began July 1, 1999.

More than 500 centers across the United States, Puerto Rico, and Canada are enrolling participants in STAR. STAR is a study of the National Surgical Adjuvant Breast and Bowel Project (NSABP) and is supported by the U.S. National Cancer Institute (NCI).

NSABP Chairman Norman Wolmark, M.D., said, "We are pleased that so many women have joined this trial to help us answer this important medical question. We encourage women to go through the risk assessment process to learn more about their breast cancer risk and about STAR. In the end, each woman who joins does so for her own reasons, but every single woman plays a vital role."

As in the BCPT, women can join STAR if they have an increased risk of developing breast cancer equivalent to the risk of an average 60-year-old woman. These women have a 1.7 percent risk of breast cancer in five years, meaning that about 17 of them in 1,000 would be expected to develop breast cancer within five years. The women who are actually choosing to join the trial, as a group, exceed that minimum requirement.

Postmenopausal women of all ethnicities and races are encouraged to participate in STAR, and about 5 percent of the first 6,000 women in STAR are minorities. In this first year of STAR, a total of 6,636 minority women went through the risk assessment process, 1,812 had an increased risk of breast cancer that would qualify them for the study, and 281 have already decided to join.

In contrast, in the entire five years of enrollment for the BCPT, a total of 8,525 minority women went through the risk assessment process, 2,979 were risk-eligible, and 486 joined the trial.

The NSABP has undertaken several novel strategies to encourage minority women to participate in STAR, which include the STAR Community Outreach Program for Education (SCOPE) under way in ten cities in the United States. The goal of SCOPE is to educate minority women about breast cancer, which may ultimately lead to their more widespread participation in clinical trials.

Moreover, STAR is supported by the National Medical Association (NMA), a network of more than 20,000 African-American physicians. As a first effort, the NSABP is working closely with Region II of the NMA, which includes members in Pennsylvania, Delaware, Maryland, Virginia, West Virginia, and the District of Columbia, to pilot a unique outreach project. The initial participation is in Philadelphia with plans to extend outreach into the rest of Region II and eventually throughout the NMA organization.

Recent analyses of the use of tamoxifen in women with breast cancer show that tamoxifen works equally well in white and African-American women. Worta McCaskill-Stevens, M.D., of the NCI's Division of Cancer Prevention, who presented this research at the May 2000 meeting of the American Society of Clinical Oncology, notes that "The benefits and risks of tamoxifen are the same in African-American and white women. Women of all races can feel comfortable about considering STAR if they are at increased risk of breast cancer."

Women who participate in STAR must be postmenopausal, at least age 35, and have an increased risk of breast cancer as determined by their age, family history of breast cancer, personal medical history, age at first menstrual period, and age at first live birth. They will also go through a process known as informed consent, during which they will learn about the potential benefits and risks of tamoxifen and raloxifene before deciding whether to participate in STAR.

Tamoxifen and raloxifene may also increase a woman's chances of developing several rare, but potentially life-threatening health problems: deep vein thrombosis (blood clot in a large vein) and pulmonary embolism (blood clot in the lung). Tamoxifen use may also increase a woman's risk of stroke and endometrial cancer (cancer of the lining of the uterus) at a rate similar to estrogen replacement therapy. In ongoing studies, raloxifene has not been associated with an increased risk of endometrial cancer. STAR will help further define the risks and benefits of tamoxifen and raloxifene therapy.

Once a woman decides to participate, she is randomly assigned to receive either 20 mg tamoxifen or 60 mg raloxifene daily for five years and has regular follow-up examinations, including mammograms and gynecologic exams.

The maker of tamoxifen, AstraZeneca Pharmaceuticals, Wilmington, Delaware, and the maker of raloxifene, Eli Lilly and Company, Indianapolis, Indiana, are providing their drugs for the trial without charge. Eli Lilly and Company has also given NSABP a $36 million five-year grant to defray recruitment costs at the participating centers.

First Year Recruitment Data

- During the first year of the trial, which started enrolling women on July 1, 1999, 47,114 women went through the risk assessment process. Of these women, 29,303 were eligible for the trial based on breast cancer risk alone. Of those risk-eligible women, 6,139 chose to participate.

- In the first year, 3,786 African-American women went through the risk assessment process, 739 were risk-eligible, and 103 joined STAR. About 1.7 percent of the women on STAR are African-American.

- In the first year, 1,688 Hispanic/Latina women went through the risk assessment process, 464 were risk-eligible, and 81 joined STAR. About 1.3 percent of the women on STAR are Hispanic/Latina.

- In the first year, 1,162 women who defined themselves as representing another minority population, such as Native American or Asian American, went through the risk assessment process, 609 were risk-eligible, and 97 joined STAR. About 1.6 percent of the women on STAR are ethnic minorities other than African-American or Hispanic/Latina.

- Of the 6,139 women joining STAR, 1,126 were from the placebo group of the Breast Cancer Prevention Trial.

- More than half of the women joining STAR had had a hysterectomy prior to enrolling (52.3 percent). Women who have had a hysterectomy are not at risk for endometrial cancer.

- The breast cancer risk of women joining STAR in the first year has been above the minimum 1.7 percent risk of developing the disease within the next five years. (see Table 61.1.)

- Women joining STAR must be postmenopausal and at least 35 years of age. The ages of women joining STAR in the first year is shown in Table 61.2.

- In the first year, 7.9 percent of the women joining STAR had had a diagnosis of lobular carcinoma in situ (LCIS), a condition that is not cancer, but which indicates an increased chance of developing invasive breast cancer.

- Number of women who joined STAR by U.S. state and Canadian province is shown in Table 61.3.

Table 61.1. Cancer Risk among STAR participants

Five-Year Breast Cancer RiskPercent of women in STAR

1.7- 2.0 percent	10.3 percent
2.0-2.9 percent	30.3 percent
3.0-4.9 percent	32.2 percent
Greater than 5.0 percent	27.2 percent

Table 61.2. Age of STAR participants

Age	Percent of women in STAR
35-49	9.4 percent
50-59	50.2 percent
60+	40.4 percent

Table 61.3. Residence of STAR participants.

U.S. States (including District of Columbia and Puerto Rico)

Alabama	20	Montana	41
Arizona	77	Nebraska	63
Arkansas	8	Nevada	38
California	359	New Hampshire	24
Colorado	110	New Jersey	98
Connecticut	96	New Mexico	44
Delaware	31	New York	231
District of Columbia	23	North Carolina	168
Florida	159	North Dakota	49
Georgia	55	Ohio	250
Hawaii	41	Oklahoma	94
Idaho	26	Oregon	63
Illinois	333	Pennsylvania	415
Indiana	119	Puerto Rico	15
Iowa	136	Rhode Island	10
Kansas	132	South Carolina	131
Kentucky	83	South Dakota	47
Louisiana	76	Tennessee	114
Maine	27	Texas	520
Maryland	72	Utah	5
Massachusetts	155	Vermont	33
Michigan	259	Virginia	54
Minnesota	151	Washington	154
Mississippi	27	West Virginia	18
Missouri	255	Wisconsin	136

Canadian Provinces

Alberta	41
British Columbia	37
Manitoba	68
Ontario	93
Quebec	254
Saskatchewan	1

- Tamoxifen (trade name Nolvadex®) was proven in the BCPT to reduce breast cancer incidence by 49 percent in women at increased risk of the disease. The FDA approved the use of tamoxifen to reduce the incidence of breast cancer in women at increased risk of the disease in October 1998. Tamoxifen has been approved by the FDA to treat women with breast cancer for more than 20 years and has been in clinical trials for about 30 years.

- Raloxifene (trade name Evista®) was shown to reduce the incidence of breast cancer in a large study of its use to prevent and treat osteoporosis. This drug was approved by the FDA to prevent osteoporosis in postmenopausal women in December 1997 and to treat osteoporosis in postmenopausal women in September 1999. It has been under study for about seven years.

Contact Information

- Postmenopausal women in the United States and Puerto Rico who are interested in participating in STAR can call the NCI's Cancer Information Service at 1-800-4-CANCER (1-800-422-6237) for information in English or Spanish. The number for callers with TTY equipment is 1-800-332-8615.

- Postmenopausal women in Canada who are interested in participating in STAR can call the Canadian Cancer Society's Cancer Information Service at 1-888-939-3333 for information in English or French.

- For more information via the Internet, visit NSABP's Web site at http://www.nsabp.pitt.edu or NCI's clinical trials Web site at http://cancertrials.nci.nih.gov.

Part Nine

Coping Strategies

Chapter 62

Home Care for Cancer Patients

Cancer patients often feel more comfortable and secure being cared for at home. Many patients want to stay at home so that they will not be separated from family, friends, and familiar surroundings. Home care can help patients achieve this desire. It often involves a team approach that includes doctors, nurses, social workers, physical therapists, family members, and others. Home care can be both rewarding and demanding for patients and caregivers. It can change relationships and require families to address new issues and cope with all aspects of patient care. To help prepare for these changes, patients and caregivers are encouraged to ask questions and get as much information as possible from the home care team or organizations devoted to home care. A doctor, nurse, or social worker can provide information about patients' specific needs, the availability of home care services, and a list of local home care agencies.

Services provided by home care agencies may include access to medical equipment; visits from registered nurses, physical therapists, and social workers; help with running errands, meal preparation, and personal hygiene; and delivery of medication. The state or local health department is another important resource in finding home care services. The health department should have a registry of licensed home care agencies.

Public and private resources of financial assistance are available to patients to pay for home care. Government-sponsored programs,

Fact Sheet 8.5, Cancer Info. Service, National Cancer Institute, June 2000.

such as Medicare, Medicaid, the Older Americans Act, and the Veterans Administration, cover home care for those who meet their criteria.

Some people may qualify for Medicare, a health insurance program for the elderly or disabled that is administered by the Health Care Financing Administration (HCFA). Medicare may offer reimbursement for some home care services. Cancer patients who qualify for Medicare may also be eligible for coverage of hospice services if they are accepted into a Medicare-certified hospice program. Information about Medicare services and coverage is available from the toll-free Medicare Hotline at 1-800-MEDICARE (1-800-633-4227), or by writing to 6325 Security Boulevard, Baltimore, MD 21207. Deaf and hard of hearing callers with TTY equipment may call 1-877-486-2048. Medicare information can also be accessed at http:www.medicare.gov on the Internet.

Medicaid, a jointly funded, Federal-State health insurance program for people who need financial assistance for medical expenses, is also coordinated by HCFA. At a minimum, states must provide home care services to people who receive Federal income assistance such as Social Security Income and Aid to Families with Dependent Children. Medicaid coverage includes part-time nursing, home care aide services, and medical supplies and equipment. Information about coverage is available from local state welfare offices, state health departments, state social services agencies, or the state Medicaid office. Information about specific state locations is also available on the HCFA website at http://cis.nci.nih.gov/asp/disclaimernew.asp?p= www.hcfa.gov/medicaid/medicaid.htm on the Internet.

The Older Americans Act provides Federal funds for state and local social service programs that help frail and disabled people age 60 and older remain independent. This funding covers home care aide, personal care, escort, meal delivery, and shopping services. Older persons, their caregivers, or anyone concerned about the welfare of an older person can contact their local Area Agency on Aging (AAA) for information and referrals to services and benefits in the community. AAAs are usually listed in the white pages of the phone book under the city or county government headings. A nationwide toll-free hotline operated by the Administration on Aging provides information about AAAs and other assistance for older people; the number is 1-800-677-1116.

Veterans who are disabled as a result of military service can receive home care services from the Veterans Administration (VA). Only home care services provided by VA hospitals may be used. More information about veterans benefits is available by calling 1-800-827-1000.

Information can also be found on the VA's website at http://cis.nci.nih. gov/asp/disclaimernew.asp?p=www.va.gov/vbs/ on the Internet.

Private health insurance policies may cover some home care or hospice services, but benefits vary from plan to plan. Policies generally pay for services given by skilled professionals, but the patient may be responsible for a deductible or copayment. Many health maintenance organizations require that home care or hospice services be given by authorized agencies. It is best to contact the insurance company to see which services are covered.

Many national organizations such as the American Cancer Society (ACS) offer a variety of services to cancer patients and their families. The ACS has free fact sheets and publications about home care. These materials can be obtained at http://cis.nci.nih.gov/asp/disclaimernew.asp?p=www.cancer.org on the Internet, or by calling 1-800-ACS-2345 (1-800-227-2345) for the address of a local ACS chapter. Services vary among ACS chapters. Many ACS chapters can provide home care equipment (or suggest other organizations that do). Other voluntary agencies, such as the Red Cross and those affiliated with churches or social service organizations, may provide free or low-cost transportation. These agencies may also be able to lend home care equipment.

With so many home care organizations and services available, it is sometimes difficult to decide which to use. In addition to the local health department, information about home care services is available from such organizations as the National Association for Home Care (NAHC). To obtain a copy of the publication *How to Choose a Home Care Provider*, contact the NAHC at 228 Seventh Street, SE., Washington, DC 20003. The telephone number is 202-547-7424. Information about the NAHC is also available at http://cis.nci.nih.gov/asp/disclaimernew.asp?p=www.nahc.org on the Internet. An affiliate of the NAHC, the Hospice Association of America, offers publications such as *All About Hospice: A Consumer's Guide*. For a copy of this publication, send a self-addressed, stamped, business envelope to the NAHC address mentioned above.

The Joint Commission on Accreditation of Healthcare Organizations (JCAHO), an independent, not-for-profit organization that evaluates and accredits health care organizations and programs in the United States, also offers information for the general public. The JCAHO can be contacted at One Renaissance Boulevard, Oakbrook Terrace, IL 60181-4294; their telephone number is 630-792-5800. The JCAHO website is located at http://cis.nci.nih.gov/asp/disclaimernew.asp?p=www.jcaho.org on the Internet.

Chapter 63

When Mom Has Cancer: Helping Children Understand

Some of the most common reactions of children to their mother's cancer are fear and insecurity, anger, sadness, isolation, and curiosity.

Fear

Fears can take many forms: fear of death of their parent, fear because their parents have fear, fear of separation, fear cancer is contagious and that they will catch it, fear that they caused the cancer, fear that the life they know will change.

Fear of death. Because our society frequently hides the diagnosis of cancer, often a child's or teen's only exposure to cancer is people who have died. Therefore cancer means death. This may be the first time that the possibility of death of someone close has ever become a consideration. They may sense your fear of death. A younger child may think death is near at hand, an older child may interpret therapies as only postponing death.

Taken from "Breast Cancer: Common Reactions of Children and How to Help," by Jane Brazy, MD and Mary Ircink, RN, Breast Problem Clinic, University of Wisconsin Medical School, January 2000; reprinted with permission. This document is available online at http://www2.medsch.wisc. edu/childrenshosp/childrens.html. The University of Wisconsin-Madison, Department of Surgery's Website is available online at http://www. surgery.wisc.edu.

Fear because their parents have fear: Children of all age groups can sense a parent's anxiety and fear. In turn they can then become more afraid and insecure. Smaller children may cling to you and want more than usual attention.

Fear of separation. When small children realize that their mother may be hospitalized, they have fear that they will be separated from you. They have little sense of time and they live in the "now." A few days may be interpreted as permanent. They may also experience separation frequently when you have radiation treatments or chemotherapy as these take up a significant fraction of their day.

Fear cancer is contagious. Many children think cancer is contagious, that they can catch it from you. After all, most of the colds and illnesses that they have had they did get from someone else. It is very important to assure children of all ages that cancer of all kinds is *not* contagious, that they can't catch it. Their friends may also think cancer is contagious and may stop playing with your child because of the fear of catching it or spreading it to their mother.

Fear that they caused cancer. Magical thinking is normal in children, and is extremely common in preschool and grade school children. Magical thinking is the idea that they can make their thoughts and wishes come true. Last week they may have been mad at you and thought, "I'm mad at Mommy; I want to hurt her." Now you have cancer and you hurt, more than they ever thought possible. They fear they caused the cancer and the impact of their wishes is now beyond their control. They feel very guilty and afraid.

Fear that their life will change. Children derive a great deal of security in knowing what to expect day by day and in the future. Suddenly their life is upset and they don't know what to expect today or from now on. Their family security is at risk of disappearing.

Anger

Anger can also take on many forms: anger at you for getting cancer, anger at the cancer for attacking you, anger at what this event is doing to their life now and what it might do to them in the future. Since anger is a normal response for you too, they may sense or see your anger and frustration.

Often the anger is misplaced. They are angry at what this event is doing to their life and take it out on you or other family members. Sometimes children act out and become more demanding and unruly. They may do less well in school or do things they would not do otherwise. There may be more conflict between siblings. We always teach children to be fair...they therefore expect life to be fair. This may be their first exposure to the unfairness in life and they respond with anger.

Sadness

Because you may cry often when you are holding your young children, they may think they are causing you to be sad. Acknowledge that you are sad because of your illness, but be sure they understand that they did not make you sad.

Occasionally older children will share in your sadness or grief and openly cry with you, but often they do not. Some will try to be cheerful when around you, but express their sadness/grief when they are alone or with friends. Others will not appear to express any sadness or emotion; for them the whole ordeal is too overwhelming and they will appear to ignore it.

Isolation/Separation

You and you spouse or other support person need to and will spend time together to work out your feelings and provide mutual support. Your children may feel left out. Your children may also feel isolated because other kids avoid them, either because they are afraid of the concept of cancer or because they think they might catch it. Small children may experience separation from you. These feelings of isolation become realities when you go to the hospital, and again each day that you have radiation treatments or chemotherapy.

Curiosity

Most children will be very curious about your surgery. Usually what they imagine is far worse than the reality. The time to address questions with small children is when they ask them. Try to make comparisons with their past experiences. For example, the incision can be compared to cuts that they have had on their fingers or knees. This may not seem as a valid comparison to you but to them little cuts on their bodies are very important. Assure them that cut edges will grow back together again. When they ask about drains and drainage, show how the fluid goes down the tube and then to the bulb. After it gets to the bulb, you measure it and throw it out. It is a way to get rid of the extra fluid that you don't need. It is good to get rid of it.

If your children are older, you can pick a time that is more suitable to you and when you perceive they are ready to handle it. Very early after surgery (especially mastectomy) may not always be the best time, first because you may not be ready and are unadjusted to its appearance, second, because it looks worse with drains in, and third, the early drainage is bloody and the sight of blood is often scary and/ or repulsive to school age children. If you show it to them early, then be sure to show it again when the drains are out and it is healing. If you feel uncomfortable showing your own body to your son or daughter, you may want to show him/her a picture or diagram from a book. Don't be surprised, however, if someday your son or daughter sneaks a peek by coming into your bedroom when you are dressing to ask a question which could have easily waited. Just act natural, don't get angry and don't be too quick to cover up (let them get their peek); their timing was probably not an accident.

Approaches

Preschool, Early Grade School

This is a time of family stress when your children need extra love and attention. It is difficult to meet all the additional needs of children when you have many unmet needs yourself. Try to find someone else who can help give your children special attention. This should be someone who is very familiar to them. If possible have their dad spend more time with them. Studies have shown that increased time with the non-ill parent helps in the child's adjustment to cancer. You may want to have their favorite baby-sitter come over for the sole purpose of entertaining them and giving them extra attention. If grandparents or close relatives live nearby, they can be of great help in this respect. If your child has a special friend, try to arrange for his mother to have your child over to play during this period. Interrupt your children's normal routine as little as possible. Do activities together as a family. Let your children do things for you if they wish, but don't force tasks on them. If your child is in day care or school, be sure to let the teacher know about your cancer. Suggest that she/he alert you to changes in your child's behavior that are of concern. If you are having radiation therapy or chemotherapy, let the teacher know that you will not be available for classroom projects or field trips. Ask her to alert you if contagious diseases (such as chicken pox) begin circulating in your child's classroom.

If your children are too young to understand the concept of cancer refer to it as "my sickness." Be sure that your children understand that they had nothing to do with your sickness (or you getting cancer), and that wishes and thoughts cannot make people sick (or get cancer). If your child seems angry, anxious or frustrated, encourage him/her to play with a toy that will allow expression of anger, for example, a pound-the-peg-board, a drum, or a fierce animal puppet or toy (tiger, shark etc.). Encourage them to draw pictures. Ask them to tell you about their pictures. Observe when your children draw or play with stuffed animals or dolls. Things that they say or do may give you clues to their thinking and emotions. Don't criticize if they have aggressive play toward their toys, but if they are doing unacceptable things, help them redirect their energies to more acceptable activities. Assure them that its okay to be sad or mad (if they are); you are sad and feel angry too. But, continue to be consistent in your parenting approach. You may find that your children regress to more immature behavior. This is normal. When they feel secure again, they will return to more age appropriate behavior.

Answer questions that they have simply. Don't offer explanations that are more complicated than the questions they ask. Keep it at their level. Let them know that Mommy will be gone to the hospital for a few days. Be sure they know who will care for them when you're not there. If possible have them visit when you are in the hospital. Make their visit as entertaining and positive as possible. Show them how to adjust the bed by pushing the buttons and make you more comfortable. A TV suspended from the wall may be novel. Answer their curiosity questions about equipment simply. Have them bring in special pictures for you, including things that they have drawn or made for you. Be sure that they bring a photo of them and a photo of the whole family for you to have in your room. See if they can think of other things to bring you to make you feel better, like a small bouquet of flowers from your garden or even dandelions from the lawn. These tokens of love will make both of you feel better and important. *But, be sure they keep their own security object at home, not with you; they will need it.*

If you are having radiation or chemotherapy, you may want to take them to visit the facility so they know where you go and what it is like. You might want to select a day that you do not have treatments so it is just a short trip and you are with them the whole time. You might want to give them a picture of you or something from your purse to keep with them and care for while you are away. Tell them you will be back for them and provide a time frame that is meaningful to them, for example, after a specific activity or TV show.

Junior High, Teens, Early 20's

The responses of older children to their mothers diagnosis of breast cancer are highly variable. Almost all children feel some anger, fear, a sense of unfairness, loss and insecurity. For some the whole thing is too overwhelming and they will choose to deal with it by trying to ignore it. They may show little or no emotion and will appear to go about their activities as if nothing happened. This may be hard for you because they seem very unfeeling to you. Some will share your sadness openly, but others will keep their sadness to themselves or share it only with their friends or other relatives and not with you. Regardless of the response, acknowledge that cancer is difficult to deal with, offer to answer questions, and be supportive. Suggest that they might want to share their feelings with some other person(s); make suggestions such as an adult relative, teacher, coach, school nurse, pediatrician or one of their peers, but let them choose who and let them regulate their closeness or distance from you and from cancer. Encourage activities that might help them vent anger and frustration safely such as shoot-the-object computer games, shooting baskets, or playing other sports. Provide for family time together, every day if possible. As soon as you are able, do your favorite family activities together.

Try to be honest with your children but don't force more information on them than they are ready to handle. Sometimes leaving age-appropriate information out on the counter for them will let them get information at a time and in amounts that they can handle. Let them know it is there for them to read if they want to and that you want to be sure they get answers to any questions that they might have. It is often a good idea to have a family discussion of your cancer. During this time you could go over some of the basic information regarding breast cancer. It is a good time to share mutual feelings. You may want to discuss the data on your own case with your children. Be optimistic. Be sure your children know what is being planned for you in the near future (therapy) and how that will effect your life (tiredness, possible loss of hair, other side effects, etc.) and most important, how it might effect their lives. However, one should strive to interrupt their life style and activities as little as possible.

A few studies have investigated children's reactions to their mother's cancer. Most mother-child relationships stayed strong or became stronger, but some mother-child relationships deteriorated. Problems were more common if the mother had a poor prognosis, if there was extensive surgery, or if there was a prior history of poor relations between the mother and child. Mother's relationships with daughters were more stressed than relationships with their sons. Pre-adolescent daughters were more likely to show signs of fearfulness. Daughters in their later teens and early 20's sometimes showed the most dramatic responses characterized by being distant, aversive to discussions of cancer, and demonstrating signs of rejection of their mother. The authors speculated that perhaps the greater reactions in daughters arose from greater fears of developing the disease themselves and the greater responsibilities placed on them. Another study identified the following factors as increasing anxiety in children when a parent had cancer: inability to discuss the diagnosis with the parents, decreased time with their friends, decreased time available for sports and leisure activity, and deterioration of their schoolwork. Stress makes it difficult to concentrate. If your child's school work is deteriorating, make the teacher aware of the situation at home so that the teacher can provide extra help and support for your child.

Teenagers, especially daughters, are very image conscious. Aspects of your therapy may embarrass them, especially in the presence of their friends. These include baldness, going without a prosthesis, or even such a minor thing as not having your "breasts" perfectly even when going out in public. Try discussing these things openly with your children and come to some agreement about what is acceptable to both of you in the presence of their friends or when out in public with them. Also, although you and other close adults may use a little humor as a way to deal with your situation, teenagers may find this very disturbing. They are likely to view it as "gross" or disgusting and not see it as a way of coping and adjusting.

Daughters and the Future Risk of Breast Cancer

As a group, daughters of women with breast cancer are at increased risk of sometime developing breast cancer. Actually, only a few daughters are at very high risk and the rest are at nearly the same risk as the general public. Risk increases if the mother developed breast cancer before menopause, had breast cancer in both breasts, and/or had the combination of ovarian cancer and breast cancer. There are several genes related to breast cancer risk. Unfortunately all the tests are not yet available that can tell you into which group your daughter falls. This is an area of very active research and within the next several years such tests will be more available. Pay attention to news regarding breast cancer genes, and the risks and benefits of screening. There are potential hidden risks in screening such as ability to get health or life insurance, guilt, etc. Discuss all aspects of screening with a professional before you decide about it.

It is *very important* that all daughters with breast development learn to correctly perform a self-breast examination. Be sure that your daughter learns it by the time she gets out of high school. There are pamphlets and tapes that can provide her with the basics. Then it is important that a health professional *show* her how to perform the examination correctly on herself. This can be your regular physician, her pediatrician, or one of your cancer specialists. Help your daughter get into the habit of performing it once a month, just after her period.

Summary for Helping Your Children

1. Be sure your children have adequate opportunities to discuss your cancer and express their feelings. You may or may not be the person they feel most comfortable talking to. They may prefer expressing their thoughts and feelings to a close friend, your spouse, a teacher, or a relative. Don't isolate them by not letting them talk to the person they feel most comfortable with, even if it is a peer. If you don't feel comfortable with too many people knowing about your cancer, help them select which friend(s) they may want to tell.

2. Be honest with them; provide them with the amount of information that they seek. Keep it at their level of education and understanding. Be sure someone answers their questions, even if you have to write them down and ask your doctor.

3. Don't be afraid to show your emotions in their presence. This will demonstrate to them that it is okay for everyone to have and show emotions.

4. Provide more family time. Do things together. Talk about activities and ideas. Discuss your cancer and your feelings as a family.

5. Be sure that they understand that cancer is not contagious; cancer can be cured; and it is normal for them to be frightened, angry, and sad.

6. Try to change their daily routine as little as possible. Encourage them to play with their friends, participate in their usual activities. If possible don't put extra work demands on them at home. But, if they volunteer to do things to help you or make you more comfortable, accept them gratefully.

7. Have your spouse or another significant person spend more time with them.

8. Once your daughter is past puberty, be sure she learns self breast examination.

Internet Resources

Kidscope—a site to help children cope with a parent's cancer
http://www.kidscope.org

Breast Cancer: Help Me Understand It!
http://www.surgery.wisc.edu/breast_info/laybreastca.html

Dr. Wolberg's Breast Tutorial—information about breast cancer and other breast problems
http://www.surgery.wisc.edu/wolberg

References

Armsden GC and Lewis FM. Behavioral adjustment and self-esteem of school-age children of women with breast cancer. *Oncol Nurs Forum* 21:39-45, 1994.

Christ GH, Siegel K, Greund B, Lanosch D, Hendersen S, Sperber D and Weinstein L. Impact of parental terminal cancer on latency-age children. *Amer J Orthopsychiatr* 63:417-425, 1993.

Issel LM, Ersek M Lewis FM. How children cope with mother's breast cancer. *Oncology Nursing Forum* 17:15-13, 1990.

Lichtman RR, Taylor SE, Wood JV, Bluming AZ, Dosik GM and Leibowitz RL. Relations with children after breast cancer: The mother-daughter relationship at risk. *Journal of Psychosocial Oncology* 2:1-19, 1985.

Nelson E, Sloper P, Charlton A and While D. Children who have a parent with cancer: A pilot study. *J Cancer Edu* 9:30-36, 1994.

Wellisch DK, Gritz ER, Schain W, Wang HJ, and Siau J. Psychological functioning of daughters of breast cancer patients. Part II: Characterizing the distressed daughter of the breast cancer patient. *Psychosomatics* 32:324-336, 1991.

Additional Resources

McCue K. and Bonn R. (1994). *How to Help Children through a Parent's Serious Illness*, St. Martin's Press, New York, NY.

Stearns Parkinson V. (1991) *My Mommy Has Cancer*, (booklet for children) Solace Publishing, Inc., Box 567 Folson, CA, 95763-0567 1-800-984-9015.

Torrey L. (1999). *Michael's Mommy has Breast Cancer* (book for children 5-10 years) Hibiscus Press, PO Box 770666, Corel Springs, FL 33077-0666 1-800-468-4004.

Resources for Children whose Parent has a Terminal Illness

Fernside: A Center for Grieving Children. http//fernside.org

Brisson, Pat. (1999) *Sky Memories,* Random House Children's Books, New York, NY. Story of 10-year-old Emily, whose mother is diagnosed with cancer and how the two find a way to ready themselves for the coming loss while celebrating life and cherishing their time left together. Comes with parent-child discussion guide. Ages 8 and up.

Goldman L. (1994). *Life and Loss, A Guide to Help Grieving Children.* Accelerated Development, A member of the Taylor and Francis Groups, Accelerated Development, Inc. Bristol, PA.

Jewell Jarratt C, (1982). *Helping Children Cope with Separation and Loss*, The Harvard Common Press, Boston, Massachusetts.

Papenbrock P and Voss R. (1988). *Children's Grief, How to Help the Child Whose Parent Has Died*, (booklet) Medic Publishing Company, Box 89 Redmond, WA. 98073. 206-881-2883.

Other Books for Children about Parents Dying

From the bibliography of *Life and Loss, A Guide to Help Grieving Children* (see above)

Blume J. (1981). *Tiger Eyes*. New York, NY: Macmillan Children's Group. Fifteen-year-old Davey works through the feelings of his father's murder in a store hold-up. Ages 11 and up.

Douglas, E. (1990). *Rachel and the Upside Down Heart*. Los Angeles, CA: Price Stern Sloan. The true story of four-year-old Rachel, and how her father's death affects her life. Ages 5-9.

Frost, D. (1991). *DAD! Why'd You Leave Me?* Scottdale, PA; Herald Press. This is a story about ten-year-old Ronnie who can't understand why his dad died. Ages 8-12.

Greenfield E. (1993). *Nathanial Talking*. New York, NY: Black Butterfly Children's Group. Nathanial, an energetic nine-year-old, helps us understand a black child's world after his mom dies. He uses rap and rhyme to express his feelings. Ages 7-11.

Krementz J. (1981). *How It Feels When a Parent Dies*. New York, NY: Knoph Publishing Co. Eighteen children (ages 7-16) speak openly about their feelings and experiences after the death of a parent.

Lanton, S. (1991). *Daddy's Chair*. Rockville, MD: Kar-Ben Copies, Inc., Michael's dad died. This follows the Shiva, the Jewish week of mourning. He doesn't want anyone to sit in Daddy's chair. Ages 5-10.

LeShan, E. (1975). *Learning to Say Goodbye When a Parent Dies*. New York, NY: Macmillan Publishing Co. Written directly to children about problems to be recognized and overcome when a parent dies. Ages 8 and up.

Levine J. (1992). *Forever in My Heart*. Burnsville, NC: Mt. Rainbow Publications. A story and workbook that helps children participate in life when their parent is dying. Ages 5-9.

Powell S. (1990). *Geranium Morning*. Minneapolis, MN: Carol Rhoda Books, Inc. A boy's dad is killed in a car accident and a girl's mom is dying. These children share their feelings within a special friendship. Ages 6 and up.

Tiffault, B. (1992). *A Quilt for Elizabeth*. Omaha, NE: Centering Cooperation, Inc. Elizabeth's grandmother helps her understand her feelings after her father dies. This is a good story to initiate an open dialogue with children. Ages 7 and up.

Thaut P. (1991). *Spike and Ben*. Deerfield Beach, FCL; Health Communication, Inc. The story of a boy whose friend's mom dies. Ages 5-9.

Vigna J. (1991). *Saying Goodbye to Daddy*. Niles, IL: Albert Whitman and Co. A sensitive story about a dad's death and the healing that takes place in the weeks that follow. Ages 5-8.

—Jane Brazy, MD and Mary Ircink, RN

Dr. Brazy is Professor of Pediatrics, University of Wisconsin. Her speciality is Newborn Intensive Care. Ms. Ircink is a pediatric nurse who works with Dr. Brazy in patient care and in research. Both are mothers and developed breast cancer before age 50. They are authors of another web site, *For Parents of Preemies: Answers to Commonly Asked Questions* at http://www2.medsch.wisc/edu/childrenshosp/parents_of_premies/index.html

Chapter 64

Nutrition during Cancer Treatment

Introduction

This patient summary on nutrition is adapted from the summary written for health professionals by cancer experts. This and other credible information about cancer treatment, screening, prevention, supportive care, and ongoing clinical trials, is available from the National Cancer Institute. Cancer and its treatment can lead to malnutrition, a common problem in cancer patients. This brief summary describes the effects of cancer and its therapy on nutrition, as well as methods for maintaining nutrition in cancer patients.

Overview

Cancer patients frequently have problems getting enough nutrition. Malnutrition is a major cause of illness and death in cancer patients. Malnutrition occurs when too little food is eaten to continue the body's functions. Progressive wasting, weakness, exhaustion, lower resistance to infection, problems tolerating cancer therapy, and finally, death may result.

Anorexia (the loss of appetite or desire to eat) is the most common symptom in people with cancer. Anorexia may occur early in the disease or later, when the tumor grows and spreads. Some patients may have anorexia when they are diagnosed with cancer; and almost all patients who have widespread cancer will develop anorexia. Anorexia

CancerNet, National Cancer Institute (www.nci.nih.gov), November 2000.

is the most common cause of malnutrition and deterioration in cancer patients.

Cachexia is a wasting syndrome characterized by weakness and a noticeable continuous loss of weight, fat, and muscle. Anorexia and cachexia often occur together. Cachexia can occur in people who are eating enough, but who cannot absorb the nutrients. Cachexia is not related to the tumor size, type, or extent. Cancer cachexia is not the same as starvation. A healthy person's body can adjust to starvation by slowing down its use of nutrients, but in cancer patients, the body does not make this adjustment.

Some cancer patients may die of the effects of malnutrition and wasting.

Effects of the Tumor

Many malnutrition problems are caused directly by the tumor. Tumors growing in the stomach, esophagus, or intestines can cause blockage, nausea and vomiting, poor digestion, slow movement through the digestive system, or poor absorption of nutrients. Cancer of the ovaries or genital and urinary organs can cause ascites (excess fluid in the abdomen), leading to feelings of early fullness, worsening malnutrition, or fluid and electrolyte imbalances. Pain caused by the tumor can result in severe anorexia and a decrease in the amount of foods and liquids consumed. Central nervous system tumors (such as brain cancer) can cause confusion or sleepiness; patients may lose interest in food or forget to eat.

Changes in the body's metabolism can also cause nutritional problems. Tumor cells often convert nutrients to energy in different, less efficient ways than do other cells.

Tumors may produce chemicals or other products that can cause anorexia and cachexia. For example, tumors can produce a substance that changes a person's sense of taste, so that the patient does not want to eat. Tumors can affect the receptors in the brain that tell the stomach if it is full. Tumors can also produce hormone substances, which can change the amount of nutrients eaten, the way they are absorbed, and the way they are used by the body.

Effect of Cancer Therapies

Nutrition problems can be caused by cancer therapies and their side effects. The treatment may have a direct effect, such as poor protein and fat absorption after certain types of surgeries, or an indirect effect, such as an increased need for energy due to infection and fever. Severe malnutrition is defined in two ways: as an increased risk of illness and/or death and as a defined amount of weight loss over a specified amount of time.

Surgery

Head and neck surgery may cause chewing and swallowing problems or may cause mental stress due to the amount of tissue removed during surgery. Surgery to the esophagus may cause stomach paralysis and poor absorption of fat. Poor absorption of protein and fat, dumping syndrome (rapid emptying of the stomach) with low blood sugar, and early feelings of fullness may follow stomach surgery. Surgery to the pancreas may also cause poor protein and fat absorption, poor absorption of vitamins and minerals, or diabetes. Small bowel and colon surgery may cause poor absorption of protein and fat, vitamin and mineral shortages, diarrhea, and severe fluid and electrolyte losses. Surgery to the urinary tract can cause electrolyte imbalances. Other side effects of surgery that can affect nutrition include infection, fistulas (holes between two organs or between an organ and the surface of the body), or short-bowel syndrome. After a colostomy, patients may decrease the amount they eat and drink.

Chemotherapy

Chemotherapy can cause anorexia, nausea and/or vomiting, diarrhea or constipation, inflammation and sores in the mouth, changes in the way food tastes, or infections. Symptoms that affect nutrition and last longer than two weeks are especially critical. The frequency and severity of these symptoms depends on the type of chemotherapy drug, the dosage, and the other drugs and treatments given at the same time. Nutrition may be seriously affected when a patient has a fever for an extended period of time since fevers increase the number of calories needed by the body.

Radiation Therapy

Radiation therapy to the head and neck can cause anorexia, taste changes, dry mouth, inflammation of the mouth and gums, swallowing problems, jaw spasms, cavities, or infection. Radiation to the chest can cause infection in the esophagus, swallowing problems, esophageal reflux (a backwards flow of the stomach contents into the esophagus), nausea, or vomiting. Radiation to the abdomen or pelvis may cause diarrhea, nausea and vomiting, inflammation of the intestine or rectum, or fistula formation. Radiation therapy may also cause tiredness, which may lead to a decrease in appetite and a reduced desire to eat. Long-term effects can include narrowing of the intestine, chronic inflamed intestines, poor absorption, or blockage of the gastrointestinal tract.

Immunotherapy

Immunotherapy (for example, biological response modifier therapy) can cause fever, tiredness, and weakness, and can lead to loss of appetite and an increased need for protein and calories.

Mental and Social Effects

Eating is an important social activity. Anorexia and food avoidance lead to social isolation when people cannot be with others during meal times. Many mental and social factors can affect a person's desire and willingness to eat. Depression, anxiety, anger, and fear are often felt by cancer patients and can lead to anorexia. Feeling a loss of control or helplessness can also reduce the desire to eat. Refusing to eat even when begged to eat by family, friends, and care givers may be one way a patient (who may not feel able to refuse treatment) feels able to have some control in life. Learned food dislikes may also cause less eating or drinking, nausea, and/or vomiting. People who have an unpleasant experience after eating a certain food may avoid that food in the future.

Factors such as living alone, an inability to cook or prepare meals, or an inability to walk to the kitchen because of physical disabilities may lead to eating problems. A social worker or nurse can evaluate the patient's home and recommend changes to help improve eating habits.

Diagnosing the cancer and treating it often means that the patient has to spend much time away from home and the normal routine, including having meals. Favorite foods may not be available in the hospital, or may not be tolerated well because of treatment side effects. For example, a person who enjoys hot, spicy food and has inflammation of the esophagus may not like the taste of bland food and may eat very little. Changes in taste can affect a person's appetite and desire for food.

The less a cancer patient eats, the weaker he or she becomes, and the more it seems that the cancer is progressing. This wasting is a constant reminder to the patient, family, and care givers of the cancer diagnosis and expected poor outcome. This can affect quality of life, social participation, and attitude. Also, with continued wasting, and the resulting tiredness, the person socializes even less. Since food and eating have such an important role in society, the inability to eat well and the consequences of inadequate nutrition isolate the patient even more.

Exercise (such as walking or mild aerobics) has a positive effect on the patient's sense of well-being, alleviating nausea and vomiting, and the patient's ability to eat. Patients who must have artificial feeding methods may show depression, changes in body image, and stress caused by feeding tubes and equipment. To cancer patients, problems with nutrition are more important to their sense of well-being than their sexuality and their ability to remain employed.

Nutritional Assessment

The patient's medical history and physical examination are the most important factors in determining the nutritional status of a cancer patient. This assessment should include a weight history; any changes in eating and drinking; symptoms affecting nutrition (including anorexia, nausea, vomiting, diarrhea, constipation, inflammation and sores in the mouth, dry mouth, taste/smell changes, or pain); medications that affect eating and the way the body uses nutrients; other illnesses or conditions that could affect nutrition or nutritional treatment; and the patient's level of functioning. The cancer patient should be asked about changes in eating and drinking compared to what is normal for him or her, and how long this change has lasted. The physical examination should look for weight loss, loss of fat under the skin, muscle wasting, fluid collection in the legs, and the presence of ascites.

Finding out how much the person likes to eat, as well as what he or she likes to eat, can help when making changes to a cancer patient's diet. Knowing the patient's specific food likes, dislikes, and allergies is also helpful.

General Treatment Guidelines

The type of treatment needed to improve a cancer patient's nutrition is chosen based on the following factors:

- The presence of a working gastrointestinal tract.

- The type of cancer therapy, such as where and how much surgery has been done, the type of chemotherapy used, where and how much of the body was irradiated, the use of biological response modifiers, and the combinations of therapies used.

• The quality of life, how well the patient is functioning, and the expected outcome of the cancer.

• The cost of the care.

Keeping the body looking well and maintaining good nutrition can help the cancer patient feel and look better and help improve his or her daily functioning. It may also help patients tolerate cancer therapy. The type of treatment chosen for nutritional problems depends on the cause of the problems. Problems caused by the tumor may end when the tumor responds to therapy.

Food odor frequently causes anorexia in cancer patients. Patients with anorexia should avoid odors caused by food preparation. Cancer patients may be able to tolerate food with little odor. For example, they may be able to eat at breakfast, since many breakfast foods have little odor.

The following suggestions can help cancer patients manage anorexia:

1. Eat small frequent meals (every 1-2 hours).

2. Eat high-protein and high-calorie foods (including snacks).

3. Avoid foods low in calories and protein and avoid empty calories (like soda).

4. Avoid liquids with meals (unless needed to help dry mouth or swallowing) to keep from feeling full early.

5. Try to eat when feeling best; use nutritional supplements when not feeling like eating. (Cancer patients usually feel better in the morning and have better appetites at that time.)

6. Try several different brands of nutritional supplements or high-calorie, high-protein drinks or pudding recipes. If it tastes too sweet or has a bitter aftertaste, adding the juice of half a freshly-squeezed lemon may help.

7. Work up an appetite with light exercise (such as, walking), a glass of wine or beer if allowed, or appetite stimulants.

8. Add extra calories and protein to food (such as butter, skim milk powder, honey, or brown sugar).

9. Take medications with high-calorie fluids (like nutritional supplements) unless the medication must be taken on an empty stomach.

10. Make eating a pleasant experience (for example, try new recipes, eat with friends, vary color and texture of foods).

11. Experiment with recipes, flavorings, spices, types, and consistencies of food. This is important, since food likes and dislikes may change from day to day.

12. Avoid strong odors. Use boiling bags, cook outdoors on the grill, use a kitchen fan when cooking, serve cold food instead of hot (since odors are in the rising steam), and take off any food covers to release the odors before entering a patient's room. Small portable fans can be used to blow food odors away from patients. Order take-out food, to avoid preparing food at home.

Suggestions for helping cancer patients manage taste changes include:

1. Use plastic utensils if the patient complains of a metallic taste while eating.

2. Cook poultry, fish, eggs, and cheese instead of red meat.

3. Marinate meats with sweet marinades or sauces.

4. Serve meats cool instead of hot.

5. Use extra seasonings, spices, and flavorings, but avoid flavorings that are very sweet or very bitter. A higher sensitivity to the taste of food may cause them to taste flavorless or boring.

6. Substitute milk shakes, puddings, ice cream, cheese, and other high protein foods for meats if the patient does not want to eat meat.

7. Rinse the mouth before eating.

8. Use lemon-flavored drinks to stimulate saliva and taste, but do not use artificial lemon and use very little sweetener.

To prevent the development of taste dislikes:

1. Try new foods and supplements when feeling well.

2. Eat lightly on the morning of, or several hours before receiving chemotherapy.

3. Do not introduce new tastes when bad odors are present.

To help dry mouth or trouble swallowing:

1. Eat soft or moist foods.

2. Process foods in a blender.

3. Moisten foods with creams, gravies, or oils.

4. Avoid rough, irritating foods.

5. Avoid hot or cold foods.

6. Avoid foods that stick to the roof of the mouth.

7. Take small bites and chew completely.

The cancer patient should be encouraged to keep a positive attitude towards treatment and try to take in enough calories and protein. Individual calorie and protein requirements can be calculated so that realistic goals can be set with the patient and his or her care givers. The actual amount of calories and protein needed by each cancer patient varies. The following formula can be used to determine how many calories are needed to maintain a cancer patient's body weight:

General guidelines of calories required (assuming light activity):

- Underweight adults—multiply weight in pounds by 18

- Normal weight adults—multiply weight in pounds by 16

- Overweight adults—multiply weight in pounds by 13

Some cancer patients need more calories and protein. A cancer nutritionist (dietician, diet technician, nurse, or doctor with special training in nutrition) can help determine the nutritional needs and options of each patient. General guidelines for grams of protein needed by cancer patients: multiply weight in pounds by 0.5.

Enteral/Parenteral Support

Sometimes it may be necessary to maintain nutrition using other methods than eating. Enteral nutrition (infusions through the intestinal tract, usually the stomach) may be used. The factors that indicate enteral nutrition is needed are:

1. Upper gastrointestinal blockage that prevents eating or drinking (difficulty swallowing, esophageal narrowing, tumor, stomach weakness or paralysis).

2. Treatment with both chemotherapy and radiation therapy (especially with radiation therapy to the esophagus) with side effects that limit eating or drinking.

3. Anorexia and/or other problems such as severe depression, confusion, or disorientation that keep the patient from eating or drinking sufficiently.

4. Problems eating or drinking (for example, pain when eating).

Enteral nutrition should not be used when the following are present:

1. Bowel obstruction.

2. Nausea and vomiting that does not respond to standard treatment.

3. Severe short gut (inability of the large or small intestine to absorb nutrients due to its removal or damage) with diarrhea that does not respond to standard treatment.

4. Fistula (a hole) in the stomach or esophagus.

Parenteral nutrition (usually an infusion into a vein) should be given for the following reasons:

1. The gastrointestinal tract is not working because of:
   - Temporary problems with oral or enteral nutrition for longer than 10 days, especially if nutritional problems were already present.
   - Obstruction or other problems caused by the tumor that are expected to get better after chemotherapy or surgery.
   - Multiple and/or uncorrectable obstructions or other problems caused by a slow-growing cancer.

2. Severe short gut (see #3 above) following surgery, radiation side effects, fistula, and problems maintaining body weight and muscle with enteral nutrition.

3. Severe and/or continuous decline in nutrition in a person with a slow-growing cancer or any cancer in which malnutrition, not the cancer, is the main problem.

Parenteral nutrition should not be used when the following are present:

1. Functioning digestive system.

2. The patient is not expected to live at least 40 days.

3. There are no good veins to use.

4. There is no severe nutritional problem (for example, a temporary problem eating after surgery).

It is believed that cancer patients who have enough nutrition are better able to stand therapy and its side effects. The type of nutritional support used should be chosen based on the patient's physical needs, degree of nutritional problem, disease, the amount of time that support will be needed, and the resources available. If the gastrointestinal tract is working and will not be affected by the cancer therapy, then enteral support is best. Enteral nutrition can be given through a tube in the nose or by tubes placed during surgery.

Medications can also be used to improve nutrition. Medications may include those for pain management, treatment of constipation or diarrhea, stimulation of the stomach, or the use of appetite stimulants.

Chapter 65

Cancer Fatigue

Overview

Fatigue occurs in 78% to 96% of people with cancer, especially those receiving treatment for their cancer. Fatigue is complex, and has biological, psychological, and behavioral causes. Fatigue is difficult to describe and people with cancer may express it in different ways, such as saying they feel tired, weak, exhausted, weary, worn-out, fatigued, heavy, or slow. Health professionals may use terms such as asthenia, fatigue, lassitude, prostration, exercise intolerance, lack of energy, and weakness to describe fatigue.

Fatigue can be described as a condition that causes distress and decreased ability to function due to a lack of energy. Specific symptoms may be physical, psychological, or emotional. To be treated effectively, fatigue related to cancer and cancer treatment needs to be distinguished from other kinds of fatigue.

Fatigue may be acute or chronic. Acute fatigue is normal tiredness with occasional symptoms that begin quickly and last for a short time. Rest may alleviate fatigue and allow a return to a normal level of functioning in a healthy individual, but this ability is diminished in people who have cancer. Chronic fatigue is long lasting. Chronic fatigue syndrome describes prolonged debilitating fatigue that may persist or relapse. This illness is sometimes diagnosed in people who do not have cancer. Although many treatment- and disease-related factors may cause fatigue, the exact process of fatigue in people with cancer is not known.

PDQ, National Cancer Institute (www.nci.nih.gov), November 2000.

Fatigue can become a very important issue in the life of a person with cancer. It may affect how the person feels about him- or herself, his or her daily activities and relationships with others, and whether he or she continues with cancer treatment. Patients receiving some cancer treatments may miss work, withdraw from friends, need more sleep, and, in some cases, may not be able to perform any physical activities because of fatigue. Finances can become difficult if people with fatigue need to take disability leave or stop working completely. Job loss may result in the loss of health insurance or the inability to get medical care. Understanding fatigue and its causes is important in determining effective treatment and in helping people with cancer cope with fatigue. Tests that measure the level of fatigue have been developed.

Causes

The causes of fatigue in people with cancer are not known. Fatigue commonly is an indicator of disease progression and is frequently one of the first symptoms of cancer in both children and adults. For example, parents of a child diagnosed with acute lymphocytic leukemia or non-Hodgkin's lymphoma frequently seek medical care because of the child's extreme fatigue. Tumors can cause fatigue directly or indirectly by spreading to the bone marrow, causing anemia, and by forming toxic substances in the body that interfere with normal cell functions. People who are having problems breathing, another symptom of some cancers, may also experience fatigue.

Fatigue can occur for many reasons. The extreme stress that people with cancer experience over a long period of time can cause them to use more energy, leading to fatigue. However, there may be other reasons that cancer patients suffer from fatigue. The central nervous system (the brain and spinal cord) may be affected by the cancer or the cancer therapy (especially biological therapy) and cause fatigue. Medication to treat pain, depression, vomiting, seizures, and other problems related to cancer may also cause fatigue. Tumor necrosis factor (TNF) is a substance that can be produced by a tumor, or may be given to a patient as a treatment for some types of cancer. TNF may cause a decrease in protein stores in muscles causing the body to work harder to perform normal functions, and therefore causing fatigue.

Factors Related to Fatigue

It is not always possible to determine the factors that cause fatigue in patients with cancer. Possible factors include cancer treatment, anemia, medications, weight loss and loss of appetite, changes in metabolism, decreased levels of hormones, emotional distress, difficulty sleeping, inactivity, difficulty breathing, loss of strength and muscle coordination, pain, infection, and having other medical conditions in addition to cancer.

Cancer Treatment

Fatigue is a common symptom following radiation therapy or chemotherapy. It may be caused by anemia, or the collection of toxic substances produced by cells. In the case of radiation, it may be caused by the increased energy needed to repair damaged skin tissue.

Several factors have been linked with fatigue caused by chemotherapy. Some people may respond to the diagnosis and treatment of cancer with mood changes and disrupted sleep patterns. Nausea, vomiting, chronic pain, and weight loss can also cause fatigue.

Fatigue has long been associated with radiation therapy although the connection between them is not well understood. Fatigue usually lessens after the therapy is completed, although not all patients return to their normal level of energy. Patients who are older, have advanced disease, or receive combination therapy (for example, chemotherapy plus radiation therapy) are at a higher risk for developing long-term fatigue.

Biological therapy frequently causes fatigue. In this setting, fatigue is one of a group of side effects known as "flu-like" syndrome. This syndrome also includes fever, chills, muscle pain, headache, and a sense of generally not feeling well. Some patients may also experience problems with their ability to think clearly. The type of biological therapy used may determine the type and pattern of fatigue experienced.

Many people with cancer undergo surgery for diagnosis or treatment. Fatigue is a problem following surgery, but fatigue from surgery improves with time. It can be made worse, however, when combined with the fatigue caused by other cancer treatments.

Anemia

Anemia may be a major factor in cancer-related fatigue and quality of life in people with cancer. Anemia may be caused by the cancer, cancer treatment, or may be related to other medical causes.

Nutrition Factors

Fatigue often occurs when the body needs more energy than the amount being supplied from the patient's diet. In people with cancer,

3 major factors may be involved: a change in the body's ability to process food normally, an increased need by the body for energy (due to tumor growth, infection, fever, or problems with breathing), and a decrease in the amount of food eaten (due to lack of appetite, nausea, vomiting, diarrhea, or bowel obstruction).

Emotional Factors

The moods, beliefs, attitudes, and reactions to stress of people with cancer can contribute to the development of fatigue. Approximately 40% to 60% of the cases of fatigue among all patients (cancer patients as well as other patients) are not caused by disease or other physical reasons. Anxiety and depression are the most common psychological disorders that cause fatigue.

Depression may be a disabling illness that affects approximately 15% to 25% of people who have cancer. When patients experience depression (loss of interest, difficulty concentrating, mental and physical tiredness, and feelings of hopelessness), the fatigue from physical causes can become worse and last longer than usual, even after the physical causes are gone. Anxiety and fear associated with a cancer diagnosis, as well as its impact on a person's physical, mental, social, and financial well-being are sources of emotional stress.

Psychological Factors

Decreased attention span and difficulty understanding and thinking are often associated with fatigue. Attention problems are common during and after cancer treatment. Attention may be restored by activities that encourage rest. Sleep is also necessary for relieving attention problems but it is not always enough.

Breathing Impairment

Breathing problems may also cause fatigue. People with advanced disease and/or lung cancer have more distress than other cancer patients. Major symptoms of breathing distress are fatigue, sleeplessness, pain, and cough.

Medications

Medications other than those used in chemotherapy may also contribute to fatigue. Opioids used in treating cancer-related pain often cause drowsiness, the extent of which may vary depending on the individual. Other types of medications such as tricyclic antidepressants and antihistamines may also produce the side effect of drowsiness. Taking several medications may compound fatigue symptoms.

Assessment

To determine the cause and best treatment for fatigue, the person's fatigue pattern must be determined, and all of the factors causing the fatigue must be identified. The following factors must be included:

- Fatigue pattern, including how and when it started, how long it has lasted, and its severity, plus any factors that make fatigue worse or better.

- Type and degree of disease and of treatment-related symptoms and/or side effects.

- Treatment history.

- Current medications.

- Sleep and/or rest patterns and relaxation habits.

- Eating habits and appetite or weight changes.

- Effects of fatigue on activities of daily living and lifestyle.

- Psychological profile, including an evaluation for depression.

- Complete physical examination.

- How well the patient is able to follow the recommended treatment.

- Job performance.

- Financial resources.

- Other factors (for example, anemia, breathing problems, decreased muscle strength).

Underlying factors that contribute to fatigue should be evaluated and treated when possible. Contributing factors include anemia, depression, anxiety, pain, dehydration, nutritional deficiencies, sedating medications, and therapies that may have poorly tolerated side effects. Patients should tell their doctors when they are experiencing fatigue and ask for information about fatigue related to underlying causes and treatment side effects.

Anemia Evaluation

There are different kinds of anemia. A medical history, a physical examination, and blood tests may be used to determine the kind and extent of anemia that a person may have. In people with cancer there may be several causes.

Treatment

Most of the treatments for fatigue in cancer patients are for treating symptoms and providing emotional support because the causes of fatigue that are specifically related to cancer have not been determined. Some of these symptom-related treatments may include adjusting the dosages of pain medications, administering red blood cell transfusions or blood cell growth factors, diet supplementation with iron and vitamins, and antidepressants or psychostimulants.

Psychostimulant Drugs

Although fatigue is one of the most common symptoms in cancer, few medications are effective in treating it. A health care provider may prescribe medication in low doses that may help patients who are depressed, unresponsive, tired, distracted, or weak. These drugs (psychostimulants) can give a sense of well-being, decrease fatigue, and increase appetite. They are also helpful in reversing the sedating effects of morphine, and they work quickly. However, these drugs can also cause sleeplessness, euphoria, and mood changes. High doses and long-term use may cause loss of appetite, nightmares, sleeplessness, euphoria, paranoid behavior, and possible heart problems.

Treatment for Anemia

Treatment for fatigue that is related to anemia may include red blood cell transfusions. Transfusions are an effective treatment for anemia, however, possible side effects include infection, immediate transfusion reaction, graft- versus-host disease, and changes in immunity. Treatment for anemia related fatigue, in patients undergoing chemotherapy, may also include drugs that stimulate the production of blood cells such as epoetin alfa.

Exercise

Exercise (including light- to moderate-intensity walking programs) helps many people with cancer. People with cancer who exercise may have more physical energy, improved ability to function, improved quality of life, improved outlook, improved sense of well being, enhanced sense of commitment, and improved ability to meet the challenges of cancer and cancer treatment.

Exercise may also help patients with advanced cancer, even those in hospice care. More benefit may result when family members are involved with the patient in the physical therapy program.

Activity and Rest

Any changes in daily routine require the body to use more energy. People with cancer should set priorities and keep a reasonable schedule. Health professionals can help patients by providing information about support services to help with daily activities and responsibilities. An activity and rest program can be developed with a health care professional to make the most of a patient's energy.

Patient Education

Treating chronic fatigue in cancer patients means accepting the condition and learning how to cope with it. People with cancer may find that fatigue becomes a chronic disability. Although fatigue is frequently an expected, temporary side effect of treatment, other factors may cause it to continue.

Since fatigue is the most common symptom in people receiving outpatient chemotherapy, patients should learn ways to manage the fatigue. Patients should be taught the following:

- The difference between fatigue and depression

- Possible medical causes of fatigue (not enough fluids, electrolyte imbalance, breathing problems, anemia)

- To observe their rest and activity patterns during the day and over time

- To engage in attention-restoring activities (walking, gardening, bird-watching)

- To recognize fatigue that is a side effect of certain therapies

- To participate in exercise programs that are realistic

- To identify activities which cause fatigue and develop ways to avoid or modify those activities

- To identify environmental or activity changes that may help decrease fatigue

- The importance of eating enough food and drinking enough fluids

- Physical therapy may help with nerve or muscle weakness

- Respiratory therapy may help with breathing problems

- To schedule important daily activities during times of less fatigue, and cancel unimportant activities that cause stress

- To avoid or change a situation that causes stress

- To observe whether treatments being used to help fatigue are working

Post-treatment Considerations

This section is for patients who have had no cancer treatment for at least 6 months. The causes of fatigue are different for patients who are receiving therapy compared to those who have completed therapy. Also, the treatment for fatigue may be different for patients who are no longer receiving treatment for cancer.

Fatigue in people who have completed treatment for cancer and who are considered to be disease-free is a different condition than the fatigue experienced by patients receiving therapy. Fatigue may significantly affect the quality of life of cancer survivors. Studies show that some patients continue to have moderate to severe fatigue for up to 18 years after bone marrow transplantation. Long-term therapies such as tamoxifen can also cause fatigue. Fatigue can cause poor school performance years later in children who were treated for brain tumors and cured. Long-term follow-up care is important for patients after cancer therapy. Physical causes should be ruled out when trying to determine the cause of fatigue in cancer survivors.

Chapter 66

Cancer Patients and Depression

People who face a diagnosis of cancer will experience different levels of stress and emotional upset. Fear of death, interruption of life plans, changes in body image and self-esteem, changes in the social role and lifestyle, and money and legal concerns are important issues in the life of any person with cancer, yet serious depression is not experienced by everyone who is diagnosed with cancer.

Sadness and grief are normal reactions to the crises faced during cancer, and will be experienced at times by all people. Since sadness is common, it is important to distinguish between "normal" levels of sadness and depression. An important part of cancer care is the recognition of depression that needs to be treated. Major depression is not simply sadness or a blue mood. Major depression affects about 25% of patients and has common symptoms that can be diagnosed and treated.

When people find out they have cancer, they often have feelings of disbelief, denial, or despair. They may also experience difficulty sleeping, loss of appetite, anxiety, and a preoccupation with worries about the future. These symptoms and fears usually lessen as a person adjusts to the diagnosis. Signs that a person has adjusted to the diagnosis include an ability to maintain active involvement in daily life activities, and an ability to continue functioning as spouse, parent, employee, or other roles by incorporating treatment into his or her

Excerpted from "Depression (PDQ®) Supportive Care—Patients," National Cancer Institute (NCI), November 2000. Full text available at http://cancernet.nci.nih.gov.

schedule. A person who cannot adjust to the diagnosis after a long period of time, and who loses interest in usual activities, may be depressed. Mild symptoms of depression can be distressing and may be helped with counseling. Even patients without obvious symptoms of depression may benefit from counseling. However, when symptoms are intense and long-lasting, or when they keep coming back, more intensive treatment is important.

Diagnosis

The symptoms of major depression include having a depressed mood for most of the day and on most days; loss of pleasure and interest in most activities; changes in eating and sleeping habits; nervousness or sluggishness; tiredness; feelings of worthlessness or inappropriate guilt; poor concentration; and constant thoughts of death or suicide. To make a diagnosis of depression, these symptoms should be present for at least 2 weeks. The diagnosis of depression can be difficult to make in people with cancer due to the difficulty of separating the symptoms of depression from the side effects of medications or the symptoms of cancer. This is especially true in patients undergoing active cancer treatment or those with advanced disease. Symptoms of guilt, worthlessness, hopelessness, thoughts of suicide, and loss of pleasure are the most useful in diagnosing depression in people who have cancer.

The most common type of depression in people with cancer is called reactive depression. This shows up as feeling moody and being unable to perform usual activities. The symptoms last longer and are more pronounced than a normal and expected reaction but do not meet the criteria for major depression. When these symptoms greatly interfere with a person's daily activities, such as work, school, shopping, or caring for a household, they should be treated in the same way that major depression is treated (such as crisis intervention, counseling, and medication, especially with drugs that can quickly relieve distressing symptoms). Basing the diagnosis on just these symptoms can be a problem in a person with advanced disease since the illness may be causing decreased functioning. In more advanced illness, focusing on despair, guilty thoughts, and a total lack of enjoyment of life is helpful in diagnosing depression.

Medical factors may also cause depression in cancer patients. Medication usually helps this type of depression more effectively than counseling, especially if the medical factors cannot be changed (for example, dosages of the medications that are causing the depression cannot be changed or stopped). Some medical causes of depression in cancer patients include uncontrolled pain; abnormal levels of calcium, sodium, or potassium in the blood; anemia; vitamin B_{12} or folate deficiency; fever; and abnormal levels of thyroid hormone or steroids in the blood.

Treatment

Major depression may be treated with a combination of counseling and medications, such as antidepressants. A primary care doctor may prescribe medications for depression and refer the patient to a psychiatrist or psychologist for the following reasons: a physician or oncologist is not comfortable treating the depression (for example, the patient has suicidal thoughts); the symptoms of depression do not improve after 2-4 weeks of treatment; the symptoms are getting worse; the side effects of the medication keep the patient from taking the dosage needed to control the depression; and/or the symptoms are interfering with the patient's ability to continue medical treatment.

Antidepressants are safe for cancer patients to use and are usually effective in the treatment of depression and its symptoms. Unfortunately, antidepressants are not often prescribed for cancer patients. About 25% of all cancer patients are depressed, but only about 2% receive medication for the depression. The choice of antidepressant depends on the patient's symptoms, potential side effects of the antidepressant, and the person's individual medical problems and previous response to antidepressant drugs.

St. John's wort (*Hypericum perforatum*) has been used as an over-the-counter herbal antidepressant. How it works is unclear, and it is not known if it may cause adverse reactions when taken with other medications. Since it is an herb, it is not required to undergo testing by the Federal Drug Administration (FDA), and therefore product safety and purity is not known. Patients with symptoms of depression should be evaluated by a health professional and not self treat with St. John's wort.

Most antidepressants take 3 to 6 weeks to begin working. The side effects must be considered when deciding which antidepressant to use. For example, a medication that causes sleepiness may be helpful in an anxious patient who is having problems sleeping, since the drug is both calming and sedating. Patients who cannot swallow pills may be able to take the medication as a liquid or as an injection. If the antidepressant helps the symptoms, treatment should continue for at least 6 months. Electroconvulsive therapy (ECT) is a useful and safe therapy when other treatments have been unsuccessful in relieving major depression.

Several psychiatric therapies have been found to be beneficial for the treatment of depression related to cancer. These therapies are often used in combination and include crisis intervention, psychotherapy, and thought/behavior techniques. These therapies usually consist of 3 to 10 sessions and explore methods of lowering distress, improving coping and problem-solving skills; enlisting support; reshaping negative and self-defeating thoughts; and developing a close personal bond with an understanding health care provider. Talking with a clergy member may also be helpful for some people.

Cancer support groups may also be helpful in treating depression in cancer patients, especially adolescents. Support groups have been shown to improve mood, encourage the development of coping skills, improve quality of life, and improve immune response. Support groups can be found through the wellness community, the American Cancer Society, and many community resources, including the social work departments in medical centers and hospitals.

Evaluation and Treatment of Suicidal Cancer Patients

The incidence of suicide in cancer patients may be as much as 10 times higher than the rate of suicide in the general population. Passive suicidal thoughts are fairly common in cancer patients. The relationships between suicidal tendency and the desire for hastened death, requests for physician-assisted suicide, and/or euthanasia are complicated and poorly understood. Overdosing with pain killers and sedatives is the most common method of suicide by cancer patients, with most cancer suicides occurring at home.

General risk factors for suicide in a person with cancer include a history of mental problems, especially those associated with impulsive behavior (such as, borderline personality disorders); a family history of suicide; a history of suicide attempts; depression; substance abuse; recent death of a friend or spouse; and having little social support.

Cancer-specific risk factors for suicide include a diagnosis of oral, pharyngeal, or lung cancer (often associated with heavy alcohol and tobacco use); advanced stage of disease and poor prognosis; confusion/delirium; poorly controlled pain; or physical impairments, such as loss of mobility, loss of bowel and bladder control, amputation, loss of eyesight or hearing, paralysis, inability to eat or swallow, tiredness, or exhaustion.

Patients who are suicidal require careful evaluation. The risk of suicide increases if the patient reports thoughts of suicide and has a plan to carry it out. Risk continues to increase if the plan is "lethal," that is, the plan is likely to cause death. A lethal suicide plan is more likely to be carried out if the way chosen to cause death is available to the person, the attempt cannot be stopped once it is started, and help is unavailable. When a person with cancer reports thoughts of death, it is important to determine whether the underlying cause is depression or a desire to control unbearable symptoms. Prompt identification and treatment of major depression is important in decreasing the risk for suicide. Risk factors, especially hopelessness (which is a better predictor for suicide than depression) should be carefully determined. The assessment of hopelessness is not easy in the person who has advanced cancer with no hope of a cure. It is important to determine the basic reasons for hopelessness, which may be related to cancer symptoms, fears of painful death, or feelings of abandonment.

Talking about suicide will not cause the patient to attempt suicide; it actually shows that this is a concern and permits the patient to describe his or her feelings and fears, providing a sense of control. A crisis intervention-oriented treatment approach should be used which involves the patient's support system. Contributing symptoms, such as pain, should be aggressively controlled and depression, psychosis, anxiety, and underlying causes of delirium should be treated. These problems are usually treated in a medical hospital or at home. Although not usually necessary, a suicidal cancer patient may need to be hospitalized in a psychiatric unit.

The goal of treatment of suicidal patients is to attempt to prevent suicide that is caused by desperation due to poorly controlled symptoms. Patients close to the end of life may not be able to stay awake without a great amount of emotional or physical pain. This often leads to thoughts of suicide or requests for aid in dying. Such patients may need sedation to ease their distress.

Other treatment considerations include using medications that work quickly to alleviate distress (such as antianxiety medication or stimulants) while waiting for the antidepressant medication to work; limiting the quantities of medications that are lethal in overdose; having frequent contact with a health care professional who can closely observe the patient; avoiding long periods of time when the patient is alone; making sure the patient has available support; and determining the patient's mental and emotional response at each crisis point during the cancer experience.

Pain and symptom treatment should not be sacrificed simply to avoid the possibility that a patient will attempt suicide. Patients often have a method to commit suicide available to them. Incomplete pain and symptom treatment might actually worsen a patient's suicide risk.

Frequent contact with the health professional can help limit the amount of lethal drugs available to the patient and family. Infusion devices that limit patient access to medications can also be used at home or in the hospital. These are programmable, portable pumps with coded access and a locked cartridge containing the medication. These pumps are very useful in controlling pain and other symptoms. Some pumps can give multiple drug infusions, and some can be programmed over the phone. The devices are available through home care agencies, but are very expensive. Some of the expense may be covered by insurance.

Chapter 67

Managing Cancer Pain

Overview

Cancer pain can be managed effectively in most patients with cancer or with a history of cancer. Although cancer pain cannot always be relieved completely, therapy can lessen pain in most patients. Pain management improves the patient's quality of life throughout all stages of the disease.

Flexibility is important in managing cancer pain. As patients vary in diagnosis, stage of disease, responses to pain and treatments, and personal likes and dislikes, management of cancer pain must be individualized. Patients, their families, and their health care providers must work together closely to manage a patient's pain effectively.

Assessment

To treat pain, it must be measured. The patient and the doctor should measure pain levels at regular intervals after starting cancer treatment, at each new report of pain, and after starting any type of treatment for pain. The cause of the pain must be identified and treated promptly.

Excerpted from "Pain (PDQ®) Supportive Care—Patients," National Cancer Institute (NCI), November 2000. Full text available at http://cancernet.nci.nih.gov.

Patient Self-Report

To help the health care provider determine the type and extent of the pain, cancer patients can describe the location and intensity of their pain, any aggravating or relieving factors, and their goals for pain control, as follows:

- **Pain:** The patient can describe the pain, when it started, how long it lasts, and whether it is worse during certain times of the day or night.

- **Location:** The patient can show exactly where the pain is on his or her body or on a drawing of a body and where the pain goes if it travels.

- **Intensity or severity:** The patient can keep a diary of pain intensity.

- **Aggravating and relieving factors:** The patient can identify factors that increase or decrease the pain.

- **Goals for pain control:** With the health care provider, the patient can decide how much pain she can tolerate and how much improvement she may achieve.

Assessment of the Outcomes

Improvement of pain management is measured as decreased pain intensity and improvement in social functioning. Monitoring the amount of medication needed for pain is also important in this assessment process.

Pain Management with Drugs

Pain management begins with drug therapy. It is effective, relatively low risk, inexpensive, and usually works quickly. People respond differently to drugs, even those within the same family of drugs. Different drugs within a category should be tried before switching therapy.

Acetaminophen and NSAIDs

NSAIDs are effective for relief of mild pain. They may be given with opioids for the relief of moderate to severe pain. Acetaminophen also relieves pain, although it does not have the anti-inflammatory effect that aspirin and NSAIDs do.

Opioids

Opioids are very effective for the relief of moderate to severe pain. Under-treatment results when concerns about addiction (psychological dependence) to these drugs is confused with tolerance and physical dependence. Many patients with cancer pain become tolerant to opioids during long-term therapy. Therefore, increasing doses are necessary to continue to relieve pain, even at the risk of side effects.

Some commonly used opioids are morphine, codeine, methadone, and fentanyl. The correct dose is the amount of opioid that controls pain with the fewest side effects. The need for higher doses of opioids often indicates the progression of disease, not drug tolerance. If opioid tolerance does occur, it can be overcome by increasing the dose or changing to another opioid.

Route of Administration

Medications for pain may be given in several ways. The preferred method is by mouth, since medications given orally are convenient and usually inexpensive. When patients cannot take medications by mouth, other less invasive methods may be used, such as rectally or through medication patches placed on the skin. Intravenous methods are used only when simpler, less demanding, and less costly methods are inappropriate or ineffective. Patient-controlled analgesia (PCA) pumps are sometimes used to allow the patient to deliver the drug as needed for pain. Drugs may be delivered into veins, skin, or the spine by this method. Intraspinal administration is especially helpful for patients who do not respond to pain medications delivered by the other methods or who experience extreme side effects.

Side Effects

Common side effects of opioids include constipation, nausea and vomiting, sleepiness, difficulty in thinking clearly, problems with breathing, gradual overdose, and problems with sexual function. Some of the milder side effects may be avoided by adjusting the time when doses are taken, such as taking them after a meal, or at bedtime if a person is experiencing nausea or sleepiness. Constipation may be helped by drinking more fluids, eating foods higher in fiber, or taking a laxative (which should be approved or prescribed by the patient's doctor). Patients should talk to their doctor about side effects that become too bothersome or severe.

Patients may find that they develop "tolerance" to opioid pain medications and may need to have their doses increased to relieve pain symptoms. Tolerance has not been shown to lead to drug addiction or drug abuse problems in patients who take opioid drugs for medical reasons. Physical dependence on opioid pain medications does not seem to occur in patients with cancer. In these patients, once the pain disappears (usually through the effective treatment of cancer) the pain medicine can be stopped without difficulty.

Adjuvant Drugs

Other drugs may be given at the same time as the pain medication. This is done to increase the effectiveness of the pain medication, treat symptoms, and relieve specific types of pain. These drugs include corticosteroids, anticonvulsants, antidepressants, local anesthetics, and stimulants.

Physical and Psychosocial Interventions

Noninvasive physical and psychological methods can be used along with drugs and other treatments to manage pain during all phases of cancer treatment. The effectiveness of the pain interventions depends on the patient's participation in treatment and his or her ability to tell the health care provider which methods work best to relieve pain.

Physical Interventions

Weakness, muscle wasting, and muscle/bone pain may be treated with heat (hot pack or heating pad); cold (flexible ice packs); massage, pressure, and vibration (to improve relaxation); exercise (to strengthen weak muscles, loosen stiff joints, help restore coordination and balance, and strengthen the heart); changing the position of the patient; restricting the movement of painful areas or broken bones; stimulation; controlled low-voltage electrical stimulation; or acupuncture.

Psychosocial Interventions

Thinking and behavior interventions are also important in treating pain. These interventions help give patients a sense of control and help them develop coping skills to deal with the disease and its symptoms. Beginning these interventions early in the course of the disease

500

is useful so that patients can learn and practice the skills while they have enough strength and energy. Several methods should be tried, and one or more should be used regularly.

- **Relaxation and imagery:** Simple relaxation techniques may be used for episodes of brief pain (for example, during cancer treatment procedures). Brief, simple techniques are suitable for periods when the patient's ability to concentrate is limited by severe pain, high anxiety, or fatigue.

- **Hypnosis:** Hypnotic techniques may be used to encourage relaxation and may be combined with other thinking/behavior methods. Hypnosis is effective in relieving pain in people who are able to concentrate and use imagery and who are willing to practice the technique.

- **Redirecting thinking:** Focusing attention on triggers other than pain or negative emotions that come with pain may involve distractions that are internal (for example, counting, praying, or saying things like "I can cope") or external (for example, music, television, talking, listening to someone read, or looking at something specific). Patients can also learn to monitor and evaluate negative thoughts and replace them with more positive thoughts and images.

- **Patient education:** Health care providers can give patients information and instructions about pain and pain management and assure them that most pain can be controlled effectively. Health care providers should also discuss the major barriers that interfere with effective pain management.

- **Psychological support:** Short-term psychological therapy helps some patients. Patients who develop clinical depression or adjustment disorder may see a psychiatrist for diagnosis.

- **Support groups and religious counseling:** Support groups help many patients. Religious counseling may also help by providing spiritual care and social support.

Anticancer Interventions

Radiation Therapy

Local or whole-body radiation therapy may increase the effectiveness of pain medication and other noninvasive therapies by directly affecting the cause of the pain (for example, by reducing tumor size). A single injection of a radioactive agent may relieve pain when cancer spreads extensively to the bones.

Surgery

Surgery may be used to remove part or all of a tumor to reduce pain directly, relieve symptoms of obstruction or compression, and improve outcome, even increasing long-term survival.

Invasive Interventions

Less invasive methods should be used for relieving pain before trying invasive treatment. However, some patients may need this type of therapy.

Nerve Blocks

A nerve block is the injection of either a local anesthetic or a drug that inactivates nerves to control otherwise uncontrollable pain. Nerve blocks can be used to determine the source of pain, to treat painful conditions that respond to nerve blocks, to predict how the pain will respond to long-term treatments, and to prevent pain following procedures.

Neurologic Interventions

Surgery can be performed to implant devices that deliver drugs or electrically stimulate the nerves. In rare cases, surgery may be done to destroy a nerve or nerves that are part of the pain pathway.

Management of Procedural Pain

Many diagnostic and treatment procedures are painful. Pain related to procedures may be treated before it occurs. Local anesthetics and short-acting opioids can be used to manage procedure-related pain, if enough time is allowed for the drug to work. Anti-anxiety drugs and sedatives may be used to reduce anxiety or to sedate the patient. Treatments such as imagery or relaxation are useful in managing procedure-related pain and anxiety.

Patients usually tolerate procedures better when they know what to expect. Having a relative or friend stay with the patient during the procedure may help reduce anxiety.

Patients and family members should receive written instructions for managing the pain at home. They should receive information regarding who to contact for questions related to pain management.

To Learn More

For more information, call the National Cancer Institute's Cancer Information Service at 1-800-4-CANCER (1-800-422-6237); TTY at 1-800-332-8615. The call is free and a trained information specialist is available to answer your questions.

The National Cancer Institute has booklets and other materials for patients, health professionals, and the public. These publications discuss types of cancer, methods of cancer treatment, coping with cancer, and clinical trials. Some publications provide information on tests for cancer, cancer causes and prevention, cancer statistics, and NCI research activities. NCI materials on these and other topics may be ordered online from the NCI Publications Locator Service at http://publications.nci.nih.gov/ or by telephone from the Cancer Information Service toll free at 1-800-4-CANCER.

For more information from the National Cancer Institute, please write to this address:

National Cancer Institute
Office of Communications
31 Center Drive, MSC 2580
Bethesda, MD 20892-2580

Chapter 68

Cancer Treatment and Vaginal Discomfort during Intercourse

Vaginal discomfort during intercourse is a common complaint of women after radiation therapy to the pelvis, chemotherapy induced menopause, or postmenopausal women who can not use estrogen replacement. This discomfort may be caused by vaginal dryness or loss of stretch of the vaginal tissues that may make penetration uncomfortable. Patients who receive radiation therapy to the pelvic region or radiation implants may need to use vaginal dilators on a regular basis to prevent scar tissue and closure of the vagina. Patients who are postmenopausal may experience a decrease in natural lubrication of the vagina. There are some effective treatments available. These include:

- Using extra lubrication to reduce pain.

- Use only water based lubricants.

- Many women prefer lubricants such as Astroglide, Moist Again, the Women's Health Institutes Lubricating Gel, and Probe over other products because they spread easily and last longer.

"Dealing with Vaginal Discomfort during Intercourse after Cancer Treatment." Excerpted from James M. Metz, MD, *CancerTips: A Handbook for Cancer Prevention and Management*, p. 51–52 (Lippincott Williams & Wilkins, October 2001). Text available online at http://www.oncolink.com/templates/oncotips/article.cfm?c=1&s=3&ss=3&id=20; reprinted with permission of the author and of Lippincott Williams and Wilkins.

- Avoid petroleum based lubricants, particularly if your partner is using condoms that can be damaged with this type of lubrication.

- Avoid scented lubricants as these may irritate the genital tissues.

- Use lubricants during foreplay and spread generously over labia, clitoris, and into vagina. Also spread lubrication on any object that will enter the vagina.

- Keep lubricants close to the bed or anywhere sexual activity may occur.

- Consider using Replens which is designed to moisturize the walls of the vagina. It is used about 3 times per week at bedtime.

- If your radiation oncologist has prescribed vaginal dilators, make sure you use them as instructed.

Chapter 69

Quality of Life and Sexuality during Cancer Treatment

Summary

When a woman is diagnosed with a gynecologic cancer, it impacts her life in many ways. The three major treatment modalities: surgery, chemotherapy, and radiation therapy, can produce numerous side effects. The side effects in turn can harm a woman's sense of self worth and sexuality. Nurses working with women during treatment need to be knowledgeable regarding the physical and emotional side effects that are likely to have an impact on their patients. Through teaching, advocacy, and support the oncology nurse plays an important role in helping women retain their sexuality and the highest quality of life possible.

Introduction

Gynecologic malignancies are the fourth most common form of cancer among women (Anderson and Lutgendorf, 1997). This type of cancer includes the ovaries, uterus, endometrium, cervix, vagina, and vulva and may involve the adjacent pelvic structures and lymph nodes. Surgery, chemotherapy, radiotherapy, or a combination of these modalities may be used to treat gynecologic cancers.

The diagnosis of cancer is an overwhelming experience for a woman and her family. Then, before the woman has had time to work through her feelings of shock and grief, she must begin treatment. The short- and long-term side effects of treatment may also impact on a woman's self worth and sexuality. Many recent studies on the impact of gynecologic cancer on a woman's quality of life find that an important outcome criterion has become measuring survival without significant morbidity [complications] (Anderson and Lutgendorf, 1997). The oncology nurse has an important role in patient education and managing side effects, thereby helping each woman maintain her sexuality and quality of life.

Pre- and Post-Operative Surgical Considerations

Surgery is often used to diagnose, stage, and treat gynecologic cancer. A total abdominal hysterectomy or a radical hysterectomy is used to treat ovarian, uterine, or cervical cancer. These procedures carry the usual surgical risks of pain, infection, hemorrhage, and pulmonary complications. In addition, a hysterectomy can affect a woman's psychological and emotional well-being. Women of childbearing age have been found to experience sadness and anger at the loss of fertility, and women of all ages view the loss of female organs as a loss of femininity (Steginga and Dunn, 1997). Radical vulvectomy and pelvic exenteration are two extensive surgeries that dramatically change a woman's physical appearance and alter her sexuality.

Women who are scheduled to have surgery for gynecologic cancer require careful preoperative needs assessment and teaching. The oncology nurse must help the woman and her partner to understand the surgical procedure and prepare for the postoperative phase. The staff nurse can lessen the likelihood of postoperative complications by encouraging pulmonary hygiene [proper care of the lungs] and ambulation [walking]. Women are better able to learn and more willing to participate in self-care if their pain is well controlled. The nurse's knowledge of pain medication and nonpharmacologic pain control techniques can increase the patient's comfort, decrease anxiety, and help ease recovery (Mann, 1996).

During the postoperative period the patient will need help adjusting to her altered body image. Many women will have to learn to care for a new colostomy or how to catheterize a continent urostomy.

Women who have had a vulvectomy will need sensitive counseling to understand that she can still respond sexually. Patients who have had a vaginectomy with reconstruction as part of a pelvic exenteration will need extensive teaching to help them achieve successful sexual functioning.

Gynecologic surgeries can be very painful and disfiguring. The oncology nurse must be willing to consult the enterostomal therapist, licensed sex therapist, psyche liaison nurse, or any member of the health care team to ensure the woman the highest quality of life possible.

Chemotherapy

Chemotherapy also has an impact on a woman's quality of life and sexuality. Many women find it difficult to respond sexually when they are feeling the fatigue, nausea, and diarrhea that are common side effects of some chemotherapeutic agents. As part of the ongoing assessment of a patient, the nurse should ask if the treatments are interfering with the woman's relationship with her family and partner or her ability to respond sexually. Using this information, the nurse can intervene appropriately by obtaining pain medication, antiemetics, or antidiarrheals. If fatigue is a hindrance to sexual activity, the nurse may suggest a rest period before sex, the avoidance of a large meal or alcohol, or positioning that requires less exertion (Lamb and Wood, 1996.) The nurse may also suggest alternate forms of loving such as cuddling, kissing, and massage.

Many chemotherapeutic agents cause bone marrow suppression. When appropriate, the nurse must instruct the patient on neutropenic and thrombocytopenic [conditions related to white blood cells and blood platelets, respectively] precautions. If a woman is instructed to avoid people with colds or infections because of neutropenia or to avoid vaginal/anal penetration due to risk of thrombocytopenia, it can increase her feelings of isolation (Boyle, Bertin, and Bratschi, 1994). Again the nurse can suggest alternate forms of lovemaking. It may also help the couple to let the partner know that handwashing and wearing a mask will allow them to be close while still protecting the woman from infection.

Alopecia is another common side effect of chemotherapy. The loss of hair is a constant reminder to a woman that she is living with cancer. She may also feel embarrassed because she appears "different." The nurse can provide information about wigs, and many cancer centers have information about local suppliers that are knowledgeable in working with cancer patients. When doing chemotherapy teaching, the nurse should suggest choosing hats and wigs before the woman begins to lose her hair. Also, nurses may direct patients to support groups that provide classes in choosing colors and make-up to help cancer patients feel more self-confident. It is important for the nurse to let the woman discuss her feelings regarding her loss of hair and the reactions of those around her.

Radiation Therapy

Radiation therapy can be used to cure or control gynecological malignancies. Radiation is usually delivered as 6-7 weeks of external beam treatments. It is important for the nurse to reassure the woman and her partner that the patient is not radioactive and the partner cannot be contaminated by close physical contact. Some women require brachytherapy. This procedure consists of an implanted radioactive source at the tumor site for a period usually lasting 1–4 days. The patient is hospitalized with minimal contact with family or staff. Again, it is important for the nurse to stress that after the implant is removed there is no risk of contamination.

The primary function of the oncology nurse in the radiotherapy setting continues to be patient education, support and symptom management. Fatigue is the primary side effect the radiation patient will experience (Baumann, 1992). The nurse encourages patients to take frequent rest periods to conserve energy for their most important activities.

Radiation causes irritation to the intestinal lining, which causes diarrhea. Women receiving pelvic radiation are encouraged to modify their diets to bland and low residue while on treatment and for one month to six weeks after treatments end. Prescriptions for anti-diarrheals are often given to help maintain normal elimination. Careful weekly assessment will also aid in the early detection of cystitis and vaginitis and will lead to prompt treatment.

Radiation also causes changes to occur in the vagina. External beam radiation and implants damage both the vaginal epithelium and the basal layer of the mucosa. It also diminishes the size and number of small blood vessels in the vagina. All of these factors lead to vaginal stenosis [narrowing] and much drier, friable [brittle] tissue (Bruner, Lanciano, Keegan, Corn, Martin, and Hanks, 1993; Keegan and Lanciano, 1992).

Vaginal stenosis and scarring can lead to long-term sexual dysfunction and painful pelvic examinations. To help prevent these complications, the oncology nurse should obtain a sexual assessment as early as possible. If the patient has a partner, it is beneficial to involve them in the counseling.

As a means to preventing vaginal stenosis, all patients are given a vaginal dilator and instructions for use. Patients who are sexually active may continue to have intercourse throughout treatment. Couples are instructed to use a water based personal lubricant to protect the dry vaginal tissues. Also, adjusting positions for the woman's increased comfort may be suggested. Vaginal penetration with either the dilator or intercourse has been found to significantly decrease the occurrence of vaginal stenosis and dyspareunia [painful intercourse] (Bruner, et al., 1993).

Many women do experience vulvar and vaginal inflammation to such a degree toward the end of treatment that intercourse may be too painful. The nurse should reassure the patient that healing will take place and, in the meantime, she and her partner may want to use other forms of lovemaking.

Conclusion

Gynecologic cancers and treatments have many emotional as well as physical side effects that can greatly change a woman's sexuality and quality of life. One Australian study found that 52% of the study participants reported persistent physical difficulties after cancer treatment. The same study demonstrated that the amount of teaching, counseling, and practical support made a difference in the quality of life of cancer survivors (Steginga and Dunn, 1997). Oncology nurses need to be knowledgeable in the management of the physical side effects of surgery, chemotherapy, and radiotherapy. Nurses must also be comfortable with their own sexuality, so that they are better able to help women overcome fears related to body image and sexual function.

References

Anderson, B., and Lutgendorf, S. (1997). Quality of life in gynecologic cancer survivors. *CA: A Journal for Clinicians*, 47, 218-225.

Baumann, L. A. (1992). Radiation therapy and the gynecologic oncology patient. *Gynecologic Oncology Nursing*, 2(3), 1-3.

Boyle, N., Bertin, K., and Bratschi, A. (1994). A patient's guide to taxol. *Oncology Nursing Forum*, 21, 1569-1572.

Bruner, D. W., Lanciano, R., Keegan, M., Corn, B., Martin, E., and Hanks, G. E. (1993). Vaginal stenosis and sexual function following intracavitary radiation for the treatment of cervical and endometrial carcinoma. *International Journal of Radiation Oncology, Biology, Physics*, 27, 825-830.

Keegan, M. and Lanciano, R. (1992). Interstitial brachytherapy for gynecologic malignancies. *Gynecologic Oncology Nursing*, 2(4-5).

Lamb, M. A. and Wood, N. F. (1996). Sexuality and the cancer patient. *Gynecologic Oncology Nursing*, 6(3), 38-45.

Mann, D. (1996). Postoperative pain management: A professional nurse's obligation. *Gynecologic Oncology Nursing*, 6(1), 13-14.

Steninga, S. K. and Dunn, J. (1997). Women's experiences following treatment for gynecologic cancer. *Oncology Nursing Forum*, 24, 1403-1408.

— by Polly Sacco Ezzell RN, OCN
Radiation Oncology Nurse
University of Pennsylvania

Chapter 70

Questions about Fertility after Cancer

Introduction

A person is never ready to hear she has cancer. The diagnosis of cancer can bring on many emotions as well as questions. Time and careful thought are needed to sort through all the questions you may have about your disease, as well as the treatment and how it affects you.

People diagnosed with cancer are being treated with more intense treatments and living longer. Questions about starting a family may come up. After cancer treatment the chances of having children may be decreased or eliminated due to the effects of treatment. As difficult as it might be, the best time to discuss options for starting a family is at the beginning of your treatment. Questions like "Am I going to live?" and "When do I start treatment?" take priority over "Does my future allow for me to start a family?" Cancer can be a life-threatening illness and may need to be treated as soon as possible, but in many cases it is possible to take the steps needed to plan for future reproduction. Your doctor or health care team will help to guide you in your decisions. Be open and honest with your doctor and nurses about all your concerns and questions, They are there to help meet your needs.

Excerpted from "Fertility After Cancer... Options for Starting a Family," *Iowa Health Book: University of Iowa Cancer Center*, © 1997 The University of Iowa Hospitals and Clinics. Full text available at www.vh.org/Patients/IHB/Cancer/Fertility/Fertilitytext.html. Copyrighted material used with permission from University of Iowa Hospitals & Clinics Department of Nursing and Virtual Hospital, www.vh.org.

The Process of Pregnancy

Fertilization of a female's egg by a male's sperm is a complex process. It takes careful timing along with a functioning reproductive and hormonal system. Once the egg is fertilized it may implant in the woman's uterus (womb), where it should continue to develop and grow until birth.

Female Reproductive System

The egg (ovum) is produced by the ovaries. Each month an ovary releases a ripe egg. A gland that is close to the brain called the pituitary gland produces the hormone FSH (follicle stimulating hormone) and LH (luteinizing hormone). These hormones help the body make estrogen so the ovary can release the ripe egg. After the egg is released from the ovary it moves through the fallopian tube where the egg can be fertilized by a sperm. The egg is only ready for fertilization for about one day during the woman's cycle. If the egg is not fertilized during this time, the woman will not become pregnant. When the unfertilized egg travels into the uterus, the lining of the uterus will be shed and it will pass through the cervix with the menstrual flow. If the egg is fertilized, it travels into the uterus where it may implant into the lining of the uterus. The lining is rich with nutrients, blood and oxygen and feeds the growing baby and placenta (protective pouch around the baby).

Cancer Treatments and How They Affect the Ability to Have Children

The type of cancer you have may change the way your reproductive system works even before you receive treatment. Treatment can also affect your fertility or ability to have children. Following are treatments that may alter your ability to have children.

Chemotherapy

Cancer treatment with chemotherapy may affect your fertility. The effects of chemotherapy depend on: your age, the types of drugs, the amounts of the drugs you receive, and how many months your treatment lasts.

Women who receive chemotherapy may have a change in their periods or menstrual cycles. Periods may become irregular, and flow may decrease or stop altogether. Some women develop symptoms of menopause such as vaginal dryness and hot flashes. Women older than forty years of age are more likely to have a loss of menstrual cycles for life. Younger women may have irregular periods during chemotherapy and may resume normal periods following treatment. Women who resume normal cycles after treatment may still be at risk for early menopause. Birth control methods need to be discussed with your physician before treatment begins. Pregnancy during treatment must be avoided and some type of birth control should be used. Chemotherapy can be harmful to the unborn child. If you are pregnant or think you may be, you need to tell your doctor right away.

Sometimes hormones will be given with chemotherapy to stop women from cycling during treatment. This may improve the chances of having children after the treatment is completed. It may not be an option that you take hormones or become pregnant due to the effects it may have on the cancer. Talk with your doctor about the best options for you.

Some chemotherapy drugs cause more damage to reproductive cells than others. A class of chemotherapy drugs called "alkylating agents" are known to be damaging. Table 70.1. is a list including some of the chemotherapy drugs that are especially damaging.

Radiation Therapy

Women may stop having menstrual cycles and experience other symptoms of menopause during radiation treatment to the pelvic area. Sometimes the damage is short term but often it is for life. Radiation may cause damage to the fetus (unborn child), so pregnancy should be avoided during treatment. Radiation therapy should not be considered as adequate birth control. Women should immediately discuss all birth control matters with their physicians. If you are pregnant before treatment, special care should be taken to protect the fetus from the radiation. This should be discussed with your doctor. The use of radiation in the pelvic area along with chemotherapy increases your chances of being unable to have children. As with chemotherapy, hormones are sometimes given along with treatment to improve the chances of having children when treatment is completed. Questions or concerns about radiation treatments can be directed to your doctors.

Surgical Treatment

To understand how surgery may affect a woman's ability to give birth, it may help to review parts of the female anatomy and their roles in reproduction.

Table 70.1. Chemotherapies Damaging to Reproductive Cells and the Common Cancers Treated

Cytoxan*	leukemias, aplastic anemia, lymphomas, breast and ovarian cancer
Ifosfamide*	sarcomas, breast and urologic cancers
L-Pam*	multiple myeloma
Nitrogen Mustard*	Hodgkin's disease
Thiotepa*	breast cancer
Busulfan*	leukemias
BCNU*	brain tumors
Chlorambucil*	leukemias
ARA-C*	leukemias, lymphomas
Cisplatin*	head/neck tumors, lung cancer, breast and ovarian cancer, lymphomas, testicular cancer
Adriamycin	breast/ovarian cancer, lymphomas, Hodgkin's disease, sarcomas, small cell lung cancer
Procarbazine	Hodgkin's disease
Velban	Hodgkin's disease, lymphomas, breast, and testicular cancer

Other chemotherapy drugs may cause damage to reproductive cells as well.

*Alkylating Agents

The uterus is where the egg settles after it is fertilized with sperm. The cervix is the entrance to the uterus at the top of the vagina. The vagina is a muscular tube that connects the external and internal parts of the reproductive tract. The clitoris is involved with sexual pleasure for a woman. The outer and inner lips (labia) pad and protect the clitoris, urethra (tube that urine passes through from the bladder), and the vagina. They also are responsible for the external appearance of a woman's genitals.

If the ovaries or uterus are removed, there are likely to be changes in hormones. If a woman is still having her menstrual cycles, and has her ovaries removed, she may have symptoms of menopause, such as hot flashes, mood swings, and irritability. If there is no uterus, child-birth is no longer possible.

If a surgery is done which removes the ovaries but not the uterus, cervix, or vagina, the ability to carry and deliver a baby remains. In this situation, in vitro fertilization with donor eggs may be an option.

There are some surgical procedures which may affect a woman's sensations related to sexual intimacy including intercourse. Some surgeries may alter the sensation of arousal from physical touch. Other surgeries may decrease vaginal lubrication which may make intercourse uncomfortable. If you have questions about how a surgery may affect your sensations or ability to have children, be sure to discuss this with your doctor before the surgery.

Any surgery which involves removal of the uterus, ovaries, clitoris, labia, vagina, colon, rectum, or bladder may after a woman's sexual pleasure or ability to have a baby. Some cancer surgeries which will alter a woman's ability to have a child are:

- oophorectomy (removal of the ovaries);

- hysterectomy (removal of the uterus);

- pelvic exenteration (removal of the uterus, cervix, ovaries, fallopian tubes, vagina, bladder, urethra, and rectum);

- radical cystectomy (removal of the bladder, uterus, ovaries, fallopian tubes, cervix, urethra, and part of the vagina).

Having Children after Cancer: Medically Assisted Ways to Achieve a Pregnancy

The options to start a family have been improved through recent advances in technology. Success is not guaranteed, but it allows women the chance to contribute to the genetic make-up of their child.

Freezing Embryos (Fertilized Eggs)

At this time a safe way to freeze unfertilized eggs has not been found. However it is possible to freeze fertilized eggs (early embryos). Women who need cancer treatment may choose to freeze their own eggs, fertilized by their husband's sperm before beginning treatment. It takes three to ten weeks to stimulate the ovaries to produce mature eggs and to retrieve the egg. If the woman's menstrual cycle is at the right stage, an unstimulated "natural cycle" may allow for the collection of an egg.

If time is not a factor, the couple may choose ovarian stimulation and retrieval of eggs. The ovaries are stimulated with hormone injections to ripen several eggs (oocytes). After about two weeks of careful monitoring of blood levels and ultrasound imaging of the ovaries, the eggs are retrieved. This is done with a minor surgical procedure using the guidance of ultrasound, and needle aspiration. Medications are given through your veins to help you to be comfortable. Sometimes medication (anesthesia) is given in your spine to help to prevent pain. It may not be possible to get hormone injections, due to the adverse effects they can have on certain types of cancers. If you are interested in freezing embryos (fertilized eggs), talk with your doctor to see if it is an option for you.

Fertilization takes place when the eggs are placed with sperm in a laboratory. These early embryos (fertilized eggs) are frozen and stored. After recovery from the cancer, transfer of these frozen fertilized eggs into your uterus can be an option for pregnancy.

In Vitro Fertilization

In vitro fertilization assists the natural reproductive process, by combining the sperm and egg in a small amount of fluid outside of the body. This is done in a laboratory. A fertilized egg is transferred to either the fallopian tube or uterus 24 to 48 hours after the egg is fertilized. There are a variety of insemination and embryo transfer methods available. The costs for an assisted fertilization procedure can range in the thousands of dollars. The amount covered by insurance may vary.

Donor Eggs and Embryos

When the time before cancer treatment does not allow for the weeks of preparation needed to preserve fertilized eggs, in vitro fertilization using donor eggs may be an option.

The donor will get hormone shots to stimulate development of several eggs. The person who will receive the egg will get medications to prepare the uterus for a pregnancy and to get her cycle on the same schedule as the donor.

Timing of the donor's egg retrieval is determined by careful monitoring of blood levels, and ultrasound imaging of the growth and number of the eggs. After the eggs are retrieved they are combined with the sperm from the husband of the woman receiving the donor egg. This is done in a laboratory. The early embryos (fertilized eggs) are then transferred to the uterus through the cervix, or into a fallopian tube. Careful medical, psychological, and genetic screening is required of both the donor and the recipient.

Couples who have been treated with in vitro fertilization often freeze some of their fertilized eggs (embryos). If they find that they cannot use their frozen embryos they may decide to donate them to a couple that cannot have children. Donated embryos will be offered first to couples who have no living children, or both partners have a problem that interferes with having children.

Medical evaluation including sexually transmitted disease testing and genetic screening will be required of donor participants. Recipients are also prepared by counseling, medical history and examination, and blood tests. Many weeks of hormone medications are given to the woman receiving the donor embryo, to prepare the uterus for a pregnancy.

Emotional Support

The decision to attempt a medically assisted reproductive procedure is one that carries a lot of emotion. There are difficult questions that a couple must think about and discuss before they can come to a decision. What is the prognosis of the partner with the diagnosis of cancer? Is the healthy partner prepared or willing to accept the responsibilities of being a single parent if their partner should relapse or die? What effects will this have on the children and their future? These are very tough questions to think about, but are questions that should be discussed. Counseling is a part of the process if you decide to pursue a medically assisted reproductive procedure. You can also discuss any concerns or questions you have with your doctor before making a decision.

Some people may feel that they are in a conflict with their religious beliefs if they choose medically assisted reproduction. These feelings need to be explored with your clergy or religious leader and resolved before you make your final decision.

There may be difficult legal and ethical issues to think about before you plan a medically assisted reproductive technique. Couples who have frozen embryos (fertilized eggs) for future use need to discuss what would be done with the embryos if something happened to one of the partners, or if the marriage was ended before they were used. If there are embryos stored and the couple divorce, should one person be awarded custody rights? These are legally and ethically charged questions that are very difficult to discuss. If it comes at a time when treatment for cancer is a concern, it is sometimes harder to talk about.

Using donated sperm or donated eggs brings with it a different set of concerns. Will it be more comforting to know the donor or is it better not to know? What will the child need to or want to know about the donor? What should family and friends know about the donor that was involved in your child's birth? All questions need to be answered before deciding to participate in medically assisted reproduction.

There are no guarantees with medically assisted reproduction, but it does allow a chance to have a child. It may take several tries to become pregnant and for some couples it may never happen. Couples should be prepared to handle the feelings of disappointment that may come if they are unable to conceive a child, as well as the feelings experienced when a pregnancy is achieved. Following a pregnancy the possibilities of a miscarriage or birth defects are the same as with a "naturally" conceived pregnancy. Being well informed and prepared to make a decision on the options of medically assisted reproduction will allow you to feel that you have some control over the decision to have a child.

Costs

Financial concerns may decide what options you are able to pursue. Health insurance coverage for the diagnosis and treatment of infertility varies from plan to plan. Some insurance providers pay for both diagnosis and treatment, some pay diagnosis only, and some pay nothing for infertility procedures. It is important for patients to write to insurance providers or call and confirm infertility benefits.

For More Information

For more information about fertility after cancer treatment, contact:

The University of Iowa Hospitals and Clinics
Center for Advanced Reproductive Care
Department of Obstetrics and Gynecology
Iowa City, Iowa 52242-1009
Phone: (319) 356-1767

Part Ten

Additional Help and Information

Chapter 71

Glossary of Gynecologic and Cancer Terms

A

Abdomen: The part of the body that contains the pancreas, stomach, intestines, liver, gallbladder, and other organs.

Abnormal: Not normal. May be cancerous or premalignant.

Adjuvant therapy: Treatment given after the primary treatment to make it work better. Adjuvant therapy may include chemotherapy, radiation therapy, or hormone therapy.

Alteration, altered: Change; different from original.

Anesthesia: Drugs or gases given before and during surgery so the patient won't feel pain. The patient may be awake or asleep.

Anesthesiologist: A doctor who gives drugs or gases that keep you comfortable during surgery.

Areola: The area of dark-colored skin on the breast that surrounds the nipple.

Ascites: Abnormal buildup of fluid in the abdomen.

Aspirate: Fluid withdrawn from a lump, often a cyst.

Definitions provided in this glossary were compiled from National Institutes of Health (NIH) Pub. Nos. 95-2047, 98-1556, 98-1562, 98-4251, 00-1556, 00-1561, and 00-1566.

Aspiration: Removal of fluid from a lump, often a cyst, with a needle and a syringe.

Atypical hyperplasia: A benign (noncancerous) condition in which cells have abnormal features and are increased in number.

Autologous bone marrow transplantation: A procedure in which bone marrow is removed from a person, stored, and then given back to the person following intensive treatment.

Axilla: The underarm or armpit.

Axillary: Having to do with the armpit.

Axillary lymph node dissection: Surgery to remove lymph nodes found in the armpit region.

B

Barium enema: A procedure in which a liquid with barium in it is put into the rectum and colon by way of the anus. Barium is a silver-white metallic compound that helps to show the image of the lower gastrointestinal tract on an x-ray.

Benign: Not malignant; does not invade nearby tissue or spread to other parts of the body.

Biological therapy: Treatment that uses the body's immune system to fight cancer or to lessen the side effects that may be caused by some cancer treatments. Also known as immunotherapy.

Biopsy: A procedure used to remove cells or tissues in order to look at them under a microscope to check for signs of disease. When an entire tumor or lesion is removed, the procedure is called an excisional biopsy. When only a sample of tissue is removed, the procedure is called an incisional biopsy or core biopsy. When a sample of tissue or fluid is removed with a needle, the procedure is called a needle biopsy or fine-needle aspiration.

Bladder: The organ that stores urine.

Bone marrow: The soft material inside bones. Blood cells are produced in the bone marrow.

Brachytherapy: A procedure in which radioactive material sealed in needles, seeds, wires, or catheters is placed directly into or near a tumor. Also called internal radiation, implant radiation, or interstitial radiation therapy.

Breast cancer in situ: Very early or noninvasive abnormal cells that are confined to the ducts or lobules in the breast. Also known as DCIS or LCIS.

Breast reconstruction: Surgery to rebuild a breast's shape after a mastectomy.

Breast-conserving surgery: An operation to remove the breast cancer but not the breast itself. Types of breast-conserving surgery include lumpectomy (removal of the lump), quadrantectomy (removal of one quarter of the breast), and segmental mastectomy (removal of the cancer as well as some of the breast tissue around the tumor and the lining over the chest muscles below the tumor).

C

CA-125: Substance sometimes found in an increased amount in the blood, other body fluids, or tissues and that may suggest the presence of some types of cancer.

Cancer: A term for diseases in which abnormal cells divide without control or order. Cancer cells can invade nearby tissues and can spread through the bloodstream and lymphatic systems to other parts of the body.

Carcinogen: Any substance that causes cancer.

Carcinoma: Cancer that begins in the lining or covering of an organ.

Carcinoma in situ: Cancer that involves only the cells in which it began and has not spread to neighboring tissues.

Catheter: A flexible tube used to deliver fluids into or withdraw fluids from the body.

Cauterization: The destruction of tissue with a hot instrument, an electrical current, or a caustic substance.

Cell: The individual unit that makes up all of the tissues of the body. All living things are made up of one or more cells.

Central nervous system (CNS): The brain and spinal cord.

Cerebrospinal fluid (CSF): The fluid flowing around the brain and spinal cord. Cerebrospinal fluid is produced in the ventricles in the brain.

Cervical intraepithelial neoplasia (CIN): A general term for the growth of abnormal cells on the surface of the cervix. Numbers from 1 to 3 may be used to describe how much of the cervix contains abnormal cells.

Cervix: The lower, narrow end of the uterus that forms a canal between the uterus and vagina.

Chemotherapy: Treatment with drugs to kill or slow the growth of cancer cells; also used to shrink tumors before surgery.

Clavicle: Collarbone.

Clear margins: An area of normal tissue that surrounds cancerous tissue, as seen during examination under a microscope.

Clinical trials: Research studies, where patients help scientist find the best way to prevent, detect, diagnose or treat diseases.

Colon: The long, coiled, tubelike organ that removes water from digested food. The remaining material, solid waste called stool, moves through the colon to the rectum and leaves the body through the anus.

Colonoscope: A thin, lighted tube used to examine the inside of the colon.

Colonoscopy: An examination of the inside of the colon using a thin, lighted tube (called a colonoscope) inserted into the rectum. If abnormal areas are seen, tissue can be removed and examined under a microscope to determine whether disease is present.

Colony-stimulating factors: Substances that stimulate the production of blood cells. Colony-stimulating factors include granulocyte colony-stimulating factors (also called G-CSF and filgrastim), granulocyte-macrophage colony-stimulating factors (also called GM-CSF and sargramostim), and promegapoietin.

Colposcopy: Examination of the vagina and cervix using a lighted magnifying instrument called a colposcope.

Computed tomography: A series of detailed pictures of areas inside the body; the pictures are created by a computer linked to an x-ray machine. Also called computed tomography (CT) scan or computerized axial tomography (CAT) scan.

Condylomata acuminata: Genital warts caused by certain human papillomaviruses (HPVs).

Conization: Surgery to remove a cone-shaped piece of tissue from the cervix and cervical canal. Conization may be used to diagnose or treat a cervical condition. Also called cone biopsy.

Corpus: The body of the uterus.

Cryosurgery: Treatment performed with an instrument that freezes and destroys abnormal tissues. This procedure is a form of cryotherapy.

Cyst: A sac or capsule filled with fluid.

Cystoscopy: Examination of the bladder and urethra using a thin, lighted instrument (called a cystoscope) inserted into the urethra. Tissue samples can be removed and examined under a microscope to determine whether disease is present.

D

Diagnosis: The process of identifying a disease by the signs and symptoms.

Diathermy: The use of heat to destroy abnormal cells. Also called cauterization or electrodiathermy.

Diethylstilbestrol: DES. A synthetic hormone that was prescribed from the early 1940s until 1971 to help women with complications of pregnancy. DES has been linked to an increased risk of clear cell carcinoma of the vagina in daughters of women who used DES. DES may also increase the risk of breast cancer in women who used DES.

Digital rectal examination (DRE): An examination in which a doctor inserts a lubricated, gloved finger into the rectum to feel for abnormalities.

Dilation and curettage (D&C): A minor operation in which the cervix is expanded enough (dilation) to permit the cervical canal and uterine lining to be scraped with a spoon-shaped instrument called a curette (curettage).

Dilator: A device used to stretch or enlarge an opening.

Douche: A procedure in which water or a medicated solution is used to clean the vagina and cervix.

Duct: A small channel in the breast through which milk passes from the lobes to the nipple.

Ductal carcinoma in situ (DCIS; intraductal carcinoma): Abnormal cells that involve only the lining of a milk duct.

Dysplasia: Cells that look abnormal under a microscope but are not cancer.

E

Endocervical curettage: The scraping of the mucous membrane of the cervical canal using a spoon-shaped instrument called a curette.

Endometriosis: A benign condition in which tissue that looks like endometrial tissue grows in abnormal places in the abdomen.

Endometrium: The layer of tissue that lines the uterus.

Epithelial carcinoma: Cancer that begins in the cells that line an organ.

Erythrocytes: Red blood cells that carry oxygen from the lungs to cells in all parts of the body, and carry carbon dioxide from the cells back to the lungs.

Estrogen receptor test: Lab test to determine if breast cancer depends on estrogen for growth.

Estrogen replacement therapy (ERT): Hormones (estrogen, progesterone, or both) given to postmenopausal women or to women who have had their ovaries surgically removed. Hormones are given to replace the estrogen no longer produced by the ovaries.

Estrogens: A family of hormones that promote the development and maintenance of female sex characteristics.

Excisional biopsy: A surgical procedure in which an entire lump or suspicious area is removed for diagnosis. The tissue is then examined under a microscope.

External radiation: Radiation therapy that uses a machine to aim high-energy rays at the cancer. Also called external-beam radiation.

F

Fallopian tubes: Part of the female reproductive tract. The long slender tubes through which eggs pass from the ovaries to the uterus.

Fecal occult blood test: A test to check for blood in stool. (Fecal refers to stool; occult means hidden.)

Fertility: The ability to produce children.

Fibroid: A benign smooth muscle tumor, usually in the uterus or gastrointestinal tract. Also called leiomyoma.

Fine-needle aspiration: The removal of tissue or fluid with a needle for examination under a microscope. Also called needle biopsy.

Fundus: The larger part of a hollow organ that is farthest away from the organ's opening. The bladder, gallbladder, stomach, uterus, eye, and cavity of the middle ear all have a fundus.

G

Gene: The functional and physical unit of heredity passed from parent to offspring. Genes are pieces of DNA, and most genes contain the information for making a specific protein.

Germ cell tumors: Tumors that begin in the cells that give rise to sperm or eggs. They can occur virtually anywhere in the body and can be either benign or malignant.

Grade: The grade of a tumor depends on how abnormal the cancer cells look under a microscope and how quickly the tumor is likely to grow and spread. Grading systems are different for each type of cancer.

Graft-versus-host disease (GVHD): A reaction of donated bone marrow or peripheral stem cells against a person's tissue.

Gynecologic oncologist: A doctor who specializes in treating cancers of the female reproductive organs.

Gynecologist: A doctor who specializes in the care and treatment of women's reproductive systems.

H

Herpes virus: A member of the herpes family of viruses.

Hormone receptor tests: Lab tests that determine if a breast cancer depends on female hormones (estrogen and progesterone) for growth.

Hormone replacement therapy (HRT): Hormones (estrogen, progesterone, or both) given to postmenopausal women or women who have had their ovaries surgically removed, to replace the estrogen no longer produced by the ovaries.

Hormone therapy: Treatment of cancer by removing, blocking, or adding hormones. Also called endocrine therapy.

Hormones: Chemicals produced by glands in the body and circulated in the bloodstream. Hormones control the actions of certain cells or organs.

Human papillomavirus (HPV): A virus that causes abnormal tissue growth (warts) and is often associated with some types of cancer.

Hyperplasia: An abnormal increase in the number of cells in an organ or tissue.

Hysterectomy: An operation in which the uterus is removed.

I

Imaging: Tests that produce pictures of areas inside the body.

Immune system: The complex group of organs and cells that defends the body against infection or disease.

Immunotherapy: Treatment to stimulate or restore the ability of the immune system to fight infection and disease. Also used to lessen side effects that may be caused by some cancer treatments. Also called biological therapy or biological response modifier (BRM) therapy.

Implant: A silicone gel-filled or saline-filled sac inserted under the chest muscle to restore breast shape.

Incision: A cut made in the body during surgery.

Incisional biopsy: A surgical procedure in which a portion of a lump or suspicious area is removed for diagnosis. The tissue is then examined under a microscope.

Infertility: The inability to produce children.

Infiltrating breast cancer: Cancer that has spread to nearby tissue, lymph nodes under the arm, or other parts of the body. Also called invasive breast cancer.

Inflammatory breast cancer: A type of breast cancer in which the breast looks red and swollen, and feels warm. The skin of the breast may also show the pitted appearance called peau d'orange (like the skin of an orange). The redness and warmth occur because the cancer cells block the lymph vessels in the skin.

Interferon: A biological response modifier (a substance that can improve the body's natural response to disease). Interferons interfere with the division of cancer cells and can slow tumor growth. There are several types of interferons, including interferon-alpha, -beta, and -gamma. These substances are normally produced by the body. They are also made in the laboratory for use in treating cancer and other diseases.

Interleukin-2 (IL-2): A type of biological response modifier (a substance that can improve the body's natural response to disease) that stimulates the growth of certain disease-fighting blood cells in the immune system. These substances are normally produced by the body. Aldesleukin is IL-2 that is made in the laboratory for use in treating cancer and other diseases.

Internal radiation: A procedure in which radioactive material sealed in needles, seeds, wires, or catheters is placed directly into or near the tumor. Also called brachytherapy, implant radiation, or interstitial radiation therapy.

Intraductal carcinoma: Abnormal cells that are contained within the milk duct and have not spread outside the duct. Also known as DCIS (ductal carcinoma in situ).

Intraepithelial: Within the layer of cells that form the surface or lining of an organ.

Intraperitoneal chemotherapy: Treatment in which anticancer drugs are put directly into the abdominal cavity through a thin tube.

Intraperitoneal radiation therapy: Treatment in which a radioactive liquid is put directly into the abdomen through a thin tube.

Intrathecal chemotherapy: Anticancer drugs that are injected into the fluid-filled space between the thin layers of tissue that cover the brain and spinal cord.

Intravenous (IV): Injection into a vein.

Intravenous pyelogram (IVP): A series of x-rays of the kidneys, ureters, and bladder. The x-rays are taken after a dye is injected into a blood vessel. The dye is concentrated in the urine, which outlines the kidneys, ureters, and bladder on the x-rays.

Invasive cancer: Cancer that has spread beyond the layer of tissue in which it developed and is growing into surrounding, healthy tissues. Also called infiltrating cancer.

L

Laparotomy: A surgical incision made in the wall of the abdomen.

Laser: A device that concentrates light into an intense, narrow beam used to cut or destroy tissue. It is used in microsurgery, photodynamic therapy, and for a variety of diagnostic purposes.

Lesion: An area of abnormal tissue change.

Leukocytes: White blood cells that defend the body against infections and other diseases.

Lobe, lobule: Located at the end of a breast duct, the part of the breast where milk is made. Each breast contains 15 to 20 sections, called lobes, each with many smaller lobules.

Lobular carcinoma in situ (LCIS): Abnormal cells found in the lobules of the breast. This condition seldom becomes invasive cancer; however, having lobular carcinoma in situ increases one's risk of developing breast cancer in either breast.

Local therapy: Treatment that affects cells in the tumor and the area close to it.

Lower GI series: X-rays of the colon and rectum (lower gastrointestinal tract) that are taken after the person is given a barium enema.

Lubricants: Oily or slippery substances.

Lumpectomy: Surgery to remove the tumor and a small amount of normal tissue around it.

Lymph: The almost colorless fluid that travels through the lymphatic system and carries cells that help fight infection and disease.

Lymph nodes: Small bean-shaped organs (sometimes called lymph glands); part of the lymphatic system. Lymph nodes under the arm drain fluid from the chest and arm.

Lymphatic system: The tissues and organs that produce, store, and carry white blood cells that fight infection and other diseases. This system includes the bone marrow, spleen, thymus, and lymph nodes and a network of thin tubes that carry lymph and white blood cells. These tubes branch, like blood vessels, into all the tissues of the body.

Lymphedema: Swelling in the arm caused by fluid that can build up when underarm lymph nodes are removed during breast cancer surgery or damaged by radiation.

M

Magnetic resonance imaging (MRI): A procedure in which a magnet linked to a computer is used to create detailed pictures of areas inside the body.

Malignant: Cancerous; capable of invading, spreading and destroying tissue.

Mammogram: An x-ray of the breast.

Mammography: The use of x-rays to create a picture of the breast.

Mastectomy: Surgery to remove the breast (or as much of the breast tissue as possible).

Medical oncologist: A doctor who specializes in diagnosing and treating cancer using chemotherapy, hormonal therapy, and biological therapy. A medical oncologist often serves as the main caretaker of someone who has cancer and coordinates treatment provided by other specialists.

Melanocytes: Cells in the skin that produce and contain the pigment called melanin.

Melanoma: A form of skin cancer that arises in melanocytes, the cells that produce pigment. Melanoma usually begins in a mole.

Menopause: The time of life when a woman's menstrual periods stop permanently. Also called "change of life."

Menstruation: Periodic discharge of blood and tissue from the uterus. Until menopause, menstruation occurs approximately every 28 days when a woman is not pregnant.

Metastasis: The spread of cancer from one part of the body to another. Tumors formed from cells that have spread are called "secondary tumors" and contain cells that are like those in the original (primary) tumor. The plural is metastases.

Microcalcifications: Tiny deposits of calcium that can be detected by mammography. A cluster of small specks of calcium may indicate that cancer is present.

Modified radical mastectomy: Surgical procedure in which the breast, some of the lymph nodes in the armpit, and the lining over the chest muscles are removed.

Monoclonal antibodies: Laboratory-produced substances that can locate and bind to cancer cells wherever they are in the body. Many monoclonal antibodies are used in cancer detection or therapy; each one recognizes a different protein on certain cancer cells. Monoclonal antibodies can be used alone, or they can be used to deliver drugs, toxins, or radioactive material directly to a tumor.

Mutation: Any change in the DNA of a cell. Mutations may be caused by mistakes during cell division, or they may be caused by exposure to DNA-damaging agents in the environment. Mutations can be harmful, beneficial, or have no effect. If they occur in cells that make eggs or sperm, they can be inherited; if mutations occur in other types of cells, they are not inherited. Certain mutations may lead to cancer or other diseases.

Myometrium: The muscular outer layer of the uterus.

N

Negative: A lab test result that is normal; failing to show a positive result for the specific disease or condition for which the test is being done.

Neoadjuvant therapy: Treatment given before the primary treatment. Neoadjuvant therapy can be chemotherapy, radiation therapy, or hormone therapy.

Nipple discharge: Fluid coming from the nipple.

Nutritionist: A health professional with specialized training in nutrition, who can offer help and choices about the foods you eat.

O

Obstruction: Blockage of a passageway.

Omentum: A fold of the peritoneum (the thin tissue that lines the abdomen) that surrounds the stomach and other organs in the abdomen.

Oncologist: Cancer specialist; a doctor who uses chemotherapy or hormonal therapy to treat cancer.

Oncology nurse: A nurse with special training in caring for cancer patients.

Oncology pharmacy specialist: A person who prepares anticancer drugs in consultation with an oncologist.

Oophorectomy: Surgery to remove one or both ovaries.

Osteoporosis: A condition that is characterized by a decrease in bone mass and density, causing bones to become fragile.

Ovaries: The pair of female reproductive organs that produce eggs and hormones.

Ovulation: The release of an egg from an ovary during the menstrual cycle.

P

Palpation: Examination by pressing on the surface of the body to feel the organs or tissues underneath.

Pap test: The collection of cells from the cervix for examination under a microscope. It is used to detect changes that may be cancer or may lead to cancer, and can show noncancerous conditions, such as infection or inflammation. Also called a Pap smear.

Pathologist: A doctor who examines tissues and cells under a microscope to determine if they are normal or abnormal.

Pathology report: Diagnosis made by a pathologist based on microscopic evidence.

Pelvis: The lower part of the abdomen, located between the hip bones.

Peripheral stem cell transplantation: A method of replacing blood-forming cells destroyed by cancer treatment. Immature blood cells (stem cells) in the circulating blood that are similar to those in the bone marrow are given to the person after treatment to help the bone marrow recover and continue producing healthy blood cells. Transplantation may be autologous (the person's blood cells saved earlier), allogeneic (blood cells donated by someone else), or syngeneic (blood cells donated by an identical twin). Also called peripheral stem cell support.

Peritoneum: The tissue that lines the abdominal wall and covers most of the organs in the abdomen.

PDQ: National Cancer Institute's computer database that contains up-to-date cancer information for scientists, health professionals, patients, and the public.

Physical therapist: A health professional who teaches exercises that help restore arm and shoulder movement and build back strength after breast cancer surgery.

Plastic surgeon: A surgeon who specializes in reducing scarring or disfigurement that may occur as a result of accidents, birth defects, or treatment for diseases.

Platelets: The part of a blood cell that helps prevent bleeding by causing blood clots to form at the site of an injury.

Polyp: A growth that protrudes from a mucous membrane.

Positive: A lab test result that reveals the presence of a specific disease or condition for which the test is being done.

Positron emission tomography (PET) scan: A computerized image of the metabolic activity of body tissues used to determine the presence of disease.

Precancerous: A term used to describe a condition that may (or is likely to) become cancer. Also called premalignant.

Primary care doctor: A doctor who usually manages your health care and can discuss cancer treatment choices with you.

Proctosigmoidoscopy: An examination of the rectum and the lower part of the colon using a thin, lighted tube called a sigmoidoscope.

Progesterone: A female hormone.

Progesterone receptor test: Lab test to determine if a breast cancer depends on progesterone for growth.

Prognosis: The likely outcome or course of a disease; the chance of recovery.

Prosthesis: An artificial replacement of a part of the body. A breast prosthesis is a breast form that may be worn under clothing. Also, a technical name for an implant that is placed under the chest muscle in breast reconstruction.

Psychologist: A specialist who can talk with you and your family about emotional and personal matters, and can help you make decisions.

R

Radiation oncologist: A doctor who uses radiation therapy to treat cancer.

Radiation therapist: A health professional who gives radiation treatment.

Radiation therapy: The use of high-energy radiation from x-rays, neutrons, and other sources to kill cancer cells and shrink tumors. Radiation may come from a machine outside the body (external-beam radiation therapy) or from material called radioisotopes. Radioisotopes produce radiation and can be placed in or near a tumor or near cancer cells. This type of radiation treatment is called internal radiation therapy, implant radiation, or brachytherapy. Systemic radiation therapy uses a radioactive substance such as a radiolabeled monoclonal antibody that circulates throughout the body. Also called radiotherapy.

Radiologist: A doctor with special training in reading x-rays and performing specialized x-ray procedures.

Radical mastectomy: Surgery for breast cancer in which the breast, chest muscles, and all of the lymph nodes under the arm are removed. For many years, this was the operation most used, but it is used now only when the tumor has spread to the chest muscles. Also called the Halsted radical mastectomy.

Radionuclide scanning: A test that produces pictures (scans) of internal parts of the body. The person is given an injection or swallows a small amount of radioactive material; a machine called a scanner then measures the radioactivity in certain organs.

Rectum: The last 8 to 10 inches of the large intestine.

Recur: To occur again. Recurrence is the return of cancer, at the same site as the original (primary) tumor or in another location, after the tumor had disappeared.

Remission: A decrease in or disappearance of signs and symptoms of cancer. In partial remission, some, but not all, signs and symptoms of cancer have disappeared. In complete remission, all signs and symptoms of cancer have disappeared, although there still may be cancer in the body.

Risk factor: A habit, trait, condition, or genetic alteration that increases a person's chance of developing a disease.

S

Salpingo-oophorectomy: Surgical removal of the fallopian tubes and ovaries.

Sarcoma: A cancer of the bone, cartilage, fat, muscle, blood vessels or other connective or supportive tissue.

Schiller test: A test in which iodine is applied to the cervix. The iodine colors healthy cells brown; abnormal cells remain unstained, usually appearing white or yellow.

Screening: Checking for disease when there are no symptoms.

Second-look surgery: Surgery performed after primary treatment to determine whether tumor cells remain.

Segmental mastectomy: The removal of the cancer as well as some of the breast tissue around the tumor and the lining over the chest muscles below the tumor. Usually some of the lymph nodes under the arm are also taken out. Sometimes called partial mastectomy.

Sentinel lymph node: The first lymph node(s) to which cancer cells spread after leaving the area of the primary tumor. Presence of cancer cells in this node alerts the doctor that the tumor has spread to the lymphatic system.

Side effects: Problems that occur when treatment affects healthy cells. Common side effects of cancer treatment are fatigue, nausea, vomiting, decreased blood cell counts, hair loss, and mouth sores.

Silicone: A synthetic gel that is used as an outer coating on breast implants and to make up the inside filling of some implants.

Social worker: A professional who can talk with you and your family about your emotional or physical needs and can help you find support services.

Sonogram: A computer picture of areas inside the body created by bouncing sound waves off organs and other tissues. Also called ultrasonogram or ultrasound.

Speculum: An instrument used to widen an opening of the body to make it easier to look inside.

Squamous cell carcinoma: Cancer that begins in squamous cells, which are thin, flat cells resembling fish scales. Squamous cells are found in the tissue that forms the surface of the skin, the lining of the hollow organs of the body, and the passages of the respiratory and digestive tracts. Also called epidermoid carcinoma.

Squamous intraepithelial lesion (SIL): A general term for the abnormal growth of squamous cells on the surface of the cervix. The changes in the cells are described as low grade or high grade, depending on how much of the cervix is affected and how abnormal the cells appear.

Stage: The extent of a cancer, especially whether the disease has spread from the original site to other parts of the body.

Staging: Performing exams and tests to learn the extent of the cancer within the body, especially whether the disease has spread from the original site to other parts of the body.

Standard: Usual, common, customary.

Stem cell: The immature cells in blood and bone marrow from which all mature blood cells develop.

Surgeon or **surgical oncologist:** A doctor who performs biopsies and other surgical procedures such as removing a lump or a breast.

Surgery: An operation; a procedure to remove or repair a part of the body or to find out whether disease is present.

Systemic therapy: Treatment that uses substances that travel through the bloodstream, reaching and affecting cells all over the body.

T

Therapy: Treatment.

Tissue: A group or layer of cells that together perform a specific function.

Tissue flap reconstruction: A flap of tissues is surgically relocated from another area of the body to the chest, and formed into a new breast mound.

Total mastectomy: Removal of the breast. Also called simple mastectomy.

Transvaginal ultrasound: A procedure used to examine the vagina, uterus, fallopian tubes, and bladder. An instrument is inserted into the vagina, and sound waves bounce off organs inside the pelvic area. These sound waves create echoes, which a computer uses to create a picture called a sonogram. Also called TVS.

Tubal ligation: An operation to tie the fallopian tubes closed. This procedure prevents pregnancy by blocking the passage of eggs from the ovaries to the uterus.

Tumor: An abnormal mass of tissue that results from excessive cell division. Tumors perform no useful body function. They may be benign (not cancerous) or malignant (cancerous).

Tumor debulking: Surgically removing as much of the tumor as possible.

Tumor marker: A substance sometimes found in an increased amount in the blood, other body fluids, or tissues and which may mean that a certain type of cancer is in the body. Examples of tumor markers include CA 125 (ovarian cancer), CA 15-3 (breast cancer), CEA (ovarian, lung, breast, pancreas, and gastrointestinal tract cancers), and PSA (prostate cancer). Also called biomarker.

U

Ultrasound test: A test that bounces sound waves off tissues and internal organs and changes the echoes into pictures (sonograms).

Uterus: The small, hollow, pear-shaped organ in a woman's pelvis. This is the organ in which a fetus develops. Also called the womb.

V

Vagina: The muscular canal extending from the uterus to the exterior of the body. Also called the birth canal.

W

Wart: A raised growth on the surface of the skin or other organ.

White blood cell: A type of cell in the immune system that helps the body fight infection and disease. White blood cells include lymphocytes, granulocytes, macrophages, and others.

X

X-ray: A high-energy form of radiation; used in low doses for diagnosing diseases and in high doses to treat cancer.

Chapter 72

Understanding the Family and Medical Leave Act (FMLA)

The U.S. Department of Labor's Employment Standards Administration, Wage and Hour Division, administers and enforces the Family and Medical Leave Act (FMLA) for all private, state and local government employees, and some federal employees. Most Federal and certain congressional employees are also covered by the law and are subject to the jurisdiction of the U.S. Office of Personnel Management or the Congress.

FMLA became effective on August 5, 1993, for most employers. If a collective bargaining agreement (CBA) was in effect on that date, FMLA became effective on the expiration date of the CBA or February 5, 1994, whichever was earlier. FMLA entitles eligible employees to take up to 12 weeks of unpaid, job-protected leave in a 12-month period for specified family and medical reasons. The employer may elect to use the calendar year, a fixed 12-month leave or fiscal year, or a 12-month period prior to or after the commencement of leave as the 12-month period.

The law contains provisions on employer coverage; employee eligibility for the law's benefits; entitlement to leave, maintenance of health benefits during leave, and job restoration after leave; notice and certification of the need for FMLA leave; and, protection for employees who request or take FMLA leave. The law also requires employers to keep certain records.

Fact Sheet No. 28, U. S. Department of Labor.

543

Employer Coverage

FMLA applies to all:

- public agencies, including state, local and federal employers, local education agencies (schools), and

- private-sector employers who employed 50 or more employees in 20 or more workweeks in the current or preceding calendar year and who are engaged in commerce or in any industry or activity affecting commerce—including joint employers and successors of covered employers.

Employee Eligibility

To be eligible for FMLA benefits, an employee must:

1. work for a covered employer;

2. have worked for the employer for a total of 12 months;

3. have worked at least 1,250 hours over the previous 12 months; and

4. work at a location in the United States or in any territory or possession of the United States where at least 50 employees are employed by the employer within 75 miles.

Leave Entitlement

A covered employer must grant an eligible employee up to a total of 12 workweeks of unpaid leave during any 12-month period for one or more of the following reasons:

- for the birth and care of the newborn child of the employee;

- for placement with the employee of a son or daughter for adoption or foster care;

- to care for an immediate family member (spouse, child, or parent) with a serious health condition; or

- to take medical leave when the employee is unable to work because of a serious health condition.

Spouses employed by the same employer are jointly entitled to a combined total of 12 work-weeks of family leave for the birth and care of the newborn child, for placement of a child for adoption or foster care, and to care for a parent who has a serious health condition.

Leave for birth and care, or placement for adoption or foster care must conclude within 12 months of the birth or placement.

Under some circumstances, employees may take FMLA leave intermittently—which means taking leave in blocks of time, or by reducing their normal weekly or daily work schedule.

- If FMLA leave is for birth and care or placement for adoption or foster care, use of intermittent leave is subject to the employer's approval.

- FMLA leave may be taken intermittently whenever medically necessary to care for a seriously ill family member, or because the employee is seriously ill and unable to work.

Also, subject to certain conditions, employees or employers may choose to use accrued paid leave (such as sick or vacation leave) to cover some or all of the FMLA leave.

The employer is responsible for designating if an employee's use of paid leave counts as FMLA leave, based on information from the employee.

"Serious health condition" means an illness, injury, impairment, or physical or mental condition that involves either:

- any period of incapacity or treatment connected with inpatient care (i.e., an overnight stay) in a hospital, hospice, or residential medical-care facility, and any period of incapacity or subsequent treatment in connection with such inpatient care; or

- Continuing treatment by a health care provider which includes any period of incapacity (i.e., inability to work, attend school or perform other regular daily activities) due to:

    1. A health condition (including treatment therefor, or recovery therefrom) lasting more than three consecutive days, and any subsequent treatment or period of incapacity relating to the same condition, that also includes:

        - treatment two or more times by or under the supervision of a health care provider; or

        - one treatment by a health care provider with a continuing regimen of treatment; or

2. Pregnancy or prenatal care. A visit to the health care provider is not necessary for each absence; or

3. A chronic serious health condition which continues over an extended period of time, requires periodic visits to a health care provider, and may involve occasional episodes of incapacity (e.g., asthma, diabetes). A visit to a health care provider is not necessary for each absence; or

4. A permanent or long-term condition for which treatment may not be effective (e.g., Alzheimer's, a severe stroke, terminal cancer). Only supervision by a health care provider is required, rather than active treatment; or

5. Any absences to receive multiple treatments for restorative surgery or for a condition which would likely result in a period of incapacity of more than three days if not treated (e.g., chemotherapy or radiation treatments for cancer).

"Health care provider" means:

- doctors of medicine or osteopathy authorized to practice medicine or surgery by the state in which the doctors practice; or

- podiatrists, dentists, clinical psychologists, optometrists and chiropractors (limited to manual manipulation of the spine to correct a subluxation as demonstrated by X-ray to exist) authorized to practice, and performing within the scope of their practice, under state law; or

- nurse practitioners, nurse-midwives and clinical social workers authorized to practice, and performing within the scope of their practice, as defined under state law; or

- Christian Science practitioners listed with the First Church of Christ, Scientist in Boston, Massachusetts; or

- Any health care provider recognized by the employer or the employer's group health plan benefits manager.

Maintenance of Health Benefits

A covered employer is required to maintain group health insurance coverage for an employee on FMLA leave whenever such insurance was provided before the leave was taken and on the same terms as if the employee had continued to work. If applicable, arrangements will need to be made for employees to pay their share of health insurance premiums while on leave.

In some instances, the employer may recover premiums it paid to maintain health coverage for an employee who fails to return to work from FMLA leave.

Job Restoration

Upon return from FMLA leave, an employee must be restored to the employee's original job, or to an equivalent job with equivalent pay, benefits, and other terms and conditions of employment.

In addition, an employee's use of FMLA leave cannot result in the loss of any employment benefit that the employee earned or was entitled to before using FMLA leave, nor be counted against the employee under a "no fault" attendance policy.

Under specified and limited circumstances where restoration to employment will cause substantial and grievous economic injury to its operations, an employer may refuse to reinstate certain highly-paid "key" employees after using FMLA leave during which health coverage was maintained. In order to do so, the employer must:

- notify the employee of his/her status as a "key" employee in response to the employee's notice of intent to take FMLA leave;

- notify the employee as soon as the employer decides it will deny job restoration, and explain the reasons for this decision;

- offer the employee a reasonable opportunity to return to work from FMLA leave after giving this notice; and

- make a final determination as to whether reinstatement will be denied at the end of the leave period if the employee then requests restoration.

A "key" employee is a salaried "eligible" employee who is among the highest paid ten percent of employees within 75 miles of the work site.

Notice and Certification

Employees seeking to use FMLA leave are required to provide 30-day advance notice of the need to take FMLA leave when the need is foreseeable and such notice is practicable.

Employers may also require employees to provide:

- medical certification supporting the need for leave due to a serious health condition affecting the employee or an immediate family member;

- second or third medical opinions (at the employer's expense) and periodic recertification; and

- periodic reports during FMLA leave regarding the employee's status and intent to return to work.

When intermittent leave is needed to care for an immediate family member or the employee's own illness, and is for planned medical treatment, the employee must try to schedule treatment so as not to unduly disrupt the employer's operation.

Covered employers must post a notice approved by the Secretary of Labor explaining rights and responsibilities under FMLA. An employer that willfully violates this posting requirement may be subject to a fine of up to $100 for each separate offense.

Also, covered employers must inform employees of their rights and responsibilities under FMLA, including giving specific written information on what is required of the employee and what might happen in certain circumstances, such as if the employee fails to return to work after FMLA leave.

Unlawful Acts

It is unlawful for any employer to interfere with, restrain, or deny the exercise of any right provided by FMLA. It is also unlawful for an employer to discharge or discriminate against any individual for opposing any practice, or because of involvement in any proceeding, related to FMLA.

Enforcement

The Wage and Hour Division investigates complaints. If violations cannot be satisfactorily resolved, the U.S. Department of Labor may bring action in court to compel compliance. Individuals may also bring a private civil action against an employer for violations.

Other Provisions

Special rules apply to employees of local education agencies. Generally, these rules provide for FMLA leave to be taken in blocks of time when intermittent leave is needed or the leave is required near the end of a school term.

Salaried executive, administrative, and professional employees of covered employers who meet the Fair Labor Standards Act (FLSA) criteria for exemption from minimum wage and overtime under Regulations, 29 CFR Part 541, do not lose their FLSA-exempt status by using any unpaid FMLA leave. This special exception to the "salary basis" requirements for FLSA's exemption extends only to "eligible" employees' use of leave required by FMLA.

The FMLA does not affect any other federal or state law which prohibits discrimination, nor supersede any state or local law which provides greater family or medical leave protection. Nor does it affect an employer's obligation to provide greater leave rights under a collective bargaining agreement or employment benefit plan. The FMLA also encourages employers to provide more generous leave rights.

Further Information

The final rule implementing FMLA is contained in the January 6, 1995, Federal Register. For additional information, visit the Wage-Hour Website: http://www.dol.gov/dol/esa/public/whd_org.htm and/or call our Wage-Hour toll-free information and helpline, available 8am to 5pm in your time zone, 1-866-4USWAGE (1-866-487-9243).

Chapter 73

Resources for Women with Cancer

Alliance for Lung Cancer Advocacy, Support, and Education (ALCASE)
P. O. Box 849
Vancouver, WA 98666
Toll-Free: 800-298-2436
Phone: 360-696-2436 U.S.
Internet: http://www.alcase.org
E-Mail: info@alcase.org

American Association for Cancer Education
9500 Euclid Avenue
Cleveland, Ohio 44195
Phone: 216-444-9827
Fax: 216-444-8685
Internet: http://
www.aaceonline.com

American Association for Cancer Research
Public Ledger Building
Suite 826
150 South Independence Mall W
Philadelphia, PA 19106
Phone: 215-440-9300
Fax: 215-440-9313
Internet: http://www.aacr.org
E-Mail: membership@aacr.org

American Brain Tumor Association (ABTA)
2720 River Road, Suite 146
Des Plaines, IL 60018
Toll-Free: 800-886-ABTA (800-886-2282)
Phone: 847-827-9910
Internet: http://www.abta.org
E-Mail: mailto:abta@aol.com

Resources listed in this chapter were compiled from many sources deemed accurate; all contact information was verified and updated in November 2001.

American Cancer Society (ACS)
1599 Clifton Road, NE
Atlanta, GA 30329-4251
Toll-Free: 800-ACS-2345 (800-227-2345)
Phone: 404-320-3333
Internet: http://www.cancer.org

American Foundation for Urologic Disease (AFUD)
1128 North Charles Street
Baltimore, MD 21201
Phone: 410-468-1800
Fax: 410-468-1808
Internet: http://www.afud.org
E-Mail: admin@afud.org

American Institute for Cancer Research (AICR)
1759 R Street, NW
Washington, DC 20009
Toll-Free: 800-843-8114
Phone: 202-328-7744
Internet: http://www.aicr.org
E-Mail: aicrweb@aicr.org

American Society of Breast Disease
P.O. Box 140186
Dallas, TX 75214
Phone: 214-368-6836
Fax: 214-368-5719
Internet: http://www.asbd.org
E-Mail: asbd1@aol.com

Association of Community Cancer Centers
11600 Nebel Street, Suite 201
Rockville, MD 20852
Phone: 301-984-9496
Fax: 301-770-1949
Internet: http://www.accc-cancer.org

Avon's Breast Cancer Awareness Campaign
Internet: http://avon.com/about/awareness/frame.html

Bloch (R.A.) Cancer Foundation, Inc.
4435 Main Street, Suite 500
Kansas City, MO 64111
Toll-Free: 800-433-0464
Phone: 816-WE-BUILD (816-932-8453)
Fax: 816- 931-7486
Internet: http://www.blochcancer.org
E-Mail: hotline@hrblock.com

The Brain Tumor Society
124 Watertown St., Suite 3H
Watertown, MA 02472
Toll-Free: 800-770-TBTS
Phone: 617-924-9997
Fax: 617-924-9998
Internet: http://www.tbts.org
E-Mail: info@tbts.org

Breast Cancer Action
55 New Montgomery Street
Suite 323
San Francisco, CA 94105
Toll Free: 877-278-6722
Phone: 415-243-9301
Fax: 415-243-3996
Internet: http://
www.bcaction.org
E-Mail: info@bcaction.org

*Breast Cancer and
Environmental Risk
Factors Program*
Cornell University
112 Rice Hall
Ithaca, NY 14853-5601
Phone: 607-254-2893
Fax: 607-255-8207
E-Mail:
breastcancer@cornell.edu
Internet: http://
www.cfe.cornell.edu/bcerf

Breast Cancer Answers
University of Wisconsin Comprehensive Cancer Center
K4/658
600 Highland Avenue
Madison, WI 53792-0001
Toll Free: 800-622- 8922
Phone: 608-263-8600
Fax: 608-263-8613
Internet: http://
www.medsch.wisc.edu/bca

*Breast Cancer Information
Clearinghouse*
Internet: http://nysernet.org/bcic

Cancer Care, Inc.
275 Seventh Avenue
New York, NY 10001
Toll-Free: 800-813-HOPE (800-813-4673)
Phone: 212- 712-8080
Fax: 212-712-8495
Internet: http://
www.cancercare.org
E-Mail: info@cancercare.org

Cancer Guide
Internet: http://
www.cancerguide.org

Cancer Hope Network
Two North Road, Suite A
Chester, NJ 07930
Phone: 877-HOPENET (877-467-3638)
Internet: http://
www.cancerhopenetwork.org
E-Mail:
info@cancerhopenetwork.org

Cancer News on the Net
Internet: http://
www.cancernews.com

*Cancer Research
Foundation of America*
1600 Duke Street, Suite 110
Alexandria, VA 22314
Toll-Free: 800-227-2732
Phone: 703-836-4412
Fax 703-836-4413
Internet: http://
www.preventcancer.org
E-Mail: info@crfa.org

Centers for Disease Control and Prevention
National Center for Chronic Disease Prevention and Health Promotion
Mail Stop K-64
4770 Buford Highway NE
Atlanta, GA 30341-3717
Toll Free Voice Information System: 888-842-6355
Phone: 770-488-4751
Fax: 770-488-4760
Internet: http://www.cdc.gov/cancer
E-Mail: cancerinfo@cdc.gov

Cure For Lymphoma Foundation (CFL)
215 Lexington Avenue
New York, NY 10016-6023
Toll-Free: 800-CFL-6848 (800-235-6848)
Phone: 212-213-9595
Internet: http://www.cfl.org
E-Mail: infocfl@cfl.org

Cyberspace Hospital Oncology Department
Internet: http://www.crc.nus.sg:80/ch/cancer.html

DES Action USA
610 16th Street, Suite 301
Oakland, CA 94612
Toll-Free: 800-DES-9288 (800-337-9288)
Phone: 510-465-4011 or
Fax: 510-465-4815
Internet: http://www.desaction.org
E-Mail: desaction@earthlink.net

DES Cancer Network
514 10th Street, NW, Suite 400
Washington, DC 20004-1403
Toll-Free: 800-DES-NET4 (800-337-6384)
Phone: 202-628-6330
Fax: 202-628-6217
Internet: http:/www.descancer.org
E-Mail: DESNETWRK@aol.com

ENCOREPlus
YWCA of the USA
Office of Women's Health Advocacy
1015 18th Street, NW, Suite 700
Washington, DC 20036
Toll-Free: 800-95E-PLUS (800-953-7587)
Phone: 202-467-0801
Internet: http://www.ywca.org

Food and Drug Administration
5600 Fishers Lane
Rockville, MD 20857
Phone: 888-463-6332
Web site: http://www.fda.gov

Gilda's Club, Inc.
195 West Houston Street
New York, NY 10014
Phone: 212-647-9700
Fax: 212-647-1151
Internet: http://www.gildasclub.org
E-Mail: info@gildasclub.org

HOSPICELINK
Hospice Education Institute
190 Westbrook Road
Essex, CT 06426-1510
Toll-Free: 800-331-1620
Phone: 860-767-1620
Internet: http://
www.hospiceworld.org
E-Mail: HOSPICEALL@aol.com

Intercultural Cancer Council
PMB-C, 1720 Dryden
Houston, TX 77030
Phone: 713-798-4617
Fax: 713-798-3990
Internet: http:www/
iccnetwork.org/who
E-Mail: info@iccnetwork.org

International Myeloma Foundation (IMF)
12650 Riverside Drive, Suite 206
North Hollywood, CA 91607
Toll-Free: 800-452-CURE (800-452-2873)
Phone: 818-487-7455
Fax: 818-487-7454
Internet: http://
www.myeloma.org
E-Mail: TheIMF@myeloma.org

Kidney Cancer Association
1234 Sherman Avenue, Suite 203
Evanston, IL 60202-1375
Toll-Free: 800-850-9132
Phone: 847-332-1051
Internet: http://www.nkca.org
E-Mail:
OFFICE@KIDNEYCANCER
ASSOCIATION.ORG

Komen (Susan G.) Breast Cancer Foundation
5005 LBJ Freeway, Suite 250
Dallas, TX 75244
Phone: 972-855-1600
Fax: 972-855-1605
Toll-Free: 800-IM-AWARE (800-462-9273)
Internet: http://www.komen.org
E-Mail: helpline@komen.org

Kushner Breast Cancer Advisory Center
P.O. Box 224
Kensington, MD 20895
Phone: 301-897-3445

The Leukemia and Lymphoma Society
1311 Mamaroneck Avenue
White Plains, NY 10605-5221
Toll-Free: 800-955-4572
Phone: 914-949-5213
Fax: 914-949-6691
Internet: http://www.leukemia-lymphoma.org
E-Mail: infocenter@leukemia-lymphoma.org

Look Good ... Feel Better
Internet: http://
www.lookgoodfeelbetter.org

Lymphoma Research Foundation of America (LRFA)
8800 Venice Boulevard, Suite 207
Los Angeles, CA 90034
Toll-Free: 800-500-9976
Phone: 310-204-7040
Fax: 310-204-7043
Internet: http://
www.lymphoma.org
E-Mail: LRFA@ lymphoma.org

Multiple Myeloma Research Foundation (MMRF)
3 Forest Street
New Canaan, CT 06840
Phone: 203-972-1250
Internet: http://
www.multiplemyeloma.org
E-Mail: themmrf@themmrf.org

National Alliance of Breast Cancer Organizations (NABCO)
Nine East 37th Street, 10th Floor
New York, NY 10016
Toll-Free: 888-80-NABCO (888-806-2226)
Phone: 212-889-0606
Internet: http://www.nabco.org
E-Mail: NABCOinfo@aol.com

National Asian Women's Health Organization (NAWHO)
250 Montgomery St., Suite 900
San Francisco, CA 94104
Phone: 415-989-9747
Fax: 415-989-9758
Internet: http://www.nawho.org
E-Mail: nawho@nawho.org

National Brain Tumor Foundation (NBTF)
414 Thirteenth Street, Suite 700
Oakland, CA 94612-2603
Toll-Free: 800-934-CURE
Phone: 510-839-9777
Fax: 510-839-9779
Internet: http://
www.braintumor.org
E-Mail: nbtf@braintumor.org

National Breast Cancer Coalition
1707 L Street NW, Suite 1060
Washington, DC 20036
Toll Free: 800-622-2838
Phone: 202-296-7477
Fax: 202-265-6854
Internet: http://www.natlbcc.org
Internet: http://
www.stopbreastcancer.org

National Cancer Institute
31 Center Drive, MSC 2580
Bethesda, MD 20892-2580
Phone: 301-435-3848
Toll-Free: 800-4-CANCER
Internet: http://www.nci.nih.gov

National Center for Complementary and Alternative Medicine
NCCAM Clearinghouse
Post Office Box 7923
Gaithersburg, MD 20898
Toll Free: 888-644-6226
Phone (301) 519-3153
TTY/TDY: 888-644-6226
Fax: 866-464-3616
Web site: http://nccam.nih.gov
E-Mail: info@nccam.nih.gov

National Coalition for Cancer Survivorship (NCCS)
1010 Wayne Avenue, Suite 770
Silver Spring, MD 20910-5600
Toll Free: 877-NCCS-YES (877-622-7937)
Phone: 301-650-9127
Fax: 301-565-9670
Internet: http://www.cansearch.org
E-Mail: info@cansearch.org

National Cosmetology Association
Internet: http://s-www.salonprofessionals.org

National Foundation for Cancer Research
4600 East-West Highway
Suite 525
Bethesda, MD 20814
Toll Free: 800-321-2873
Phone: 301-654-1250
Fax: 301-654-5824
Internet: http://www.nfcr.org

National Heart, Lung, and Blood Institute
Post Office Box 30105
Bethesda, MD 20824-0105
Phone: 301-592-8573
Fax: 301-592-8563
Internet: http://www.nhlbi.nih.gov
E-Mail: NHLBIinfo@rover.nhlbi.nih.gov

National Hospice and Palliative Care Organization (NHPCO)
1700 Diagonal Road
Suite 300
Alexandria, VA 22314
Toll-Free: 800-658-8898 (Helpline)
Phone: 703- 837-1500
Internet: http://www.nhpco.org
E-Mail: info@nhpco.org

National Institute on Aging (NIA)
Public Information Office
Building 31, Room 5C27
31 Center Drive, MSC 2292
Bethesda, MD 20892
Toll Free: 800-222-2225
Phone: 301-496-1752
Internet: http://www.nia.nih.gov

National Lymphedema Network (NLN)
1611 Telegraph Avenue
Suite 1111
Oakland, CA 94612-2138
Toll-Free: 800-541-3259
Phone: 510-208-3200
Fax: 510-208-3110
Internet: http://www.lymphnet.org
E-Mail: nln@lymphnet.org

National Marrow Donor Program

3001 Broadway St., NE,
Suite 500
Minneapolis, MN 55413
Toll-Free: 800-MARROW-2 (800-627-7692)
Office of Patient Advocacy: 888-999-6743
Phone: 612-627-5800
Internet: http://www.marrow.org

National Ovarian Cancer Coalition (NOCC)

500 Northeast Spanish River
Boulevard, Suite 14
Boca Raton, FL 33431
Toll-Free: 888-OVARIAN (888-682-7426)
Phone: 561-393-0005
Internet: http://www.ovarian.org
E-Mail: NOCC@ovarian.org

National Women's Health Resource Center

120 Albany Street, Suite 820
New Brunswick, NJ 08901
Toll Free: 877-986-9472
Internet: http://
www.healthywomen.org
E-Mail: info@healthywomen.org

OncoLink

University of Pennsylvania Cancer Center
3400 Spruce Street - 2 Donner
Philadelphia, PA 19104-4283
Fax: 215-349-5445
Internet: http://
cancer.med.upenn.edu

Ovarian Cancer National Alliance

910 17th Street, NW, Suite 413
Washington, DC 20006
Phone: 202-331-1332
Internet: http://
www.ovariancancer.org
E-Mail: ovarian@aol.com

Pancreatic Cancer Action Network (PanCAN)

Post Office Box 1010
Torrance, CA 90505
Phone: 877-2-PANCAN (877-272-6226)
Internet: http://www.pancan.org
E-Mail: information@pancan.org

Patient Advocate Foundation (PAF)

753 Thimble Shoals Boulevard,
Suite B
Newport News, VA 23606
Toll-Free: 800-532-5274
Phone: 757-873-6668
Fax: 757-873-8999
Internet: http://
www.patientadvocate.org
E-Mail:
help@patientadvocate.org

The Registry for Research on Hormonal Transplacental Carcinogenesis (Clear Cell Cancer Registry)
Department of Obstetrics and Gynecology
The University of Chicago
5841 South Maryland Avenue, MC 2050
Chicago, IL 60637
Phone: 773-702-6671
Fax number: 773-702-0840
Internet: http://cis.nci.nih.gov/asp/disclaimernew.asp?p=obgyn.bsd uchicago.edu/registry.html
E-Mail: registry@babies.bsd.uchicago.edu

Sisters Network
8787 Woodway Drive
Suite 4206
Houston, TX 77063
Phone: 713-781-0255
Fax: 713-780-8998
Internet: http://www.sistersnetworkinc.org
E-Mail: sisnet4@aol.com

The Skin Cancer Foundation
245 Fifth Avenue, Suite 1403
New York, NY 10016
Toll-Free: 800-SKIN-490 (800-754-6490)
Phone: 212-725-5176
Fax: 212-725-5751
Internet: http//:www.skincancer.org
E-Mail: info@skincancer.org

STARBRIGHT Foundation
11835 West Olympic Blvd., Suite 500
Los Angeles, CA 90064
Toll-Free: 800-315-2580
Phone: 310-479-1212
Fax 310-479-1235
Internet: http://www.starbright.org

The United Ostomy Association, Inc.
19772 MacArthur Boulevard, Suite 200
Irvine, CA 92612-2405
Toll-Free: 800-826-0826 (6:30 a.m.-4:30 p.m., Pacific time)
Phone: 949-660-8624
Internet: http://www.uoa.org
E-Mail: info@uoa.org

The University of Iowa Hospitals and Clinics
Center for Advanced Reproductive Care
Department of Obstetrics and Gynecology
200 Hawkins Drive
Iowa City, Iowa 52242-1009
Toll Free: 800-777-8442
Phone: 319-356-1767

U.S. Department of Health and Human Services

Office on Women's Health
200 Independence Ave., S.W.,
Room 718F
Washington, D.C. 20201
Toll Free: 877-696-6775
Womens Health Toll Free: 800-994-9662
Phone: 202-619-0257
Internet: http://
www.4woman.gov/napbc
E-Mail: napbcinfo@soza.com

Vital Options and "The Group Room" Cancer Radio Talk Show

Post Office Box 19233
Encino, CA 91416-9233
Toll-Free: 800-GRP-ROOM (800-477-7666)
Phone: 818-508-5657
Internet: http://
www.vitaloptions.org
E-Mail: geninfo@vitaloptions.org

The Wellness Community

35 East Seventh Street
Suite 412
Cincinnati, OH 45202
Toll-Free: 888-793-WELL (888-793-9355)
Phone: 513-421-7111
Fax: 513-421-7119
Internet: http://www.wellness-community.org
E-Mail: help@wellness-community.org

Women's Cancer Network

c/o Gynecologic Cancer Foundation
401 N. Michigan Avenue
Chicago, IL 60611
Toll-Free: 800-444-4441 (for a referral to a gynecologic cancer specialist)
Phone: 312-644-6610
Internet: www.wcn.org
E-Mail: gcf@sba.com

Women's Health Initiative (WHI)

Program Office
Suite 300 MS 7966
One Rockledge Center
6705 Rockledge Drive
Bethesda, MD 20892-7966
Phone: 301-402-2900
Fax: 301-480-5158
Internet: http://
www.nhlbi.nih.gov/whi

Y-Me National Breast Cancer Organization, Inc.

212 West Van Buren Street
Chicago, IL 60607-3908
Toll-Free: 800-221-2141 (English)
Toll-Free: 800-986-9505 (Spanish)
Phone: 312-986-8338
Fax: 312-294-8597
Internet: http://www.y-me.org
E-Mail: help@y-me.org

Index

Index

P

paclitaxel 149, 151, 383–85
PAF *see* Patient Advocate Foundation
pain management
 breast cancer treatment 20
 cancer 497–503
"Pain (PDQ) Supportive Care — Patients" (NCI) 497n
palpation, defined 535
PanCAN *see* Pancreatic Cancer Action Network
pancreatic cancer, CA 19-9 tumor marker 272
Pancreatic Cancer Action Network (PanCAN), contact information 558
Papanicolaou, George 251, 257
papillary serous adenocarcinomas 88
PAPNET 258–59
Pap smear *see* Pap test
Pap tests
 abnormal results 241–42, 263–67, 282
 accuracy 257–62
 Bethesda system, described 50
 cervical cancer 49–50, 70, 78
 clinical studies 415–19
 defined 535
 described 79, 205–6, 258–60
 endometrial cancer 90, 105
 Medicare coverage 66
 questions and answers 251–55
 racial factor 74
 statistics *275*
 uterine sarcoma 177
 vaginal cancer 182
partial mastectomy, defined 538–39
pathologist, defined 252, 536
pathology report, defined 536
Patient Advocate Foundation (PAF), contact information 558
patient-controlled analgesia (PCA) 499
PCA *see* patient-controlled analgesia
PDQ, defined 536
PDT *see* photodynamic therapy

pelvic examinations
 cervical cancer 74–75
 endometrial cancer 90
 gestational trophoblastic tumor 156
 ovarian cancer 118
pelvic exenteration 82, 517
pelvic inflammatory disease (PID) 212–13
pelvis, defined 536
penile cancer 247
penile intraepithelial neoplasia 247
PEPI *see* Postmenopausal Estrogen/Progestin Intervenions
peripheral stem cell transplantation, defined 536
peripheral T-cell lymphoma 200
peritoneum
 defined 536
 ovarian cancer 115, 135–36
PET scan *see* positron emission tomography
photodynamic therapy (PDT) 378
physical therapist, defined 536
phytoestrogens, hormone replacement therapy 303
PID *see* pelvic inflammatory disease
placental-site trophoblastic disease 155
plastic surgeon, defined 536
platelets, defined 536
PLCO *see* Prostate, Lung, Colorectal, and Ovarian Screening Trial
Podofilox (podophyllotoxin) 283
podophyllin 283
podophyllotoxin 283
polyp, defined 536
positive, defined 536
positron emission tomography (PET scan)
 breast cancer research 27
 defined 536
Postmenopausal Estrogen/Progestin Intervenions (PEPI) clinical trial 302
post-transplantation lymphoproliferative disorder 200
Post-traumatic Stress Disorder (NIMH) 315n
post-traumatic stress disorder, described 315–16

Health Reference Series
COMPLETE CATALOG

AIDS Sourcebook, 1st Edition

Basic Information about AIDS and HIV Infection, Featuring Historical and Statistical Data, Current Research, Prevention, and Other Special Topics of Interest for Persons Living with AIDS

Along with Source Listings for Further Assistance

Edited by Karen Bellenir and Peter D. Dresser. 831 pages. 1995. 0-7808-0031-1. $78.

"One strength of this book is its practical emphasis. The intended audience is the lay reader . . . useful as an educational tool for health care providers who work with AIDS patients. Recommended for public libraries as well as hospital or academic libraries that collect consumer materials."
—*Bulletin of the Medical Library Association, Jan '96*

"This is the most comprehensive volume of its kind on an important medical topic. Highly recommended for all libraries." —*Reference Book Review, '96*

"Very useful reference for all libraries."
—*Choice, Association of College and Research Libraries, Oct '95*

"There is a wealth of information here that can provide much educational assistance. It is a must book for all libraries and should be on the desk of each and every congressional leader. Highly recommended."
—*AIDS Book Review Journal, Aug '95*

"Recommended for most collections."
—*Library Journal, Jul '95*

■

AIDS Sourcebook, 2nd Edition

Basic Consumer Health Information about Acquired Immune Deficiency Syndrome (AIDS) and Human Immunodeficiency Virus (HIV) Infection, Featuring Updated Statistical Data, Reports on Recent Research and Prevention Initiatives, and Other Special Topics of Interest for Persons Living with AIDS, Including New Antiretroviral Treatment Options, Strategies for Combating Opportunistic Infections, Information about Clinical Trials, and More

Along with a Glossary of Important Terms and Resource Listings for Further Help and Information

Edited by Karen Bellenir. 751 pages. 1999. 0-7808-0225-X. $78.

"Highly recommended."
—*American Reference Books Annual, 2000*

"Excellent sourcebook. This continues to be a highly recommended book. There is no other book that provides as much information as this book provides."
—*AIDS Book Review Journal, Dec-Jan 2000*

"Recommended reference source."
—*Booklist, American Library Association, Dec '99*

"A solid text for college-level health libraries."
—*The Bookwatch, Aug '99*

Cited in *Reference Sources for Small and Medium-Sized Libraries, American Library Association, 1999*

■

Alcoholism Sourcebook

Basic Consumer Health Information about the Physical and Mental Consequences of Alcohol Abuse, Including Liver Disease, Pancreatitis, Wernicke-Korsakoff Syndrome (Alcoholic Dementia), Fetal Alcohol Syndrome, Heart Disease, Kidney Disorders, Gastrointestinal Problems, and Immune System Compromise and Featuring Facts about Addiction, Detoxification, Alcohol Withdrawal, Recovery, and the Maintenance of Sobriety

Along with a Glossary and Directories of Resources for Further Help and Information

Edited by Karen Bellenir. 613 pages. 2000. 0-7808-0325-6. $78.

"This title is one of the few reference works on alcoholism for general readers. For some readers this will be a welcome complement to the many self-help books on the market. Recommended for collections serving general readers and consumer health collections."
—*E-Streams, Mar '01*

"This book is an excellent choice for public and academic libraries."
—*American Reference Books Annual, 2001*

"Recommended reference source."
—*Booklist, American Library Association, Dec '00*

"Presents a wealth of information on alcohol use and abuse and its effects on the body and mind, treatment, and prevention." —*SciTech Book News, Dec '00*

"Important new health guide which packs in the latest consumer information about the problems of alcoholism." —*Reviewer's Bookwatch, Nov '00*

SEE ALSO *Drug Abuse Sourcebook, Substance Abuse Sourcebook*

■

Allergies Sourcebook, 1st Edition

Basic Information about Major Forms and Mechanisms of Common Allergic Reactions, Sensitivities, and Intolerances, Including Anaphylaxis, Asthma, Hives and Other Dermatologic Symptoms, Rhinitis, and Sinusitis

Along with Their Usual Triggers Like Animal Fur, Chemicals, Drugs, Dust, Foods, Insects, Latex, Pollen, and Poison Ivy, Oak, and Sumac; Plus Information on Prevention, Identification, and Treatment

Edited by Allan R. Cook. 611 pages. 1997. 0-7808-0036-2. $78.

Allergies Sourcebook, 2nd Edition

Basic Consumer Health Information about Allergic Disorders, Triggers, Reactions, and Related Symptoms, Including Anaphylaxis, Rhinitis, Sinusitis, Asthma, Dermatitis, Conjunctivitis, and Multiple Chemical Sensitivity

Along with Tips on Diagnosis, Prevention, and Treatment, Statistical Data, a Glossary, and a Directory of Sources for Further Help and Information

Edited by Annemarie S. Muth. 598 pages. 2001. 0-7808-0376-0. $78.

■

Alternative Medicine Sourcebook

Basic Consumer Health Information about Alternatives to Conventional Medicine, Including Acupressure, Acupuncture, Aromatherapy, Ayurveda, Bioelectromagnetics, Environmental Medicine, Essence Therapy, Food and Nutrition Therapy, Herbal Therapy, Homeopathy, Imaging, Massage, Naturopathy, Reflexology, Relaxation and Meditation, Sound Therapy, Vitamin and Mineral Therapy, and Yoga, and More

Edited by Allan R. Cook. 737 pages. 1999. 0-7808-0200-4. $78.

"Recommended reference source."
—Booklist, American Library Association, Feb '00

"A great addition to the reference collection of every type of library." *—American Reference Books Annual, 2000*

■

Alzheimer's, Stroke & 29 Other Neurological Disorders Sourcebook, 1st Edition

Basic Information for the Layperson on 31 Diseases or Disorders Affecting the Brain and Nervous System, First Describing the Illness, Then Listing Symptoms, Diagnostic Methods, and Treatment Options, and Including Statistics on Incidences and Causes

Edited by Frank E. Bair. 579 pages. 1993. 1-55888-748-2. $78.

"Nontechnical reference book that provides reader-friendly information."
—Family Caregiver Alliance Update, Winter '96

"Should be included in any library's patient education section." *—American Reference Books Annual, 1994*

"Written in an approachable and accessible style. Recommended for patient education and consumer health collections in health science center and public libraries." *—Academic Library Book Review, Dec '93*

"It is very handy to have information on more than thirty neurological disorders under one cover, and there is no recent source like it." *—Reference Quarterly, American Library Association, Fall '93*

SEE ALSO Brain Disorders Sourcebook

Alzheimer's Disease Sourcebook, 2nd Edition

Basic Consumer Health Information about Alzheimer's Disease, Related Disorders, and Other Dementias, Including Multi-Infarct Dementia, AIDS-Related Dementia, Alcoholic Dementia, Huntington's Disease, Delirium, and Confusional States

Along with Reports Detailing Current Research Efforts in Prevention and Treatment, Long-Term Care Issues, and Listings of Sources for Additional Help and Information

Edited by Karen Bellenir. 524 pages. 1999. 0-7808-0223-3. $78.

"Provides a wealth of useful information not otherwise available in one place. This resource is recommended for all types of libraries."
—American Reference Books Annual, 2000

"Recommended reference source."
—Booklist, American Library Association, Oct '99

■

Arthritis Sourcebook

Basic Consumer Health Information about Specific Forms of Arthritis and Related Disorders, Including Rheumatoid Arthritis, Osteoarthritis, Gout, Polymyalgia Rheumatica, Psoriatic Arthritis, Spondyloarthropathies, Juvenile Rheumatoid Arthritis, and Juvenile Ankylosing Spondylitis

Along with Information about Medical, Surgical, and Alternative Treatment Options, and Including Strategies for Coping with Pain, Fatigue, and Stress

Edited by Allan R. Cook. 550 pages. 1998. 0-7808-0201-2. $78.

". . . accessible to the layperson."
—Reference and Research Book News, Feb '99

■

Asthma Sourcebook

Basic Consumer Health Information about Asthma, Including Symptoms, Traditional and Nontraditional Remedies, Treatment Advances, Quality-of-Life Aids, Medical Research Updates, and the Role of Allergies, Exercise, Age, the Environment, and Genetics in the Development of Asthma

Along with Statistical Data, a Glossary, and Directories of Support Groups, and Other Resources for Further Information

Edited by Annemarie S. Muth. 628 pages. 2000. 0-7808-0381-7. $78.

"A worthwhile reference acquisition for public libraries and academic medical libraries whose readers desire a quick introduction to the wide range of asthma information." *—Choice, Association of College and Research Libraries, Jun '01*

"Recommended reference source."
—Booklist, American Library Association, Feb '01

◼

Back & Neck Disorders Sourcebook

Basic Information about Disorders and Injuries of the Spinal Cord and Vertebrae, Including Facts on Chiropractic Treatment, Surgical Interventions, Paralysis, and Rehabilitation

Along with Advice for Preventing Back Trouble

Edited by Karen Bellenir. 548 pages. 1997. 0-7808-0202-0. $78.

◼

Blood & Circulatory Disorders Sourcebook

Basic Information about Blood and Its Components, Anemias, Leukemias, Bleeding Disorders, and Circulatory Disorders, Including Aplastic Anemia, Thalassemia, Sickle-Cell Disease, Hemochromatosis, Hemophilia, Von Willebrand Disease, and Vascular Diseases

Along with a Special Section on Blood Transfusions and Blood Supply Safety, a Glossary, and Source Listings for Further Help and Information

Edited by Karen Bellenir and Linda M. Shin. 554 pages. 1998. 0-7808-0203-9. $78.

◼

Brain Disorders Sourcebook

Basic Consumer Health Information about Strokes, Epilepsy, Amyotrophic Lateral Sclerosis (ALS/Lou Gehrig's Disease), Parkinson's Disease, Brain Tumors, Cerebral Palsy, Headache, Tourette Syndrome, and More

Along with Statistical Data, Treatment and Rehabilitation Options, Coping Strategies, Reports on Current

Research Initiatives, a Glossary, and Resource Listings for Additional Help and Information

Edited by Karen Bellenir. 481 pages. 1999. 0-7808-0229-2. $78.

SEE ALSO Alzheimer's, Stroke & 29 Other Neurological Disorders Sourcebook, 1st Edition

◼

Breast Cancer Sourcebook

Basic Consumer Health Information about Breast Cancer, Including Diagnostic Methods, Treatment Options, Alternative Therapies, Self-Help Information, Related Health Concerns, Statistical and Demographic Data, and Facts for Men with Breast Cancer

Along with Reports on Current Research Initiatives, a Glossary of Related Medical Terms, and a Directory of Sources for Further Help and Information

Edited by Edward J. Prucha and Karen Bellenir. 580 pages. 2001. 0-7808-0244-6. $78.

SEE ALSO Cancer Sourcebook for Women, 1st and 2nd Editions, Women's Health Concerns Sourcebook

◼

Breastfeeding Sourcebook

Basic Consumer Health Information about the Benefits of Breastmilk, Preparing to Breastfeed, Breastfeeding as a Baby Grows, Nutrition, and More, Including Information on Special Situations and Concerns Such as Mastitis, Illness, Medications, Allergies, Multiple Births, Prematurity, Special Needs, and Adoption

Along with a Glossary and Resources for Additional Help and Information

Edited by Jenni Lynn Colson. 350 pages. 2002. 0-7808-0332-9. $78.

SEE ALSO Pregnancy & Birth Sourcebook

Burns Sourcebook

Basic Consumer Health Information about Various Types of Burns and Scalds, Including Flame, Heat, Cold, Electrical, Chemical, and Sun Burns

Along with Information on Short-Term and Long-Term Treatments, Tissue Reconstruction, Plastic Surgery, Prevention Suggestions, and First Aid

Edited by Allan R. Cook. 604 pages. 1999. 0-7808-0204-7. $78.

"This key reference guide is an invaluable addition to all health care and public libraries in confronting this ongoing health issue."
—*American Reference Books Annual, 2000*

"This is an exceptional addition to the series and is highly recommended for all consumer health collections, hospital libraries, and academic medical centers."
— *E-Streams, Mar '00*

"Recommended reference source."
—*Booklist, American Library Association, Dec '99*

SEE ALSO Skin Disorders Sourcebook

■

Cancer Sourcebook, 1st Edition

Basic Information on Cancer Types, Symptoms, Diagnostic Methods, and Treatments, Including Statistics on Cancer Occurrences Worldwide and the Risks Associated with Known Carcinogens and Activities

Edited by Frank E. Bair. 932 pages. 1990. 1-55888-888-8. $78.

Cited in *Reference Sources for Small and Medium-Sized Libraries, American Library Association, 1999*

"Written in nontechnical language. Useful for patients, their families, medical professionals, and librarians."
— *Guide to Reference Books, 1996*

"Designed with the non-medical professional in mind. Libraries and medical facilities interested in patient education should certainly consider adding the *Cancer Sourcebook* to their holdings. This compact collection of reliable information . . . is an invaluable tool for helping patients and patients' families and friends to take the first steps in coping with the many difficulties of cancer."
— *Medical Reference Services Quarterly, Winter '91*

"Specifically created for the nontechnical reader . . . an important resource for the general reader trying to understand the complexities of cancer."
— *American Reference Books Annual, 1991*

"This publication's nontechnical nature and very comprehensive format make it useful for both the general public and undergraduate students."
— *Choice, Association of College and Research Libraries, Oct '90*

New Cancer Sourcebook, 2nd Edition

Basic Information about Major Forms and Stages of Cancer, Featuring Facts about Primary and Secondary Tumors of the Respiratory, Nervous, Lymphatic, Circulatory, Skeletal, and Gastrointestinal Systems, and Specific Organs; Statistical and Demographic Data; Treatment Options; and Strategies for Coping

Edited by Allan R. Cook. 1,313 pages. 1996. 0-7808-0041-9. $78.

"An excellent resource for patients with newly diagnosed cancer and their families. The dialogue is simple, direct, and comprehensive. Highly recommended for patients and families to aid in their understanding of cancer and its treatment."
— *Booklist Health Sciences Supplement, American Library Association, Oct '97*

"The amount of factual and useful information is extensive. The writing is very clear, geared to general readers. Recommended for all levels."
—*Choice, Association of College and Research Libraries, Jan '97*

■

Cancer Sourcebook, 3rd Edition

Basic Consumer Health Information about Major Forms and Stages of Cancer, Featuring Facts about Primary and Secondary Tumors of the Respiratory, Nervous, Lymphatic, Circulatory, Skeletal, and Gastrointestinal Systems, and Specific Organs

Along with Statistical and Demographic Data, Treatment Options, Strategies for Coping, a Glossary, and a Directory of Sources for Additional Help and Information

Edited by Edward J. Prucha. 1,069 pages. 2000. 0-7808-0227-6. $78.

"This title is recommended for health sciences and public libraries with consumer health collections."
—*E-Streams, Feb '01*

". . . can be effectively used by cancer patients and their families who are looking for answers in a language they can understand. Public and hospital libraries should have it on their shelves."
—*American Reference Books Annual, 2001*

"Recommended reference source."
—*Booklist, American Library Association, Dec '00*

■

Cancer Sourcebook for Women, 1st Edition

Basic Information about Specific Forms of Cancer That Affect Women, Featuring Facts about Breast Cancer, Cervical Cancer, Ovarian Cancer, Cancer of the Uterus and Uterine Sarcoma, Cancer of the Vagina, and Cancer of the Vulva; Statistical and Demographic Data; Treatments, Self-Help Management Suggestions, and Current Research Initiatives

Edited by Allan R. Cook and Peter D. Dresser. 524 pages. 1996. 0-7808-0076-1. $78.

"... written in easily understandable, non-technical language. Recommended for public libraries or hospital and academic libraries that collect patient education or consumer health materials."
— *Medical Reference Services Quarterly, Spring '97*

"Would be of value in a consumer health library.... written with the health care consumer in mind. Medical jargon is at a minimum, and medical terms are explained in clear, understandable sentences."
— *Bulletin of the Medical Library Association, Oct '96*

"The availability under one cover of all these pertinent publications, grouped under cohesive headings, makes this certainly a most useful sourcebook."
— *Choice, Association of College and Research Libraries, Jun '96*

"Presents a comprehensive knowledge base for general readers. Men and women both benefit from the gold mine of information nestled between the two covers of this book. Recommended."
— *Academic Library Book Review, Summer '96*

"This timely book is highly recommended for consumer health and patient education collections in all libraries." — *Library Journal, Apr '96*

SEE ALSO *Breast Cancer Sourcebook, Women's Health Concerns Sourcebook*

■

Cancer Sourcebook for Women, 2nd Edition

Basic Consumer Health Information about Gynecologic Cancers and Related Concerns, Including Cervical Cancer, Endometrial Cancer, Gestational Trophoblastic Tumor, Ovarian Cancer, Uterine Cancer, Vaginal Cancer, Vulvar Cancer, Breast Cancer, and Common Non-Cancerous Uterine Conditions, with Facts about Cancer Risk Factors, Screening and Prevention, Treatment Options, and Reports on Current Research Initiatives

Along with a Glossary of Cancer Terms and a Directory of Resources for Additional Help and Information

Edited by Karen Bellenir. 604 pages. 2002. 0-7808-0226-8. $78.

SEE ALSO *Breast Cancer Sourcebook, Women's Health Concerns Sourcebook*

■

Cardiovascular Diseases & Disorders Sourcebook, 1st Edition

Basic Information about Cardiovascular Diseases and Disorders, Featuring Facts about the Cardiovascular System, Demographic and Statistical Data, Descriptions of Pharmacological and Surgical Interventions, Lifestyle Modifications, and a Special Section Focusing on Heart Disorders in Children

Edited by Karen Bellenir and Peter D. Dresser. 683 pages. 1995. 0-7808-0032-X. $78.

"... comprehensive format provides an extensive overview on this subject." — *Choice, Association of College and Research Libraries, Jun '96*

"... an easily understood, complete, up-to-date resource. This well executed public health tool will make valuable information available to those that need it most, patients and their families. The typeface, sturdy non-reflective paper, and library binding add a feel of quality found wanting in other publications. Highly recommended for academic and general libraries. "
— *Academic Library Book Review, Summer '96*

SEE ALSO *Healthy Heart Sourcebook for Women, Heart Diseases & Disorders Sourcebook, 2nd Edition*

■

Caregiving Sourcebook

Basic Consumer Health Information for Caregivers, Including a Profile of Caregivers, Caregiving Responsibilities and Concerns, Tips for Specific Conditions, Care Environments, and the Effects of Caregiving

Along with Facts about Legal Issues, Financial Information, and Future Planning, a Glossary, and a Listing of Additional Resources

Edited by Joyce Brennfleck Shannon. 600 pages. 2001. 0-7808-0331-0. $78.

"Recommended reference source."
— *Booklist, American Library Association, Oct '01*

"An ideal addition to the reference collection of any public library. Health sciences information professionals may also want to acquire the *Caregiving Sourcebook* for their hospital or academic library for use as a ready reference tool by health care workers interested in aging and caregiving." — *E-Streams, Jan '02*

■

Colds, Flu & Other Common Ailments Sourcebook

Basic Consumer Health Information about Common Ailments and Injuries, Including Colds, Coughs, the Flu, Sinus Problems, Headaches, Fever, Nausea and Vomiting, Menstrual Cramps, Diarrhea, Constipation, Hemorrhoids, Back Pain, Dandruff, Dry and Itchy Skin, Cuts, Scrapes, Sprains, Bruises, and More

Along with Information about Prevention, Self-Care, Choosing a Doctor, Over-the-Counter Medications, Folk Remedies, and Alternative Therapies, and Including a Glossary of Important Terms and a Directory of Resources for Further Help and Information

Edited by Chad T. Kimball. 638 pages. 2001. 0-7808-0435-X. $78.

"Will prove valuable to any library seeking to maintain a current, comprehensive reference collection of health resources.... Excellent reference."
— *The Bookwatch, Aug '01*

"Recommended reference source."
— *Booklist, American Library Association, July '01*

Communication Disorders Sourcebook

Basic Information about Deafness and Hearing Loss, Speech and Language Disorders, Voice Disorders, Balance and Vestibular Disorders, and Disorders of Smell, Taste, and Touch

Edited by Linda M. Ross. 533 pages. 1996. 0-7808-0077-X. $78.

"This is skillfully edited and is a welcome resource for the layperson. It should be found in every public and medical library." — *Booklist Health Sciences Supplement, American Library Association, Oct '97*

■

Congenital Disorders Sourcebook

Basic Information about Disorders Acquired during Gestation, Including Spina Bifida, Hydrocephalus, Cerebral Palsy, Heart Defects, Craniofacial Abnormalities, Fetal Alcohol Syndrome, and More

Along with Current Treatment Options and Statistical Data

Edited by Karen Bellenir. 607 pages. 1997. 0-7808-0205-5. $78.

"Recommended reference source."
— *Booklist, American Library Association, Oct '97*

SEE ALSO Pregnancy & Birth Sourcebook

■

Consumer Issues in Health Care Sourcebook

Basic Information about Health Care Fundamentals and Related Consumer Issues, Including Exams and Screening Tests, Physician Specialties, Choosing a Doctor, Using Prescription and Over-the-Counter Medications Safely, Avoiding Health Scams, Managing Common Health Risks in the Home, Care Options for Chronically or Terminally Ill Patients, and a List of Resources for Obtaining Help and Further Information

Edited by Karen Bellenir. 618 pages. 1998. 0-7808-0221-7. $78.

"Both public and academic libraries will want to have a copy in their collection for readers who are interested in self-education on health issues."
— *American Reference Books Annual, 2000*

"The editor has researched the literature from government agencies and others, saving readers the time and effort of having to do the research themselves. Recommended for public libraries."
— *Reference and User Services Quarterly, American Library Association, Spring '99*

"Recommended reference source."
— *Booklist, American Library Association, Dec '98*

Contagious & Non-Contagious Infectious Diseases Sourcebook

Basic Information about Contagious Diseases like Measles, Polio, Hepatitis B, and Infectious Mononucleosis, and Non-Contagious Infectious Diseases like Tetanus and Toxic Shock Syndrome, and Diseases Occurring as Secondary Infections Such as Shingles and Reye Syndrome

Along with Vaccination, Prevention, and Treatment Information, and a Section Describing Emerging Infectious Disease Threats

Edited by Karen Bellenir and Peter D. Dresser. 566 pages. 1996. 0-7808-0075-3. $78.

■

Death & Dying Sourcebook

Basic Consumer Health Information for the Layperson about End-of-Life Care and Related Ethical and Legal Issues, Including Chief Causes of Death, Autopsies, Pain Management for the Terminally Ill, Life Support Systems, Insurance, Euthanasia, Assisted Suicide, Hospice Programs, Living Wills, Funeral Planning, Counseling, Mourning, Organ Donation, and Physician Training

Along with Statistical Data, a Glossary, and Listings of Sources for Further Help and Information

Edited by Annemarie S. Muth. 641 pages. 1999. 0-7808-0230-6. $78.

"Public libraries, medical libraries, and academic libraries will all find this sourcebook a useful addition to their collections."
— *American Reference Books Annual, 2001*

"An extremely useful resource for those concerned with death and dying in the United States."
— *Respiratory Care, Nov '00*

"Recommended reference source."
— *Booklist, American Library Association, Aug '00*

"This book is a definite must for all those involved in end-of-life care." — *Doody's Review Service, 2000*

■

Diabetes Sourcebook, 1st Edition

Basic Information about Insulin-Dependent and Non-insulin-Dependent Diabetes Mellitus, Gestational Diabetes, and Diabetic Complications, Symptoms, Treatment, and Research Results, Including Statistics on Prevalence, Morbidity, and Mortality

Along with Source Listings for Further Help and Information

Edited by Karen Bellenir and Peter D. Dresser. 827 pages. 1994. 1-55888-751-2. $78.

". . . very informative and understandable for the layperson without being simplistic. It provides a comprehensive overview for laypersons who want a general understanding of the disease or who want to focus on various aspects of the disease."
— *Bulletin of the Medical Library Association, Jan '96*

Diabetes Sourcebook, 2nd Edition

Basic Consumer Health Information about Type 1 Diabetes (Insulin-Dependent or Juvenile-Onset Diabetes), Type 2 (Noninsulin-Dependent or Adult-Onset Diabetes), Gestational Diabetes, and Related Disorders, Including Diabetes Prevalence Data, Management Issues, the Role of Diet and Exercise in Controlling Diabetes, Insulin and Other Diabetes Medicines, and Complications of Diabetes Such as Eye Diseases, Periodontal Disease, Amputation, and End-Stage Renal Disease

Along with Reports on Current Research Initiatives, a Glossary, and Resource Listings for Further Help and Information

Edited by Karen Bellenir. 688 pages. 1998. 0-7808-0224-1. $78.

"This comprehensive book is an excellent addition for high school, academic, medical, and public libraries. This volume is highly recommended."
—American Reference Books Annual, 2000

"An invaluable reference." —Library Journal, May '00

Selected as one of the 250 "Best Health Sciences Books of 1999." —Doody's Rating Service, Mar-Apr 2000

"Recommended reference source."
—Booklist, American Library Association, Feb '99

"... provides reliable mainstream medical information ... belongs on the shelves of any library with a consumer health collection." —E-Streams, Sep '99

"Provides useful information for the general public."
—Healthlines, University of Michigan Health Management Research Center, Sep/Oct '99

Diet & Nutrition Sourcebook, 1st Edition

Basic Information about Nutrition, Including the Dietary Guidelines for Americans, the Food Guide Pyramid, and Their Applications in Daily Diet, Nutritional Advice for Specific Age Groups, Current Nutritional Issues and Controversies, the New Food Label and How to Use It to Promote Healthy Eating, and Recent Developments in Nutritional Research

Edited by Dan R. Harris. 662 pages. 1996. 0-7808-0084-2. $78.

"Useful reference as a food and nutrition sourcebook for the general consumer." —Booklist Health Sciences Supplement, American Library Association, Oct '97

"Recommended for public libraries and medical libraries that receive general information requests on nutrition. It is readable and will appeal to those interested in learning more about healthy dietary practices."
—Medical Reference Services Quarterly, Fall '97

"An abundance of medical and social statistics is translated into readable information geared toward the general reader." —Bookwatch, Mar '97

"With dozens of questionable diet books on the market, it is so refreshing to find a reliable and factual reference book. Recommended to aspiring professionals, librari-

ans, and others seeking and giving reliable dietary advice. An excellent compilation." —Choice, Association of College and Research Libraries, Feb '97

SEE ALSO *Digestive Diseases & Disorders Sourcebook, Gastrointestinal Diseases & Disorders Sourcebook*

Diet & Nutrition Sourcebook, 2nd Edition

Basic Consumer Health Information about Dietary Guidelines, Recommended Daily Intake Values, Vitamins, Minerals, Fiber, Fat, Weight Control, Dietary Supplements, and Food Additives

Along with Special Sections on Nutrition Needs throughout Life and Nutrition for People with Such Specific Medical Concerns as Allergies, High Blood Cholesterol, Hypertension, Diabetes, Celiac Disease, Seizure Disorders, Phenylketonuria (PKU), Cancer, and Eating Disorders, and Including Reports on Current Nutrition Research and Source Listings for Additional Help and Information

Edited by Karen Bellenir. 650 pages. 1999. 0-7808-0228-4. $78.

"This book is an excellent source of basic diet and nutrition information." —Booklist Health Sciences Supplement, American Library Association, Dec '00

"This reference document should be in any public library, but it would be a very good guide for beginning students in the health sciences. If the other books in this publisher's series are as good as this, they should all be in the health sciences collections."
—American Reference Books Annual, 2000

"This book is an excellent general nutrition reference for consumers who desire to take an active role in their health care for prevention. Consumers of all ages who select this book can feel confident they are receiving current and accurate information." —Journal of Nutrition for the Elderly, Vol. 19, No. 4, '00

"Recommended reference source."
—Booklist, American Library Association, Dec '99

SEE ALSO *Digestive Diseases & Disorders Sourcebook, Gastrointestinal Diseases & Disorders Sourcebook*

Digestive Diseases & Disorders Sourcebook

Basic Consumer Health Information about Diseases and Disorders that Impact the Upper and Lower Digestive System, Including Celiac Disease, Constipation, Crohn's Disease, Cyclic Vomiting Syndrome, Diarrhea, Diverticulosis and Diverticulitis, Gallstones, Heartburn, Hemorrhoids, Hernias, Indigestion (Dyspepsia), Irritable Bowel Syndrome, Lactose Intolerance, Ulcers, and More

Along with Information about Medications and Other Treatments, Tips for Maintaining a Healthy Digestive Tract, a Glossary, and Directory of Digestive Diseases Organizations

Edited by Karen Bellenir. 335 pages. 1999. 0-7808-0327-2. $78.

"This title would be an excellent addition to all public or patient-research libraries."
—*American Reference Books Annual, 2001*

"This title is recommended for public, hospital, and health sciences libraries with consumer health collections."
—*E-Streams, Jul-Aug '00*

"Recommended reference source."
—*Booklist, American Library Association, May '00*

SEE ALSO Diet & Nutrition Sourcebook, 1st and 2nd Editions, Gastrointestinal Diseases & Disorders Sourcebook

■

Disabilities Sourcebook

Basic Consumer Health Information about Physical and Psychiatric Disabilities, Including Descriptions of Major Causes of Disability, Assistive and Adaptive Aids, Workplace Issues, and Accessibility Concerns

Along with Information about the Americans with Disabilities Act, a Glossary, and Resources for Additional Help and Information

Edited by Dawn D. Matthews. 616 pages. 2000. 0-7808-0389-2. $78.

"A much needed addition to the Omnigraphics *Health Reference Series*. A current reference work to provide people with disabilities, their families, caregivers or those who work with them, a broad range of information in one volume, has not been available until now. . . . is recommended for all public and academic library reference collections."
—*E-Streams, May '01*

"An excellent source book in easy-to-read format covering many current topics; highly recommended for all libraries."
—*Choice, Association of College and Research Libraries, Jan '01*

"Recommended reference source."
—*Booklist, American Library Association, Jul '00*

"An involving, invaluable handbook."
—*The Bookwatch, May '00*

■

Domestic Violence & Child Abuse Sourcebook

Basic Consumer Health Information about Spousal/ Partner, Child, Sibling, Parent, and Elder Abuse, Covering Physical, Emotional, and Sexual Abuse, Teen Dating Violence, and Stalking; Includes Information about Hotlines, Safe Houses, Safety Plans, and Other Resources for Support and Assistance, Community Initiatives, and Reports on Current Directions in Research and Treatment

Along with a Glossary, Sources for Further Reading, and Governmental and Non-Governmental Organizations Contact Information

Edited by Helene Henderson. 1,064 pages. 2000. 0-7808-0235-7. $78.

"This is important information. The Web has many resources but this sourcebook fills an important societal need. I am not aware of any other resources of this type."
—*Doody's Review Service, Sep '01*

"Recommended for all libraries, scholars, and practitioners."
—*Choice, Association of College & Research Libraries, Jul '01*

"Recommended reference source."
—*Booklist, American Library Association, Apr '01*

"Important pick for college-level health reference libraries."
—*The Bookwatch, Mar '01*

"Because this problem is so widespread and because this book includes a lot of issues within one volume, this work is recommended for all public libraries."
—*American Reference Books Annual, 2001*

■

Drug Abuse Sourcebook

Basic Consumer Health Information about Illicit Substances of Abuse and the Diversion of Prescription Medications, Including Depressants, Hallucinogens, Inhalants, Marijuana, Narcotics, Stimulants, and Anabolic Steroids

Along with Facts about Related Health Risks, Treatment Issues, and Substance Abuse Prevention Programs, a Glossary of Terms, Statistical Data, and Directories of Hotline Services, Self-Help Groups, and Organizations Able to Provide Further Information

Edited by Karen Bellenir. 629 pages. 2000. 0-7808-0242-X. $78.

"Containing a wealth of information, this book will be useful to the college student just beginning to explore the topic of substance abuse. This resource belongs in libraries that serve a lower-division undergraduate or community college clientele as well as the general public."
—*Choice, Association of College and Research Libraries, Jun '01*

"Recommended reference source."
—*Booklist, American Library Association, Feb '01*

"Highly recommended." —*The Bookwatch, Jan '01*

"Even though there is a plethora of books on drug abuse, this volume is recommended for school, public, and college libraries."
—*American Reference Books Annual, 2001*

SEE ALSO Alcoholism Sourcebook, Substance Abuse Sourcebook

■

Ear, Nose & Throat Disorders Sourcebook

Basic Information about Disorders of the Ears, Nose, Sinus Cavities, Pharynx, and Larynx, Including Ear Infections, Tinnitus, Vestibular Disorders, Allergic and Non-Allergic Rhinitis, Sore Throats, Tonsillitis, and Cancers That Affect the Ears, Nose, Sinuses, and Throat

Along with Reports on Current Research Initiatives, a Glossary of Related Medical Terms, and a Directory of Sources for Further Help and Information

Edited by Karen Bellenir and Linda M. Shin. 576 pages. 1998. 0-7808-0206-3. $78.

"Overall, this sourcebook is helpful for the consumer seeking information on ENT issues. It is recommended for public libraries."
— *American Reference Books Annual, 1999*

"Recommended reference source."
— *Booklist, American Library Association, Dec '98*

■

Eating Disorders Sourcebook

Basic Consumer Health Information about Eating Disorders, Including Information about Anorexia Nervosa, Bulimia Nervosa, Binge Eating, Body Dysmorphic Disorder, Pica, Laxative Abuse, and Night Eating Syndrome

Along with Information about Causes, Adverse Effects, and Treatment and Prevention Issues, and Featuring a Section on Concerns Specific to Children and Adolescents, a Glossary, and Resources for Further Help and Information

Edited by Dawn D. Matthews. 322 pages. 2001. 0-7808-0335-3. $78.

"This volume is another convenient collection of excerpted articles. Recommended for school and public library patrons; lower-division undergraduates; and two-year technical program students."
— *Choice, Association of College & Research Libraries, Jan '02*

"Recommended reference source." — *Booklist, American Library Association, Oct 15, '01*

■

Endocrine & Metabolic Disorders Sourcebook

Basic Information for the Layperson about Pancreatic and Insulin-Related Disorders Such as Pancreatitis, Diabetes, and Hypoglycemia; Adrenal Gland Disorders Such as Cushing's Syndrome, Addison's Disease, and Congenital Adrenal Hyperplasia; Pituitary Gland Disorders Such as Growth Hormone Deficiency, Acromegaly, and Pituitary Tumors; Thyroid Disorders Such as Hypothyroidism, Graves' Disease, Hashimoto's Disease, and Goiter; Hyperparathyroidism; and Other Diseases and Syndromes of Hormone Imbalance or Metabolic Dysfunction

Along with Reports on Current Research Initiatives

Edited by Linda M. Shin. 574 pages. 1998. 0-7808-0207-1. $78.

"Omnigraphics has produced another needed resource for health information consumers."
— *American Reference Books Annual, 2000*

"Recommended reference source."
— *Booklist, American Library Association, Dec '98*

Environmentally Induced Disorders Sourcebook

Basic Information about Diseases and Syndromes Linked to Exposure to Pollutants and Other Substances in Outdoor and Indoor Environments Such as Lead, Asbestos, Formaldehyde, Mercury, Emissions, Noise, and More

Edited by Allan R. Cook. 620 pages. 1997. 0-7808-0083-4. $78.

"Recommended reference source."
— *Booklist, American Library Association, Sep '98*

"This book will be a useful addition to anyone's library." — *Choice Health Sciences Supplement, Association of College and Research Libraries, May '98*

". . . a good survey of numerous environmentally induced physical disorders . . . a useful addition to anyone's library."
— *Doody's Health Sciences Book Reviews, Jan '98*

". . . provide[s] introductory information from the best authorities around. Since this volume covers topics that potentially affect everyone, it will surely be one of the most frequently consulted volumes in the *Health Reference Series*." — *Rettig on Reference, Nov '97*

■

Ethnic Diseases Sourcebook

Basic Consumer Health Information for Ethnic and Racial Minority Groups in the United States, Including General Health Indicators and Behaviors, Ethnic Diseases, Genetic Testing, the Impact of Chronic Diseases, Women's Health, Mental Health Issues, and Preventive Health Care Services

Along with a Glossary and a Listing of Additional Resources

Edited by Joyce Brennfleck Shannon. 664 pages. 2001. 0-7808-0336-1. $78.

"Recommended for health sciences libraries where public health programs are a priority."
— *E-Streams, Jan '02*

"Recommended reference source."
— *Booklist, American Library Association, Oct '01*

"Will prove valuable to any library seeking to maintain a current, comprehensive reference collection of health resources.... An excellent source of health information about genetic disorders which affect particular ethnic and racial minorities in the U.S."
— *The Bookwatch, Aug '01*

■

Family Planning Sourcebook

Basic Consumer Health Information about Planning for Pregnancy and Contraception, Including Traditional Methods, Barrier Methods, Hormonal Methods, Permanent Methods, Future Methods, Emergency Contraception, and Birth Control Choices for Women at Each Stage of Life

Along with Statistics, a Glossary, and Sources of Additional Information

Edited by Amy Marcaccio Keyzer. 520 pages. 2001. 0-7808-0379-5. $78.

"Recommended reference source."
—*Booklist, American Library Association, Oct '01*

"Will prove valuable to any library seeking to maintain a current, comprehensive reference collection of health resources. . . . Excellent reference."
—*The Bookwatch, Aug '01*

SEE ALSO *Pregnancy & Birth Sourcebook*

■

Fitness & Exercise Sourcebook, 1st Edition

Basic Information on Fitness and Exercise, Including Fitness Activities for Specific Age Groups, Exercise for People with Specific Medical Conditions, How to Begin a Fitness Program in Running, Walking, Swimming, Cycling, and Other Athletic Activities, and Recent Research in Fitness and Exercise

Edited by Dan R. Harris. 663 pages. 1996. 0-7808-0186-5. $78.

"A good resource for general readers."   —*Choice, Association of College and Research Libraries, Nov '97*

"The perennial popularity of the topic . . . make this an appealing selection for public libraries."
—*Rettig on Reference, Jun/Jul '97*

■

Fitness & Exercise Sourcebook, 2nd Edition

Basic Consumer Health Information about the Fundamentals of Fitness and Exercise, Including How to Begin and Maintain a Fitness Program, Fitness as a Lifestyle, the Link between Fitness and Diet, Advice for Specific Groups of People, Exercise as It Relates to Specific Medical Conditions, and Recent Research in Fitness and Exercise

Along with a Glossary of Important Terms and Resources for Additional Help and Information

Edited by Kristen M. Gledhill. 646 pages. 2001. 0-7808-0334-5. $78.

"Highly recommended for public, consumer, and school grades fourth through college."
—*E-Streams, Nov '01*

"Recommended reference source."   —*Booklist, American Library Association, Oct 15, '01*

"The information appears quite comprehensive and is considered reliable. . . . This second edition is a welcomed addition to the series."
—*Doody's Review Service, Sep '01*

"This reference is a valuable choice for those who desire a broad source of information on exercise, fitness, and chronic-disease prevention through a healthy lifestyle."   —*American Medical Writers Association Journal, Fall '01*

"Will prove valuable to any library seeking to maintain a current, comprehensive reference collection of health resources. . . . Excellent reference."
—*The Bookwatch, Aug '01*

■

Food & Animal Borne Diseases Sourcebook

Basic Information about Diseases That Can Be Spread to Humans through the Ingestion of Contaminated Food or Water or by Contact with Infected Animals and Insects, Such as Botulism, E. Coli, Hepatitis A, Trichinosis, Lyme Disease, and Rabies

Along with Information Regarding Prevention and Treatment Methods, and Including a Special Section for International Travelers Describing Diseases Such as Cholera, Malaria, Travelers' Diarrhea, and Yellow Fever, and Offering Recommendations for Avoiding Illness

Edited by Karen Bellenir and Peter D. Dresser. 535 pages. 1995. 0-7808-0033-8. $78.

"Targeting general readers and providing them with a single, comprehensive source of information on selected topics, this book continues, with the excellent caliber of its predecessors, to catalog topical information on health matters of general interest. Readable and thorough, this valuable resource is highly recommended for all libraries."
—*Academic Library Book Review, Summer '96*

"A comprehensive collection of authoritative information."   —*Emergency Medical Services, Oct '95*

■

Food Safety Sourcebook

Basic Consumer Health Information about the Safe Handling of Meat, Poultry, Seafood, Eggs, Fruit Juices, and Other Food Items, and Facts about Pesticides, Drinking Water, Food Safety Overseas, and the Onset, Duration, and Symptoms of Foodborne Illnesses, Including Types of Pathogenic Bacteria, Parasitic Protozoa, Worms, Viruses, and Natural Toxins

Along with the Role of the Consumer, the Food Handler, and the Government in Food Safety; a Glossary, and Resources for Additional Help and Information

Edited by Dawn D. Matthews. 339 pages. 1999. 0-7808-0326-4. $78.

"This book is recommended for public libraries and universities with home economic and food science programs."   —*E-Streams, Nov '00*

"This book takes the complex issues of food safety and foodborne pathogens and presents them in an easily understood manner. [It does] an excellent job of covering a large and often confusing topic."
—*American Reference Books Annual, 2000*

"Recommended reference source."
—*Booklist, American Library Association, May '00*

Forensic Medicine Sourcebook

Basic Consumer Information for the Layperson about Forensic Medicine, Including Crime Scene Investigation, Evidence Collection and Analysis, Expert Testimony, Computer-Aided Criminal Identification, Digital Imaging in the Courtroom, DNA Profiling, Accident Reconstruction, Autopsies, Ballistics, Drugs and Explosives Detection, Latent Fingerprints, Product Tampering, and Questioned Document Examination

Along with Statistical Data, a Glossary of Forensics Terminology, and Listings of Sources for Further Help and Information

Edited by Annemarie S. Muth. 574 pages. 1999. 0-7808-0232-2. $78.

"Given the expected widespread interest in its content and its easy to read style, this book is recommended for most public and all college and university libraries."
— E-Streams, Feb '01

"There are several items that make this book attractive to consumers who are seeking certain forensic data. . . . This is a useful current source for those seeking general forensic medical answers."
— American Reference Books Annual, 2000

"Recommended for public libraries."
— Reference & User Services Quarterly, American Library Association, Spring 2000

"Recommended reference source."
— Booklist, American Library Association, Feb '00

"A wealth of information, useful statistics, references are up-to-date and extremely complete. This wonderful collection of data will help students who are interested in a career in any type of forensic field. It is a great resource for attorneys who need information about types of expert witnesses needed in a particular case. It also offers useful information for fiction and nonfiction writers whose work involves a crime. A fascinating compilation. All levels." — Choice, Association of College and Research Libraries, Jan 2000

∎

Gastrointestinal Diseases & Disorders Sourcebook

Basic Information about Gastroesophageal Reflux Disease (Heartburn), Ulcers, Diverticulosis, Irritable Bowel Syndrome, Crohn's Disease, Ulcerative Colitis, Diarrhea, Constipation, Lactose Intolerance, Hemorrhoids, Hepatitis, Cirrhosis, and Other Digestive Problems, Featuring Statistics, Descriptions of Symptoms, and Current Treatment Methods of Interest for Persons Living with Upper and Lower Gastrointestinal Maladies

Edited by Linda M. Ross. 413 pages. 1996. 0-7808-0078-8. $78.

". . . very readable form. The successful editorial work that brought this material together into a useful and understandable reference makes accessible to all readers information that can help them more effectively understand and obtain help for digestive tract problems."
— Choice, Association of College and Research Libraries, Feb '97

SEE ALSO Diet & Nutrition Sourcebook, 1st and 2nd Editions, Digestive Diseases & Disorders

∎

Genetic Disorders Sourcebook, 1st Edition

Basic Information about Heritable Diseases and Disorders Such as Down Syndrome, PKU, Hemophilia, Von Willebrand Disease, Gaucher Disease, Tay-Sachs Disease, and Sickle-Cell Disease, Along with Information about Genetic Screening, Gene Therapy, Home Care, and Including Source Listings for Further Help and Information on More Than 300 Disorders

Edited by Karen Bellenir. 642 pages. 1996. 0-7808-0034-6. $78.

"Recommended for undergraduate libraries or libraries that serve the public."
— Science & Technology Libraries, Vol. 18, No. 1, '99

"Provides essential medical information to both the general public and those diagnosed with a serious or fatal genetic disease or disorder." — Choice, Association of College and Research Libraries, Jan '97

"Geared toward the lay public. It would be well placed in all public libraries and in those hospital and medical libraries in which access to genetic references is limited." — Doody's Health Sciences Book Review, Oct '96

∎

Genetic Disorders Sourcebook, 2nd Edition

Basic Consumer Health Information about Hereditary Diseases and Disorders, Including Cystic Fibrosis, Down Syndrome, Hemophilia, Huntington's Disease, Sickle Cell Anemia, and More; Facts about Genes, Gene Research and Therapy, Genetic Screening, Ethics of Gene Testing, Genetic Counseling, and Advice on Coping and Caring

Along with a Glossary of Genetic Terminology and a Resource List for Help, Support, and Further Information

Edited by Kathy Massimini. 768 pages. 2001. 0-7808-0241-1. $78.

"Recommended for public libraries and medical and hospital libraries with consumer health collections."
— E-Streams, May '01

"Recommended reference source."
— Booklist, American Library Association, Apr '01

"Important pick for college-level health reference libraries." — The Bookwatch, Mar '01

∎

Head Trauma Sourcebook

Basic Information for the Layperson about Open-Head and Closed-Head Injuries, Treatment Advances, Recovery, and Rehabilitation

Along with Reports on Current Research Initiatives

Edited by Karen Bellenir. 414 pages. 1997. 0-7808-0208-X. $78.

Headache Sourcebook

Basic Consumer Health Information about Migraine, Tension, Cluster, Rebound and Other Types of Headaches, with Facts about the Cause and Prevention of Headaches, the Effects of Stress and the Environment, Headaches during Pregnancy and Menopause, and Childhood Headaches

Along with a Glossary and Other Resources for Additional Help and Information

Edited by Dawn D. Matthews. 350 pages. 2002. 0-7808-0337-X. $78.

■

Health Insurance Sourcebook

Basic Information about Managed Care Organizations, Traditional Fee-for-Service Insurance, Insurance Portability and Pre-Existing Conditions Clauses, Medicare, Medicaid, Social Security, and Military Health Care

Along with Information about Insurance Fraud

Edited by Wendy Wilcox. 530 pages. 1997. 0-7808-0222-5. $78.

"Particularly useful because it brings much of this information together in one volume. This book will be a handy reference source in the health sciences library, hospital library, college and university library, and medium to large public library."
— *Medical Reference Services Quarterly, Fall '98*

Awarded "Books of the Year Award"
— *American Journal of Nursing, 1997*

"The layout of the book is particularly helpful as it provides easy access to reference material. A most useful addition to the vast amount of information about health insurance. The use of data from U.S. government agencies is most commendable. Useful in a library or learning center for healthcare professional students."
— *Doody's Health Sciences Book Reviews, Nov '97*

■

Health Reference Series Cumulative Index 1999

A Comprehensive Index to the Individual Volumes of the Health Reference Series, Including a Subject Index, Name Index, Organization Index, and Publication Index

Along with a Master List of Acronyms and Abbreviations

Edited by Edward J. Prucha, Anne Holmes, and Robert Rudnick. 990 pages. 2000. 0-7808-0382-5. $78.

"This volume will be most helpful in libraries that have a relatively complete collection of the Health Reference Series."
— *American Reference Books Annual, 2001*

"Essential for collections that hold any of the numerous *Health Reference Series* titles."
— *Choice, Association of College and Research Libraries, Nov '00*

Healthy Aging Sourcebook

Basic Consumer Health Information about Maintaining Health through the Aging Process, Including Advice on Nutrition, Exercise, and Sleep, Help in Making Decisions about Midlife Issues and Retirement, and Guidance Concerning Practical and Informed Choices in Health Consumerism

Along with Data Concerning the Theories of Aging, Different Experiences in Aging by Minority Groups, and Facts about Aging Now and Aging in the Future; and Featuring a Glossary, a Guide to Consumer Help, Additional Suggested Reading, and Practical Resource Directory

Edited by Jenifer Swanson. 536 pages. 1999. 0-7808-0390-6. $78.

"Recommended reference source."
— *Booklist, American Library Association, Feb '00*

SEE ALSO *Physical & Mental Issues in Aging Sourcebook*

■

Healthy Heart Sourcebook for Women

Basic Consumer Health Information about Cardiac Issues Specific to Women, Including Facts about Major Risk Factors and Prevention, Treatment and Control Strategies, and Important Dietary Issues

Along with a Special Section Regarding the Pros and Cons of Hormone Replacement Therapy and Its Impact on Heart Health, and Additional Help, Including Recipes, a Glossary, and a Directory of Resources

Edited by Dawn D. Matthews. 336 pages. 2000. 0-7808-0329-9. $78.

"A good reference source and recommended for all public, academic, medical, and hospital libraries."
— *Medical Reference Services Quarterly, Summer '01*

"Because of the lack of information specific to women on this topic, this book is recommended for public libraries and consumer libraries."
— *American Reference Books Annual, 2001*

"Contains very important information about coronary artery disease that all women should know. The information is current and presented in an easy-to-read format. The book will make a good addition to any library."
— *American Medical Writers Association Journal, Summer '00*

"Important, basic reference."
— *Reviewer's Bookwatch, Jul '00*

SEE ALSO *Cardiovascular Diseases & Disorders Sourcebook, 1st Edition, Heart Diseases & Disorders Sourcebook, 2nd Edition, Women's Health Concerns Sourcebook*

Heart Diseases & Disorders Sourcebook, 2nd Edition

Basic Consumer Health Information about Heart Attacks, Angina, Rhythm Disorders, Heart Failure, Valve Disease, Congenital Heart Disorders, and More, Including Descriptions of Surgical Procedures and Other Interventions, Medications, Cardiac Rehabilitation, Risk Identification, and Prevention Tips

Along with Statistical Data, Reports on Current Research Initiatives, a Glossary of Cardiovascular Terms, and Resource Directory

Edited by Karen Bellenir. 612 pages. 2000. 0-7808-0238-1. $78.

"This work stands out as an imminently accessible resource for the general public. It is recommended for the reference and circulating shelves of school, public, and academic libraries."
— *American Reference Books Annual, 2001*

"Recommended reference source."
— *Booklist, American Library Association, Dec '00*

"Provides comprehensive coverage of matters related to the heart. This title is recommended for health sciences and public libraries with consumer health collections."
— *E-Streams, Oct '00*

SEE ALSO Cardiovascular Diseases & Disorders Sourcebook, 1st Edition; Healthy Heart Sourcebook for Women

Household Safety Sourcebook

Basic Consumer Health Information about Household Safety, Including Information about Poisons, Chemicals, Fire, and Water Hazards in the Home

Along with Advice about the Safe Use of Home Maintenance Equipment, Choosing Toys and Nursery Furniture, Holiday and Recreation Safety, a Glossary, and Resources for Further Help and Information

Edited by Dawn D. Matthews. 606 pages. 2001. 0-7808-0338-8. $78.

Immune System Disorders Sourcebook

Basic Information about Lupus, Multiple Sclerosis, Guillain-Barré Syndrome, Chronic Granulomatous Disease, and More

Along with Statistical and Demographic Data and Reports on Current Research Initiatives

Edited by Allan R. Cook. 608 pages. 1997. 0-7808-0209-8. $78.

Infant & Toddler Health Sourcebook

Basic Consumer Health Information about the Physical and Mental Development of Newborns, Infants, and Toddlers, Including Neonatal Concerns, Nutrition Recommendations, Immunization Schedules, Common Pediatric Disorders, Assessments and Milestones, Safety Tips, and Advice for Parents and Other Caregivers

Along with a Glossary of Terms and Resource Listings for Additional Help

Edited by Jenifer Swanson. 585 pages. 2000. 0-7808-0246-2. $78.

"As a reference for the general public, this would be useful in any library." — *E-Streams, May '01*

"Recommended reference source."
— *Booklist, American Library Association, Feb '01*

"This is a good source for general use."
— *American Reference Books Annual, 2001*

Injury & Trauma Sourcebook

Basic Consumer Health Information about the Impact of Injury, the Diagnosis and Treatment of Common and Traumatic Injuries, Emergency Care, and Specific Injuries Related to Home, Community, Workplace, Transportation, and Recreation

Along with Guidelines for Injury Prevention, a Glossary, and a Directory of Additional Resources

Edited by Joyce Brennfleck Shannon. 700 pages. 2002. 0-7808-0421-X. $78.

Kidney & Urinary Tract Diseases & Disorders Sourcebook

Basic Information about Kidney Stones, Urinary Incontinence, Bladder Disease, End Stage Renal Disease, Dialysis, and More

Along with Statistical and Demographic Data and Reports on Current Research Initiatives

Edited by Linda M. Ross. 602 pages. 1997. 0-7808-0079-6. $78.

Learning Disabilities Sourcebook

Basic Information about Disorders Such as Dyslexia, Visual and Auditory Processing Deficits, Attention Deficit/Hyperactivity Disorder, and Autism

Along with Statistical and Demographic Data, Reports on Current Research Initiatives, an Explanation of the Assessment Process, and a Special Section for Adults with Learning Disabilities

Edited by Linda M. Shin. 579 pages. 1998. 0-7808-0210-1. $78.

Named "Outstanding Reference Book of 1999."
— *New York Public Library, Feb 2000*

"An excellent candidate for inclusion in a public library reference section. It's a great source of information. Teachers will also find the book useful. Definitely worth reading."
— *Journal of Adolescent & Adult Literacy, Feb 2000*

"Readable . . . provides a solid base of information regarding successful techniques used with individuals who have learning disabilities, as well as practical suggestions for educators and family members. Clear language, concise descriptions, and pertinent information for contacting multiple resources add to the strength of this book as a useful tool." — *Choice, Association of College and Research Libraries, Feb '99*

"Recommended reference source."
— *Booklist, American Library Association, Sep '98*

"A useful resource for libraries and for those who don't have the time to identify and locate the individual publications." — *Disability Resources Monthly, Sep '98*

■

Liver Disorders Sourcebook

Basic Consumer Health Information about the Liver and How It Works; Liver Diseases, Including Cancer, Cirrhosis, Hepatitis, and Toxic and Drug Related Diseases; Tips for Maintaining a Healthy Liver; Laboratory Tests, Radiology Tests, and Facts about Liver Transplantation

Along with a Section on Support Groups, a Glossary, and Resource Listings

Edited by Joyce Brennfleck Shannon. 591 pages. 2000. 0-7808-0383-3. $78.

"A valuable resource."
— *American Reference Books Annual, 2001*

"This title is recommended for health sciences and public libraries with consumer health collections."
— *E-Streams, Oct '00*

"Recommended reference source."
— *Booklist, American Library Association, Jun '00*

■

Lung Disorders Sourcebook

Basic Consumer Health Information about Emphysema, Pneumonia, Tuberculosis, Asthma, Cystic Fibrosis, and Other Lung Disorders, Including Facts about Diagnostic Procedures, Treatment Strategies, Disease Prevention Efforts, and Such Risk Factors as Smoking, Air Pollution, and Exposure to Asbestos, Radon, and Other Agents

Along with a Glossary and Resources for Additional Help and Information

Edited by Dawn D. Matthews. 600 pages. 2002. 0-7808-0339-6. $78.

■

Medical Tests Sourcebook

Basic Consumer Health Information about Medical Tests, Including Periodic Health Exams, General Screening Tests, Tests You Can Do at Home, Findings of the U.S. Preventive Services Task Force, X-ray and Radiology Tests, Electrical Tests, Tests of Blood and Other Body Fluids and Tissues, Scope Tests, Lung Tests, Genetic Tests, Pregnancy Tests, Newborn Screening Tests, Sexually Transmitted Disease Tests, and Computer Aided Diagnoses

Along with a Section on Paying for Medical Tests, a Glossary, and Resource Listings

Edited by Joyce Brennfleck Shannon. 691 pages. 1999. 0-7808-0243-8. $78.

"A valuable reference guide."
— *American Reference Books Annual, 2000*

"Recommended for hospital and health sciences libraries with consumer health collections."
— *E-Streams, Mar '00*

"This is an overall excellent reference with a wealth of general knowledge that may aid those who are reluctant to get vital tests performed."
— *Today's Librarian, Jan 2000*

■

Men's Health Concerns Sourcebook

Basic Information about Health Issues That Affect Men, Featuring Facts about the Top Causes of Death in Men, Including Heart Disease, Stroke, Cancers, Prostate Disorders, Chronic Obstructive Pulmonary Disease, Pneumonia and Influenza, Human Immunodeficiency Virus and Acquired Immune Deficiency Syndrome, Diabetes Mellitus, Stress, Suicide, Accidents and Homicides; and Facts about Common Concerns for Men, Including Impotence, Contraception, Circumcision, Sleep Disorders, Snoring, Hair Loss, Diet, Nutrition, Exercise, Kidney and Urological Disorders, and Backaches

Edited by Allan R. Cook. 738 pages. 1998. 0-7808-0212-8. $78.

"This comprehensive resource and the series are highly recommended."
— *American Reference Books Annual, 2000*

"Recommended reference source."
— *Booklist, American Library Association, Dec '98*

■

Mental Health Disorders Sourcebook, 1st Edition

Basic Information about Schizophrenia, Depression, Bipolar Disorder, Panic Disorder, Obsessive-Compulsive Disorder, Phobias and Other Anxiety Disorders, Paranoia and Other Personality Disorders, Eating Disorders, and Sleep Disorders

Along with Information about Treatment and Therapies

Edited by Karen Bellenir. 548 pages. 1995. 0-7808-0040-0. $78.

"This is an excellent new book . . . written in easy-to-understand language."
— *Booklist Health Sciences Supplement, American Library Association, Oct '97*

". . . useful for public and academic libraries and consumer health collections."
— *Medical Reference Services Quarterly, Spring '97*

"The great strengths of the book are its readability and its inclusion of places to find more information. Especially recommended." — *Reference Quarterly, American Library Association, Winter '96*

". . . a good resource for a consumer health library."
— *Bulletin of the Medical Library Association, Oct '96*

"The information is data-based and couched in brief, concise language that avoids jargon. . . . a useful reference source." —*Readings, Sep '96*

"The text is well organized and adequately written for its target audience." — *Choice, Association of College and Research Libraries, Jun '96*

". . . provides information on a wide range of mental disorders, presented in nontechnical language." — *Exceptional Child Education Resources, Spring '96*

"Recommended for public and academic libraries." — *Reference Book Review, 1996*

■

Mental Health Disorders Sourcebook, 2nd Edition

Basic Consumer Health Information about Anxiety Disorders, Depression and Other Mood Disorders, Eating Disorders, Personality Disorders, Schizophrenia, and More, Including Disease Descriptions, Treatment Options, and Reports on Current Research Initiatives

Along with Statistical Data, Tips for Maintaining Mental Health, a Glossary, and Directory of Sources for Additional Help and Information

Edited by Karen Bellenir. 605 pages. 2000. 0-7808-0240-3. $78.

"Well organized and well written." —*American Reference Books Annual, 2001*

"Recommended reference source." —*Booklist, American Library Association, Jun '00*

■

Mental Retardation Sourcebook

Basic Consumer Health Information about Mental Retardation and Its Causes, Including Down Syndrome, Fetal Alcohol Syndrome, Fragile X Syndrome, Genetic Conditions, Injury, and Environmental Sources

Along with Preventive Strategies, Parenting Issues, Educational Implications, Health Care Needs, Employment and Economic Matters, Legal Issues, a Glossary, and a Resource Listing for Additional Help and Information

Edited by Joyce Brennfleck Shannon. 642 pages. 2000. 0-7808-0377-9. $78.

"Public libraries will find the book useful for reference and as a beginning research point for students, parents, and caregivers." —*American Reference Books Annual, 2001*

"The strength of this work is that it compiles many basic fact sheets and addresses for further information in one volume. It is intended and suitable for the general public. This sourcebook is relevant to any collection providing health information to the general public." —*E-Streams, Nov '00*

"From preventing retardation to parenting and family challenges, this covers health, social and legal issues and will prove an invaluable overview." —*Reviewer's Bookwatch, Jul '00*

Obesity Sourcebook

Basic Consumer Health Information about Diseases and Other Problems Associated with Obesity, and Including Facts about Risk Factors, Prevention Issues, and Management Approaches

Along with Statistical and Demographic Data, Information about Special Populations, Research Updates, a Glossary, and Source Listings for Further Help and Information

Edited by Wilma Caldwell and Chad T. Kimball. 376 pages. 2001. 0-7808-0333-7. $78.

"This is a very useful resource book for the lay public." —*Doody's Review Service, Nov '01*

"Well suited for the health reference collection of a public library or an academic health science library that serves the general population." —*E-Streams, Sep '01*

" Recommended pick both for specialty health library collections and any general consumer health reference collection." — *The Bookwatch, Apr '01*

"Recommended reference source." —*Booklist, American Library Association, Apr '01*

■

Ophthalmic Disorders Sourcebook

Basic Information about Glaucoma, Cataracts, Macular Degeneration, Strabismus, Refractive Disorders, and More

Along with Statistical and Demographic Data and Reports on Current Research Initiatives

Edited by Linda M. Ross. 631 pages. 1996. 0-7808-0081-8. $78.

■

Oral Health Sourcebook

Basic Information about Diseases and Conditions Affecting Oral Health, Including Cavities, Gum Disease, Dry Mouth, Oral Cancers, Fever Blisters, Canker Sores, Oral Thrush, Bad Breath, Temporomandibular Disorders, and other Craniofacial Syndromes

Along with Statistical Data on the Oral Health of Americans, Oral Hygiene, Emergency First Aid, Information on Treatment Procedures and Methods of Replacing Lost Teeth

Edited by Allan R. Cook. 558 pages. 1997. 0-7808-0082-6. $78.

"Unique source which will fill a gap in dental sources for patients and the lay public. A valuable reference tool even in a library with thousands of books on dentistry. Comprehensive, clear, inexpensive, and easy to read and use. It fills an enormous gap in the health care literature." — *Reference and User Services Quarterly, American Library Association, Summer '98*

"Recommended reference source." — *Booklist, American Library Association, Dec '97*

Osteoporosis Sourcebook

Basic Consumer Health Information about Primary and Secondary Osteoporosis and Juvenile Osteoporosis and Related Conditions, Including Fibrous Dysplasia, Gaucher Disease, Hyperthyroidism, Hypophosphatasia, Myeloma, Osteopetrosis, Osteogenesis Imperfecta, and Paget's Disease

Along with Information about Risk Factors, Treatments, Traditional and Non-Traditional Pain Management, a Glossary of Related Terms, and a Directory of Resources

Edited by Allan R. Cook. 584 pages. 2001. 0-7808-0239-X. $78.

"This would be a book to be kept in a staff or patient library. The targeted audience is the layperson, but the therapist who needs a quick bit of information on a particular topic will also find the book useful."
—*Physical Therapy, Jan '02*

"Recommended for all public libraries and general health collections, especially those supporting patient education or consumer health programs."
—*E-Streams, Nov '01*

"Will prove valuable to any library seeking to maintain a current, comprehensive reference collection of health resources. . . . From prevention to treatment and associated conditions, this provides an excellent survey."
—*The Bookwatch, Aug '01*

"Recommended reference source."
—*Booklist, American Library Association, July '01*

SEE ALSO *Women's Health Concerns Sourcebook*

■

Pain Sourcebook

Basic Information about Specific Forms of Acute and Chronic Pain, Including Headaches, Back Pain, Muscular Pain, Neuralgia, Surgical Pain, and Cancer Pain

Along with Pain Relief Options Such as Analgesics, Narcotics, Nerve Blocks, Transcutaneous Nerve Stimulation, and Alternative Forms of Pain Control, Including Biofeedback, Imaging, Behavior Modification, and Relaxation Techniques

Edited by Allan R. Cook. 667 pages. 1997. 0-7808-0213-6. $78.

"The text is readable, easily understood, and well indexed. This excellent volume belongs in all patient education libraries, consumer health sections of public libraries, and many personal collections."
—*American Reference Books Annual, 1999*

"A beneficial reference." —*Booklist Health Sciences Supplement, American Library Association, Oct '98*

"The information is basic in terms of scholarship and is appropriate for general readers. Written in journalistic style . . . intended for non-professionals. Quite thorough in its coverage of different pain conditions and summarizes the latest clinical information regarding pain treatment." —*Choice, Association of College and Research Libraries, Jun '98*

"Recommended reference source."
—*Booklist, American Library Association, Mar '98*

■

Pediatric Cancer Sourcebook

Basic Consumer Health Information about Leukemias, Brain Tumors, Sarcomas, Lymphomas, and Other Cancers in Infants, Children, and Adolescents, Including Descriptions of Cancers, Treatments, and Coping Strategies

Along with Suggestions for Parents, Caregivers, and Concerned Relatives, a Glossary of Cancer Terms, and Resource Listings

Edited by Edward J. Prucha. 587 pages. 1999. 0-7808-0245-4. $78.

"A valuable addition to all libraries specializing in health services and many public libraries."
—*American Reference Books Annual, 2000*

"Recommended reference source."
—*Booklist, American Library Association, Feb '00*

"An excellent source of information. Recommended for public, hospital, and health science libraries with consumer health collections." —*E-Streams, Jun '00*

■

Physical & Mental Issues in Aging Sourcebook

Basic Consumer Health Information on Physical and Mental Disorders Associated with the Aging Process, Including Concerns about Cardiovascular Disease, Pulmonary Disease, Oral Health, Digestive Disorders, Musculoskeletal and Skin Disorders, Metabolic Changes, Sexual and Reproductive Issues, and Changes in Vision, Hearing, and Other Senses

Along with Data about Longevity and Causes of Death, Information on Acute and Chronic Pain, Descriptions of Mental Concerns, a Glossary of Terms, and Resource Listings for Additional Help

Edited by Jenifer Swanson. 660 pages. 1999. 0-7808-0233-0. $78.

"Recommended for public libraries."
—*American Reference Books Annual, 2000*

"This is a treasure of health information for the layperson." — *Choice Health Sciences Supplement, Association of College & Research Libraries, May 2000*

"Recommended reference source."
—*Booklist, American Library Association, Oct '99*

SEE ALSO *Healthy Aging Sourcebook*

■

Podiatry Sourcebook

Basic Consumer Health Information about Foot Conditions, Diseases, and Injuries, Including Bunions, Corns, Calluses, Athlete's Foot, Plantar Warts, Hammertoes and Clawtoes, Clubfoot, Heel Pain, Gout, and More

Along with Facts about Foot Care, Disease Prevention, Foot Safety, Choosing a Foot Care Specialist, a Glossary of Terms, and Resource Listings for Additional Information

Edited by M. Lisa Weatherford. 380 pages. 2001. 0-7808-0215-2. $78.

■

Pregnancy & Birth Sourcebook

Basic Information about Planning for Pregnancy, Maternal Health, Fetal Growth and Development, Labor and Delivery, Postpartum and Perinatal Care, Pregnancy in Mothers with Special Concerns, and Disorders of Pregnancy, Including Genetic Counseling, Nutrition and Exercise, Obstetrical Tests, Pregnancy Discomfort, Multiple Births, Cesarean Sections, Medical Testing of Newborns, Breastfeeding, Gestational Diabetes, and Ectopic Pregnancy

Edited by Heather E. Aldred. 737 pages. 1997. 0-7808-0216-0. $78.

"A well-organized handbook. Recommended."
— Choice, Association of College and Research Libraries, Apr '98

"Recommended reference source."
— Booklist, American Library Association, Mar '98

"Recommended for public libraries."
— American Reference Books Annual, 1998

SEE ALSO Congenital Disorders Sourcebook, Family Planning Sourcebook

■

Prostate Cancer Sourcebook

Basic Consumer Health Information about Prostate Cancer, Including Information about the Associated Risk Factors, Detection, Diagnosis, and Treatment of Prostate Cancer

Along with Information on Non-Malignant Prostate Conditions, and Featuring a Section Listing Support and Treatment Centers and a Glossary of Related Terms

Edited by Dawn D. Matthews. 358 pages. 2001. 0-7808-0324-8. $78.

"Recommended reference source."
— Booklist, American Library Association, Jan '02

■

Public Health Sourcebook

Basic Information about Government Health Agencies, Including National Health Statistics and Trends, Healthy People 2000 Program Goals and Objectives, the Centers for Disease Control and Prevention, the Food and Drug Administration, and the National Institutes of Health

Along with Full Contact Information for Each Agency

Edited by Wendy Wilcox. 698 pages. 1998. 0-7808-0220-9. $78.

"Recommended reference source."
— Booklist, American Library Association, Sep '98

"This consumer guide provides welcome assistance in navigating the maze of federal health agencies and their data on public health concerns."
— SciTech Book News, Sep '98

■

Reconstructive & Cosmetic Surgery Sourcebook

Basic Consumer Health Information on Cosmetic and Reconstructive Plastic Surgery, Including Statistical Information about Different Surgical Procedures, Things to Consider Prior to Surgery, Plastic Surgery Techniques and Tools, Emotional and Psychological Considerations, and Procedure-Specific Information

Along with a Glossary of Terms and a Listing of Resources for Additional Help and Information

Edited by M. Lisa Weatherford. 374 pages. 2001. 0-7808-0214-4. $78.

"Recommended for health science libraries that are open to the public, as well as hospital libraries that are open to the patients. This book is a good resource for the consumer interested in plastic surgery."
— E-Streams, Dec '01

"Recommended reference source."
— Booklist, American Library Association, July '01

■

Rehabilitation Sourcebook

Basic Consumer Health Information about Rehabilitation for People Recovering from Heart Surgery, Spinal Cord Injury, Stroke, Orthopedic Impairments, Amputation, Pulmonary Impairments, Traumatic Injury, and More, Including Physical Therapy, Occupational Therapy, Speech/ Language Therapy, Massage Therapy, Dance Therapy, Art Therapy, and Recreational Therapy

Along with Information on Assistive and Adaptive Devices, a Glossary, and Resources for Additional Help and Information

Edited by Dawn D. Matthews. 531 pages. 1999. 0-7808-0236-5. $78.

"This is an excellent resource for public library reference and health collections."
— American Reference Books Annual, 2001

"Recommended reference source."
— Booklist, American Library Association, May '00

■

Respiratory Diseases & Disorders Sourcebook

Basic Information about Respiratory Diseases and Disorders, Including Asthma, Cystic Fibrosis, Pneumonia, the Common Cold, Influenza, and Others, Featuring Facts about the Respiratory System, Statistical and Demographic Data, Treatments, Self-Help Management Suggestions, and Current Research Initiatives

Edited by Allan R. Cook and Peter D. Dresser. 771 pages. 1995. 0-7808-0037-0. $78.

"Designed for the layperson and for patients and their families coping with respiratory illness. . . . an extensive array of information on diagnosis, treatment, management, and prevention of respiratory illnesses for the general reader." — *Choice, Association of College and Research Libraries, Jun '96*

"A highly recommended text for all collections. It is a comforting reminder of the power of knowledge that good books carry between their covers." — *Academic Library Book Review, Spring '96*

"A comprehensive collection of authoritative information presented in a nontechnical, humanitarian style for patients, families, and caregivers." — *Association of Operating Room Nurses, Sep/Oct '95*

■

Sexually Transmitted Diseases Sourcebook, 1st Edition

Basic Information about Herpes, Chlamydia, Gonorrhea, Hepatitis, Nongonoccocal Urethritis, Pelvic Inflammatory Disease, Syphilis, AIDS, and More

Along with Current Data on Treatments and Preventions

Edited by Linda M. Ross. 550 pages. 1997. 0-7808-0217-9. $78.

■

Sexually Transmitted Diseases Sourcebook, 2nd Edition

Basic Consumer Health Information about Sexually Transmitted Diseases, Including Information on the Diagnosis and Treatment of Chlamydia, Gonorrhea, Hepatitis, Herpes, HIV, Mononucleosis, Syphilis, and Others

Along with Information on Prevention, Such as Condom Use, Vaccines, and STD Education; And Featuring a Section on Issues Related to Youth and Adolescents, a Glossary, and Resources for Additional Help and Information

Edited by Dawn D. Matthews. 538 pages. 2001. 0-7808-0249-7. $78.

"Every school and public library should have a copy of this comprehensive and user-friendly reference book." — *Choice, Association of College & Research Libraries, Sep '01*

"This is a highly recommended book. This is an especially important book for all school and public libraries." — *AIDS Book Review Journal, Jul-Aug '01*

"Recommended pick both for specialty health library collections and any general consumer health reference collection." — *The Bookwatch, Apr '01*

"Recommended reference source." — *Booklist, American Library Association, Apr '01*

Skin Disorders Sourcebook

Basic Information about Common Skin and Scalp Conditions Caused by Aging, Allergies, Immune Reactions, Sun Exposure, Infectious Organisms, Parasites, Cosmetics, and Skin Traumas, Including Abrasions, Cuts, and Pressure Sores

Along with Information on Prevention and Treatment

Edited by Allan R. Cook. 647 pages. 1997. 0-7808-0080-X. $78.

". . . comprehensive, easily read reference book." — *Doody's Health Sciences Book Reviews, Oct '97*

SEE ALSO Burns Sourcebook

■

Sleep Disorders Sourcebook

Basic Consumer Health Information about Sleep and Its Disorders, Including Insomnia, Sleepwalking, Sleep Apnea, Restless Leg Syndrome, and Narcolepsy

Along with Data about Shiftwork and Its Effects, Information on the Societal Costs of Sleep Deprivation, Descriptions of Treatment Options, a Glossary of Terms, and Resource Listings for Additional Help

Edited by Jenifer Swanson. 439 pages. 1998. 0-7808-0234-9. $78.

"This text will complement any home or medical library. It is user-friendly and ideal for the adult reader." — *American Reference Books Annual, 2000*

"Recommended reference source." — *Booklist, American Library Association, Feb '99*

"A useful resource that provides accurate, relevant, and accessible information on sleep to the general public. Health care providers who deal with sleep disorders patients may also find it helpful in being prepared to answer some of the questions patients ask." — *Respiratory Care, Jul '99*

■

Sports Injuries Sourcebook

Basic Consumer Health Information about Common Sports Injuries, Prevention of Injury in Specific Sports, Tips for Training, and Rehabilitation from Injury

Along with Information about Special Concerns for Children, Young Girls in Athletic Training Programs, Senior Athletes, and Women Athletes, and a Directory of Resources for Further Help and Information

Edited by Heather E. Aldred. 624 pages. 1999. 0-7808-0218-7. $78.

"Public libraries and undergraduate academic libraries will find this book useful for its nontechnical language." — *American Reference Books Annual, 2000*

"While this easy-to-read book is recommended for all libraries, it should prove to be especially useful for public, high school, and academic libraries; certainly it should be on the bookshelf of every school gymnasium." — *E-Streams, Mar '00*

602

Substance Abuse Sourcebook

Basic Health-Related Information about the Abuse of Legal and Illegal Substances Such as Alcohol, Tobacco, Prescription Drugs, Marijuana, Cocaine, and Heroin; and Including Facts about Substance Abuse Prevention Strategies, Intervention Methods, Treatment and Recovery Programs, and a Section Addressing the Special Problems Related to Substance Abuse during Pregnancy

Edited by Karen Bellenir. 573 pages. 1996. 0-7808-0038-9. $78.

"A valuable addition to any health reference section. Highly recommended."
— *The Book Report, Mar/Apr '97*

". . . a comprehensive collection of substance abuse information that's both highly readable and compact. Families and caregivers of substance abusers will find the information enlightening and helpful, while teachers, social workers and journalists should benefit from the concise format. Recommended."
— *Drug Abuse Update, Winter '96/'97*

SEE ALSO *Alcoholism Sourcebook, Drug Abuse Sourcebook*

■

Transplantation Sourcebook

Basic Consumer Health Information about Organ and Tissue Transplantation, Including Physical and Financial Preparations, Procedures and Issues Relating to Specific Solid Organ and Tissue Transplants, Rehabilitation, Pediatric Transplant Information, the Future of Transplantation, and Organ and Tissue Donation

Along with a Glossary and Listings of Additional Resources

Edited by Joyce Brennfleck Shannon. 628 pages. 2002. 0-7808-0322-1. $78.

■

Traveler's Health Sourcebook

Basic Consumer Health Information for Travelers, Including Physical and Medical Preparations, Transportation Health and Safety, Essential Information about Food and Water, Sun Exposure, Insect and Snake Bites, Camping and Wilderness Medicine, and Travel with Physical or Medical Disabilities

Along with International Travel Tips, Vaccination Recommendations, Geographical Health Issues, Disease Risks, a Glossary, and a Listing of Additional Resources

Edited by Joyce Brennfleck Shannon. 613 pages. 2000. 0-7808-0384-1. $78.

"Recommended reference source."
— *Booklist, American Library Association, Feb '01*

"This book is recommended for any public library, any travel collection, and especially any collection for the physically disabled."
— *American Reference Books Annual, 2001*

Women's Health Concerns Sourcebook

Basic Information about Health Issues That Affect Women, Featuring Facts about Menstruation and Other Gynecological Concerns, Including Endometriosis, Fibroids, Menopause, and Vaginitis; Reproductive Concerns, Including Birth Control, Infertility, and Abortion; and Facts about Additional Physical, Emotional, and Mental Health Concerns Prevalent among Women Such as Osteoporosis, Urinary Tract Disorders, Eating Disorders, and Depression

Along with Tips for Maintaining a Healthy Lifestyle

Edited by Heather E. Aldred. 567 pages. 1997. 0-7808-0219-5. $78.

"Handy compilation. There is an impressive range of diseases, devices, disorders, procedures, and other physical and emotional issues covered . . . well organized, illustrated, and indexed." — *Choice, Association of College and Research Libraries, Jan '98*

SEE ALSO *Breast Cancer Sourcebook, Cancer Sourcebook for Women, 1st and 2nd Editions, Healthy Heart Sourcebook for Women, Osteoporosis Sourcebook*

■

Workplace Health & Safety Sourcebook

Basic Consumer Health Information about Workplace Health and Safety, Including the Effect of Workplace Hazards on the Lungs, Skin, Heart, Ears, Eyes, Brain, Reproductive Organs, Musculoskeletal System, and Other Organs and Body Parts

Along with Information about Occupational Cancer, Personal Protective Equipment, Toxic and Hazardous Chemicals, Child Labor, Stress, and Workplace Violence

Edited by Chad T. Kimball. 626 pages. 2000. 0-7808-0231-4. $78.

"As a reference for the general public, this would be useful in any library." —*E-Streams, Jun '01*

"Provides helpful information for primary care physicians and other caregivers interested in occupational medicine. . . . General readers; professionals."
— *Choice, Association of College and Research Libraries, May '01*

"Recommended reference source."
— *Booklist, American Library Association, Feb '01*

"Highly recommended." —*The Bookwatch, Jan '01*

■

Worldwide Health Sourcebook

Basic Information about Global Health Issues, Including Malnutrition, Reproductive Health, Disease Dispersion and Prevention, Emerging Diseases, Risky Health Behaviors, and the Leading Causes of Death

Along with Global Health Concerns for Children, Women, and the Elderly, Mental Health Issues, Research and Technology Advancements, and Economic, Environmental, and Political Health Implications, a Glossary, and a Resource Listing for Additional Help and Information

Edited by Joyce Brennfleck Shannon. 614 pages. 2001. 0-7808-0330-2. $78.

"Named an Outstanding Academic Title."
—*Choice, Association of College & Research Libraries, Jan '02*

"Yet another handy but also unique compilation in the extensive Health Reference Series, this is a useful work because many of the international publications reprinted or excerpted are not readily available. Highly recommended."
—*Choice, Association of College & Research Libraries, Nov '01*

"Recommended reference source."
—*Booklist, American Library Association, Oct '01*

Health Reference Series

Adolescent Health Sourcebook

AIDS Sourcebook, 1st Edition

AIDS Sourcebook, 2nd Edition

Alcoholism Sourcebook

Allergies Sourcebook, 1st Edition

Allergies Sourcebook, 2nd Edition

Alternative Medicine Sourcebook, 1st Edition

Alternative Medicine Sourcebook, 2nd Edition

Alzheimer's, Stroke & 29 Other Neurological Disorders Sourcebook, 1st Edition

Alzheimer's Disease Sourcebook, 2nd Edition

Arthritis Sourcebook

Asthma Sourcebook

Attention Deficit Disorder Sourcebook

Back & Neck Disorders Sourcebook

Blood & Circulatory Disorders Sourcebook

Brain Disorders Sourcebook

Breast Cancer Sourcebook

Breastfeeding Sourcebook

Burns Sourcebook

Cancer Sourcebook, 1st Edition

Cancer Sourcebook (New), 2nd Edition

Cancer Sourcebook, 3rd Edition

Cancer Sourcebook for Women, 1st Edition

Cancer Sourcebook for Women, 2nd Edition

Cardiovascular Diseases & Disorders Sourcebook, 1st Edition

Caregiving Sourcebook

Colds, Flu & Other Common Ailments Sourcebook

Communication Disorders Sourcebook

Congenital Disorders Sourcebook

Consumer Issues in Health Care Sourcebook

Contagious & Non-Contagious Infectious Diseases Sourcebook

Death & Dying Sourcebook

Diabetes Sourcebook, 1st Edition

Diabetes Sourcebook, 2nd Edition

Diet & Nutrition Sourcebook, 1st Edition

Diet & Nutrition Sourcebook, 2nd Edition

Digestive Diseases & Disorder Sourcebook

Disabilities Sourcebook

Domestic Violence & Child Abuse Sourcebook

Drug Abuse Sourcebook

Ear, Nose & Throat Disorders Sourcebook

Eating Disorders Sourcebook

Emergency Medical Services Sourcebook

Endocrine & Metabolic Disorders Sourcebook

Environmentally Induced Disorders Sourcebook

Ethnic Diseases Sourcebook

Family Planning Sourcebook

Fitness & Exercise Sourcebook, 1st Edition

Fitness & Exercise Sourcebook, 2nd Edition

Food & Animal Borne Diseases Sourcebook

Food Safety Sourcebook

Forensic Medicine Sourcebook

Gastrointestinal Diseases & Disorders Sourcebook